Mohit Agrawal
Manmohan Singhal
Amit Kumar Nayak
Shailendra Bhatt
Kamal Shah
Editors

Neurodegenerative Disorders

From Pathogenesis to Clinical Approaches

nova
science publishers
www.novapublishers.com

DOI: https://doi.org/10.52305/GQSI1551

Library of Congress Cataloging-in-Publication Data

ISBN: 979-8-89530-143-2 (Hardcover)
ISBN: 979-8-89530-312-2 (eBook)

Published by Nova Science Publishers, Inc. † New York

Dedication

This book is dedicated to Almighty God "Lord Shiva"
and all editors and authors contributing their best to research.

Contents

Foreword

It is with great pleasure that I write this foreword, not only because I have known Mohit Agrawal for several years, but also because I strongly believe in the immense value of the teaching-learning process. I am confident that students at every stage of their academic journey can greatly enhance their understanding and knowledge by engaging with and reviewing well-curated scholarly works.

In this regard, this book serves as an invaluable resource for pharmaceutical scholars, offering a thorough exploration of both theoretical and practical concepts related to neurological disorders and their treatment strategies. Neurological disorders affect millions of people worldwide, making the exploration of advanced treatment options particularly relevant and timely.

This book presents a comprehensive approach to understanding a variety of neurological conditions, providing clinically relevant insights into the signs, symptoms, and treatment strategies associated with these disorders. It offers an all-encompassing view of central nervous system (CNS) disorders and their management, making it a one-stop resource for researchers, students, and practitioners.

The volume is structured around detailed chapters that track the advancements in understanding these diseases, as well as the various treatment techniques employed in their management. Furthermore, the book explores the intricate relationships between different neurological disorders, offering readers a holistic understanding of the subject.

I personally found the content of this book to be both informative and enriching. The depth and breadth of the knowledge presented in this work will undoubtedly benefit a wide audience, including research scholars, academicians, students, and faculty members, all of whom will find valuable information that connects to the broader field of neurological disorders.

I would like to extend my heartfelt congratulations to Mohit Agrawal for editing this groundbreaking book. I also express my sincere gratitude to the researchers and contributors whose work has made this book an essential reference. I am confident that this book will prove to be an indispensable tool for anyone seeking to deepen their understanding of pharmaceutical strategies in the treatment of neurological disorders.

I wish the editor and co-editors continued success in their efforts, and I am certain that this book will have a lasting impact on readers around the world.

With Best Wishes,
Professor Hema Chaudhary
Dean
K. R. Mangalam University, India

Preface

"*Neurodegenerative Disorders: From Pathogenesis to Clinical Approaches*" offers a comprehensive exploration of various neurological and central nervous system (CNS) disorders. The discovery and development of effective treatments for these complex conditions remain a significant challenge in the field of neuroscience. With the global prevalence of neurological disorders on the rise, the need for innovative therapeutic strategies has never been more pressing. Researchers are increasingly looking to new frontiers, such as nanotechnology and advanced molecular therapies, to address the unmet needs in treating these diseases. Achieving this goal requires an in-depth understanding of the physiological mechanisms driving these disorders and how emerging treatments can target their underlying pathophysiology.

This book provides an updated and insightful look into the pathophysiology, mechanisms, and treatment strategies for neurological and CNS disorders. It aims to enhance the knowledge of researchers by shedding light on the role of various therapies, including nanotechnology and molecular-based treatments, in the progression of these diseases. The objective is not only to inform but also to inspire innovative approaches to develop new therapeutic interventions targeting neurological diseases.

The volume consists of 17 well-curated chapters that address the core aspects of neurological disorders, including basic science, pharmacology, and pathophysiological mechanisms at the molecular and ionic levels. Alongside this, the book highlights various synthetic treatment strategies designed to counteract or manage these disorders. Each chapter is crafted to provide a clear understanding of the complex relationships between molecular mechanisms and their clinical manifestations, making this an indispensable resource for researchers, students, and clinicians alike.

In addition to detailed literature reviews, the authors have enriched the content with diagrammatic pathways and tables, offering concise yet thorough explanations of the key concepts. These visual aids facilitate a deeper understanding of the material, enabling readers to absorb complex information efficiently and apply it to their own research. By covering the types of pathological changes that occur in neurological disorders, the book also explores the advanced molecules involved in triggering specific signs and symptoms, ultimately affecting the quality of life for patients.

This book is intended for a broad audience, including undergraduate and postgraduate students, researchers from academia, and professionals from the pharmaceutical industry. It serves as a valuable reference to deepen their understanding of neurological pathways and the various treatment strategies being employed to address these diseases. Furthermore, the book is designed to inspire young scientists and researchers from multidisciplinary fields to engage in innovative research with the aim of developing novel therapeutic interventions that will one day cure or alleviate the impact of neurological and CNS disorders, thereby improving human health globally.

We hope this book will not only serve as a source of knowledge but also motivate future generations of researchers to continue exploring new horizons in the quest to understand and treat neurological diseases.

Editors

Acknowledgments

"If you don't like to read, you haven't found the right book."

— J.K. Rowling

First and foremost, we express our heartfelt gratitude to the Almighty, Lord Shiva, whose divine blessings have guided us throughout the journey of completing this book. It is with deep faith and reverence that we acknowledge the grace and mercy that made this endeavor possible.

Mohit Agrawal would like to extend his sincere thanks to K.R. Mangalam University, Gurugram, for their unwavering support and for providing the necessary facilities that contributed to the successful completion of this book. His heartfelt gratitude also goes to all the contributors, whose expertise and dedication have enriched the content and made this book a valuable resource.

A special note of appreciation is due to the management of K.R. Mangalam University for its continued encouragement and invaluable support throughout the process of bringing this book to fruition.

Manmohan Singhal acknowledges DIT University, Dehradun, India, for their continuous support and motivation, which have been instrumental in completing this work.

Kamal Shah expresses his gratitude to GLA University, Mathura, for providing all the necessary facilities and for their assistance in every aspect, ensuring that this project was accomplished successfully.

We would also like to thank our families, friends, and colleagues for their understanding, patience, and constant support during the course of this work. Without their encouragement and contributions, this book would not have been possible.

Lastly, we wish to thank the readers, researchers, and students who will benefit from this book. We hope it serves as a valuable resource in the field of neurological disorders and inspires further research and innovation.

Editors

Chapter 1

Effects of Cataract Surgery on the Cognitive Decline of Elderly Patients: An Updated Review

Ahsas Goyal[1,*], PhD,
Shobhit Chaudhary[1],
Nitin Chitranshi[2], PhD,
and Amit K. Tiwari[3], PhD
[1]Institute of Pharmaceutical Research, GLA University, Mathura, Uttar Pradesh, India
[2]Macquarie Medical School, Macquarie University, Sydney, Australia
[3]University of Arkansas for Medical Sciences (UAMS) College of Pharmacy, USA

Abstract

Cataracts and cognitive decline are two distinct eye and brain disorders, mainly affecting age-related individuals. It has been demonstrated that cataract surgery is beneficial in substantially reducing the risk of dementia. Visual impairments and interventions to treat vision may improve dementia outcomes. Particularly, sensory disorders may lead to social isolation and reduce cognitive-related simulations, increasing the risk of brain structural damage, thus reducing cognitive function. We selectively considered PubMed produced published literature (1987–2022) and evaluated the references used in reputable primary articles and reviews for this literature. The findings have implications for managing older patients who are particularly at risk for cataracts and age-related dementia. Due to the remarkable correlation between cataract extraction and a lower risk of dementia, the affected patients and their families are

* Corresponding Author's Email: ahsasgoyal1990@gmail.com.

In: Neurogenerative Disorders
Editors: Mohit Agrawal, Manmohan Singhal, Amit Kumar Nayak et al.
ISBN: 979-8-89530-143-2

expected to anticipate a substantial improvement in quality of life. There is a need for more research into the pathways via which cataract removal may influence the risk of dementia.

Keywords: cognitive function, Alzheimer's disease, cataract surgery, age-related dementia

Abbreviations

ACE-R	Revised Addenbrooke's Cognitive Examination
ACT	Adult Changes in Thought
AD	Alzheimer's Disease
ARC	Age-Related Cataracts
BCVA	Best Corrected Visual Acuity
CCT	Central Corneal Thickness
ECC	Endothelial Cell Count
ELSA	English Longitudinal Study of Ageing
FTLD	Frontotemporal Lobar Degeneration
GDS	Geriatric Depression Scale
HDS-R	Revised Hasegawa Dementia Scale
HMW	High Molecular Weight
ipRGCs	Intrinsically Photosensitive Retinal Ganglion Cells
LBD	Lewy Body Dementia
MMSE	Mini-Mental State Examination
MOMSSE	Mattis Organic Mental Syndrome Screening Examination
VaD	Vascular Dementia
VCI	Vascular Cognitive Impairment

Introduction

Older people's cognitive abilities are critical to their daily functioning. Regrettably, several of these cognitive abilities (such as problem-solving activities, memory, and speed processing) deteriorate with age (Harada, 2013; Ockleford, 2009; Salthouse, 2012; Reichman., 2010). The number of elderly patients with cognitive impairment has increased as society has aged. Geriatric signs, such as probable dementia and depression, were detected in significant proportions of individuals (Lee, 2003). Nearly 50 million individuals (about twice the population of Texas) worldwide suffer from dementia, and there are no viable therapies (Livingston, 2020). The WHO estimates that by 2040, the very aged (those 85 and above) will account for more than 5.8% of the global population (https://www.who.int/ageing/publications/globalhealth.pdf).

Dementia has a significant impact on the lives of people suffering from it, as well as their family and caretakers. It is a disorder which presents numerous obstacles to health workers from prompt diagnosis to end-of-life care. There are numerous criteria for describing the clinical signs of dementia, but the underlying elements emphasise an acquired disorder represented by various cognitive deficits and a decrease from earlier function. The exclusion of depression or delirium, which can resemble cognitive impairment, is an important aspect of the screening process. Alzheimer disease (AD), vascular cognitive impairment (VCI)/vascular dementia (VaD), and dementia with Lewy bodies (LBD) are the most common underlying causes of dementia in the elderly. Neuropathological investigations are progressively revealing that dementia in old age represents more than one pathological state (Kovacs, 2008). Caring for dementia sufferers places a significant emotional and economic strain on families and society. Patients can be treated initially at home, but institutionalization is eventually required for many - about 67% expire in nursing homes (Mitchell, 2005). In 2010, the yearly per person cost attributed to dementia ranged from $41,689 to $56,290, depending on the techniques employed to value informal care. These costs are bound to rise with time (Hurd, 2013). If current demographic trends continue, the number of people with dementia is expected to triple by 2050 (Prince, 2013). There are distinct gender disparities in the prevalence of dementia. While men are more likely to get Frontotemporal Lobar Degeneration (FTLD) (before the age of 55), VaD (between the ages of 45 and 75), and LBD (through the age spectrum), women are more likely to develop AD (Dementia Report United Kingdom (2007). London; (Savica, 2013). There used to be a difference in the prevalence rates between developed countries and less developed countries, with VaD once being the most common dementia subtype in South-East Asia. However, as people lived longer and were in better physical health, the prevalence of AD - which often manifests later in life than VaD - rose in conjunction with the ageing population. Better physical health lowers the prevalence of cerebrovascular disease and, consequently, VaD. These modifications also have a tendency to tilt the sex ratio in favour of more cases involving women (Dementia Report United Kingdom (2007). London).

Visual impairment is a major risk factor for dementia (Chen, 2017; Zheng, 2018) Cataract is an opacification (either partial or total) of the crystalline lens that is usually gradual and irreversible, resulting in visual loss with medical, social, as well as economic consequences (Asbell, 2005). This is demonstrated to occur anytime the lens's refractive index alters substantially over distances close to the wavelength of the transmitted light (Benedek, 1971; Delaye and Tardieu, 1983). This shift in the refractive index can be caused by a number of factors, including alterations to lens cell structure, lens proteins, or a combination of these (Hejtmanick, 2001). Changes in the geometrical order of the lens and its protective membranes can enhance these effects, increasing light scattering. Congenital cataracts are frequently related to lens micro-architecture break down. Vacuoles can occur, causing substantial changes in optical density as well as light scattering. On the other hand, age-related cataracts are frequently characterised by light scattering and opacity caused by the accumulation of high molecular weight (HMW) protein aggregates, which are typically 1000 Å or larger in size. This can also interfere with the short-range ordered packing of lens crystallins, a process that is crucial for keeping the crystallins in a homogenous phase and has serious implications for lens transparency because they make up over 90% of soluble lens proteins (Zhang, 2004).

Cataracts can be classified based on their age of onset, though the distinctions between different forms of cataract are just approximate. If a cataract is discovered during the first year of birth, it is referred to as congenital or infantile. If the cataract appears within the first decade of life, it is called juvenile, and if it appears later but before the age of 45, it is called presenile, while senile or age-related cataracts appear after 50 or maybe 60 years of age. The situation is further entangled by the fact that fine cataracts, which can be asymptomatic, might go unnoticed to clinical attention for years. Furthermore, the age of cataract onset does not reflect a specific aetiology. Hereditary cataracts account for approximately 8.3-25% of congenital cataracts (François, 1982; Haargaard, 2005; Merin, 2005). Age-related cataracts (ARC) also have an element of genetics, though the sequence variations that contribute to ARC are likely to increase disease risk against an array of environmental insults to which all individuals are subjected to, probably by making those who have the variation more vulnerable to a variety of environmental insults built up throughout the years (McCarty and Taylor, 2001; Shiels and Hejtmancik, 2013). Although they frequently appear in a mixed pattern as they progress, age-related cataracts can be separated into three different types according to their location inside the lens: nuclear, cortical, and posterior subcapsular (Merin, 2005). Cataract surgery is also the most common ophthalmological procedure in the world (Flaxman, 2017). The most common cause of reversible vision impairment in the world is age-related cataract. Cataract surgery is amongst the most prevalent surgeries worldwide, with about 1.7 million procedures performed in the United States annually (Liu, 2017; Acklande, 2017). Cataract, being the primary cause of blindness in the world, affects more than 35 million people and blinding about 20 million (Lee and Afshari, 2017). Cataracts and cognitive impairment are considered age-related health disorders because their prevalence increases with age (Ferri, 2005). Considering that cataract is the most common cause of temporary blindness, surgical treatment may be one technique for lowering cognitive impairment (Kheirkhah, 2018).

The removal of visual impairment through cataract surgery may be linked to a lowered risk of dementia. The mechanisms underlying the association between cataract surgery and lower dementia risk have yet to be discovered, but visual impairment can cause psycho-social difficulties, social retreat, and a decrease in active lifestyle, all of which are linked to cognitive decline (Brenner, 1993; Livingston, 2020). Reversal of all of these can reduce the incidence of cognitive impairment and lower the dementia risk. The purpose of this review was to analyse, identify and summarise up-to-date information to see whether cataract surgery results in a substantial improvement in cognitive decline and dementia.

Methods

Published literature was yielded by discerning PubMed (1987-2022). A broad search approach with pertinent descriptions and keywords was utilized. These include cataract extraction, dementia, cognitive impairment, visual impairment, or a combination of these. We examined the references of recognized primary reports and reviews. Following a careful examination and discussion of the abstracts by the authors, relevant publications were thoroughly researched.

Common Causes of Dementia and Cataracts

Dementia and cataracts are both degenerative diseases that are known to have similar causal mechanisms (Harding, 1998; Goldstein, 2003). Advancement in age, smoking, and lesser education levels (possibly from a lower socioeconomic group) are all possible causes of cataract (Sperduto, 2001; Seddon, 1995; Leske, 1991), and they are also causes of dementia (Fillit et al., 2008; Qiu et al., 2009; Anstey, 2007; Schmidt e, 2008) Similarly, obesity and diabetes are also possible causes for cataract (Tan et al., 2008; Schaumberg, 2000) and dementia (Fillit, 2008). Patients with dementia are more likely to develop cataracts due to several causes (Jefferis, 2011). However, some studies discovered no link between cataracts and cognitive impairment (Grodstein, 2003; Anstey, 2006).

The Link between Cognitive Decline and Visual Impairment

According to prior research, the likelihood of cognitive impairment among the elderly with vision impairment is greater (Swenor, 2019; Lin, 2004; Fischer, 2016; Zheng, 2018). The link between visual acuity and cognitive test results is strong (Lindenberger and Baltes, 1994). Scientists have tried to investigate and explain the relationship between cognitive and perceptual decline and aging for over fifty years, yet this correlation remains unclear. This research has led to the development of various hypotheses that attempt to clarify the connection between age-related cognitive and visual impairment (Monge and Madden, 2016).

A distinct factor is related to aging, which negatively impacts both cognition and vision and adds to their decline. This hypothesis known as the Common Cause, which was supported by Lindenberger and Baltes (Baltes and Lindenberger, 1997; Lindenberger and Baltes, 1994) demonstrated that imitating elderly vision in younger patients did not affect their cognitive ability. The lack of a correlation between 'elderly vision' and 'elderly cognition' suggests that impaired vision alone cannot explain the reason for lower test scores in elderly. Drobny (Drobny, 2005) also demonstrated that patients with impaired vision scored badly on cognitive tasks lacking vision requirements, indicating that they had a genuine cognitive impairment.

A decrease in perception gradually degrades neural substrates, which influence cognition. This is the sensory deprivation theory, supported by Lindenberger and Baltes (Lindenberger and Baltes, 1994) stating that due to a nonlinear negative correlation between sensory functioning and deprivation, the association between sensory and cognitive functioning is greater at decreased levels of sensory functioning.

Regrettably, the majority of studies addressing the correlation between visual and cognitive impairment in aging have been correlational (Baltes and

Lindenberger, 1997; Lindenberger and Baltes, 1994), preventing adequate testing of these theories. Correlational analyses were unable to demonstrate if altering the visual signal strength of survey participants has immediate effects on cognitive function; an intervention or experimental manipulation is necessary to determine this (Monge and Madden, 2016).

Cognitive Performance and Effects on Dementia Following Cataract Surgery

Cognitive and visual impairment are linked and possibly related; consequently, reversing visual impairment may enhance cognitive performance. Numerous research has examined the concept of Cataract surgery improving Cognitive function with variable outcomes, which are summarised in Table 1. The conclusion of the study carried out by Tamura (Tamura, 2004) suggested that cognitive performance increases after cataract surgery, which may be due to light stimulus increasing the activity of the brain after extraction of the lens. The longitudinal study of Hall (Hall, 2005) showed that cognitive function may improve, but this can't be attributed to the surgery itself or better vision. The studies carried out by Gray (Gray, 2006) and Ishii (Ishii, 2008) also suggest that cataract surgery substantially improved elderly patients' cognitive impairment. Jefferis (Jefferis, 2015) showed that people with reduced cognition following bilateral cataract surgery benefit from cataract surgery, but not to the same extent as those with normal cognition. Miyata's (Miyata, 2018) study shows that cataract surgery may reduce the possibility of developing mild cognitive impairment regardless of visual acuity, but not dementia. Results from Kheirkhah (Kheirkhah, 2018), Maharani (Maharani, 2018), and Verdina (Verdina, 2022) exhibit an improvement in cognitive function after cataract surgery, and due to the limits of their respective studies, they proposed that additional research should be carried out to explain the concept. Later on, Lee (Lee, 2022) showed that cataract surgery was strongly connected with a reduced chance of developing dementia due to increased quality and quantity of light.

Ultimately, while there is adequate evidence to suggest that cataract surgery improves cognitive performance and reduces the risk of dementia, it is limited by various drawbacks in each of the employed study methods.

Table 1. Cataract surgery improving cognitive function with variable outcomes

Authors	Design	Representative Group	Cognitive Evaluation	Result
Tamura (Tamura, 2004)	Prospective, Observational study	20 patients with cognitive impairment (average age 82.1, range 61-90) underwent cataract surgery. 20 controls without cataract surgery (mean age 84.3, range 70-93) with cognitive impairment	Revised Hasegawa Dementia Scale (HDS-R) before and after surgery	The surgical group showed remarkable improvement postoperatively, but not the control group
Hall (Hall, 2005)	Longitudinal, Nonrandomised control study	92 patients with normal cognition and without cataract (average age 66.8 ± 5.9), 122 (mean age 70.9 ± 6.8) cataract patients who elected surgery, and 87 (mean age 71.1 ± 5.4) cataract patients who refused to have surgery	Mattis Organic Mental Syndrome Screening Examination (MOMSSE scores) at the start and 1-year follow-up after surgery	At the time of the follow-up, both the Cataract (surgery) and Cataract (without surgery) groups had higher cognitive scores
Gray (Gray, 2006)	Prospective, Observational study (no control group)	92 patients (average age 78.1 ± 6.5) with normal cognition having cataract surgery on the first eye, the second eye, or sequentially	Mini-Mental State Examination (MMSE) scores 2 weeks prior surgery with 2 and 6 months post-surgery	MMSE scores elevated at 6 months after surgery (but not 2 months post surgery)
Ishii (Ishii, 2008)	Prospective, Nonrandomised study (no control group)	102 patients (average age 75.3 ± 8.2) with normal cognition having cataract surgery	MMSE scores prior to and 2 months post-cataract surgery	A substantial increase in MMSE scores post-cataract surgery
Jefferis (Jefferis, 2015)	Longitudinal follow-up study	112 patients (age $\geq$75 years), of those, 64 (57%) had impaired cognition while 48 (43%) were having normal cognition.	Revised Addenbrooke's Cognitive Examination (ACE-R)at the start and 1 year following surgery	Patients with cognitive impairment benefited less from surgery than those with normal cognition.
Miyata (Miyata, 2018)	Cross-sectional epidemiological study	Out of 2,764 subjects (mean age 76.3 ± 4.8 years), 668 had gone through cataract surgery. Of these, 150 had dementia and 877 had mild cognitive impairment.	MMSE scores preoperatively and postoperatively and Geriatric Depression Scale (GDS-15)	Cataract surgery decreases the chances of acquiring mild cognitive impairment but not dementia

Authors	Design	Representative Group	Cognitive Evaluation	Result
Kheirkhah (Kheirkhah 2018)	Before – After a clinical trial	Out of 250 patients, 54 failed to return for the third-month follow-up. Remaining 196 (mean age 71.77 ± 8.08), 51% were females, 72.9% without any education, and 76% without diabetes	MMSE scores a day before and 3 months after cataract surgery and GDS scores difference preoperatively and postoperatively	Enhanced visual acuity has a significantly greater impact on lowering cognitive impairment
Maharani (Maharani, 2018)	A longitudinal study with treatment and control group	2,068 patients had cataract surgery (Wave 2 and 6) while 3,636 people were in the control group with no cataract.	Seven different waves of English Longitudinal Study of Ageing (ELSA) were utilized for a 13 year period from 2002 to 2015	Cataract surgery could have a positive influence on the cognitive decline pathways in old age.
Verdina (Verdina, 2022)	Prospective, Nonrandomised comparative study	Out of 78 patients (mean age 80.3 ± 6.2), 24 were very elderly (age $\geq$85 years) and 54 were elderly (age $\geq 65 < 85$ years)	Endothelial Cell Count (ECC), Best Corrected Visual Acuity (BCVA) and Central Corneal Thickness (CCT) were evaluated 90 days prior to, during, and 90 days post-surgery	Very elderly patients appear to benefit more from cataract surgery than elderly patients.
Lee (Lee, 2022)	Prospective, Longitudinal cohort study	3,038 patients (mean age 74.4 ± 6.2), among which 1800 (59%) women and 1238 (41%) men.	Data from the Adult Changes in Thought (ACT) study was collected from 1994 to 2018 and analysed from 2019 to 2021	Cataract removal was significantly connected with a lower risk of developing dementia.

Are There Any Mechanisms Responsible for Cognitive Enhancement after Cataract Surgery?

Various studies present the following possible mechanisms underlying the improvement in cognition after cataract surgery:

Light stimulus may help to slow aging of the brain. Acute lens opacity affects the majority of elderly individuals who are cognitively impaired. As a result, light stimulus following lens extraction may enhance brain activity, resulting in improved cognition (Tamura, 2004).

The quantity of light that reaches the retina after cataract surgery is significantly increased. This is essential because light is an important environmental cue for regulating the biological clock, and a disruption in the circadian rhythm can result in cognitive impairment (Kondratova and Kondratov, 2012; Coogan, 2013). By increasing light transmittance required to maintain circadian rhythms, cataract surgery increases sleep quality (Ayaki, 2013). As a result, an increase in the amount of light affecting the retina could possibly be a preventative mechanism for cognitive impairment (Miyata, 2018).

Cataract-related visual impairment might reduce neuronal input, potentially speeding up neurodegeneration or amplifying its effects through cortical atrophy. With vision loss, the visual cortex experiences structural alterations (Boucard, 2009; Hagen, 2005). According to Hanson (Hanson, 2019), vision loss was linked to visual cortex atrophy in individuals with neovascular age-related macular degeneration, and also a rise in gray matter volume was observed post-cataract surgery (Lin, 2018).

Increased quantity and quality of light may also be linked to a lower risk of dementia following cataract extraction. Cognitive function, Circadian rhythm, and Alzheimer's disease have all been linked to intrinsically photosensitive retinal ganglion cells (ipRGCs), which are extraordinarily photosensitive to blue light (Schmoll, 2011).

What Impact Does Cognitive Decline Have on Cataract Surgery Results?

With increasing age, visual acuities following cataract surgery deteriorate (Jay, 1987). Even when other ocular comorbidities are taken into consideration, older age is known to diminish the benefits of cataract surgery

(Westcott, 2000; Wong, 2001). According to a study (Jefferis, 2015), patients with both normal and poor cognition reported notable enhancements in visual outcomes following cataract surgery. However, visual improvements post-surgery may be limited by cognitive impairment. This is because cerebral alterations in the brain may play a role in reducing postoperative visual acuities in older patients after cataract surgery. Patients may also encounter visual symptoms caused by cognitive impairment that they mistake for eye diseases and expect to resolve following cataract surgery (Jefferis, 2011).

Visual Symptoms of Cataracts and Dementia: Are They Similar?

Cataract patients may encounter a lack of visual acuity, difficulties reading, recognizing people, watching television, and glaring and colour recognition issues. A study (Crabtree, 1999) examined the noticeable symptoms of cataract patients above the age of 65 but excluded patients with low MMSE scores i.e., those having mild dementia (20-24), and moderate dementia (13-20), and severe dementia (<12). All the patients had MMSE scores of 25 or above. The patient's symptoms were divided into three categories: Recognition and Perception, Sight-related mobility, and Hand-eye coordination. This procedure of differentiating symptoms based on interviews resulted in the establishment of the Cataract Symptom Scale (Crabtree, 1999).

Table 2. Visual symptoms that may be prevalent in dementia

Type of Symptoms	Visual traits of Cataract (Crabtree, 1999)	Visual traits of Dementia (Lee and Martin, 2004; Sadun, 1987b; Kiyosawa, Thomas M. Bosley, 1989)
Sight-associated Mobility	Going Downstairs Crossing Roads Getting off the pavement	Wandering around in familiar territory Colliding with objects
Recognition and Perception	Blurred Vision Recognizing someone across the street Reading newspapers and books Seeing the numbers on a bus Seeing television subtitles/Teletext	Blurred Vision Recognising objects Recognising faces Reading
Hand-eye Coordination	Glare while driving Pouring hot beverages Seeing while writing	Glaring and driving Hitting a golf ball Hitting a tennis ball

Dementia patients complained about symptoms which included difficulty in reading, driving, playing sports, blurred vision, and visual hallucinations (Kiyosawa, Thomas M Bosley, 1989; Sadun, 1987a; Lee and Martin, 2004). The visual symptoms that may be prevalent in dementia are included in Table 2, categorised similarly to cataracts for comparison.

The visual symptoms of cataract and dementia overlap substantially. This makes it difficult to discern between symptoms caused by cataract and cognitive impairment, especially in the elderly, since the majority of patients will show some level of lens opacity on evaluation (Congdon, 2004; Williams, 2006).

Are Other Diseases Associated with Cataract Surgery?

Cataract surgery may also be associated with reduced depression (Pellegrini, 2020; Kheirkhah, 2018; Miyata, 2018). However, other research has shown contradictory findings. According to a study, the decrease in depression symptoms in elderly individuals following cataract surgery had little statistical significance (Ishii, 2008). Furthermore, a study found that vision enhancement post cataract surgery had no significant effects on depression-like symptoms in older patients (McGwin, 2003). Considering the significance of the negative psychosocial effects of cataract and the contradicting information about the effect of cataract surgery on depressed symptoms in elderly individuals, Deilami (Norouzpour Deilami, 2021) sought to examine the effect of cataract surgery on depression in elderly patients.

A study showed that visual hallucinations may also be improved by cataract surgery (Chapman, 1999). Patients with pre-existing Alzheimer's disease and visual hallucinations experienced a reduction in their visual hallucinations after having their vision corrected with refraction. Patients with cataract were more likely to experience visual hallucinations, and the researchers hypothesized that cataract surgery would also alleviate these visual hallucinations (Jefferis, 2011).

Conclusion and Outlook

The main objective of this review was to see if cataract surgery and dementia are correlated. Studies exhibit that after cataract surgery, there is a reduction in the rate of cognitive impairment and also a lower risk of dementia development. This is the most comprehensive assessment to date of the effects of cataract surgery on cognition and dementia. The findings indicate that cataract surgery has a significant impact on cognitive performance. These have implications for the management of elderly individuals who are particularly at risk for both cataract and age-related dementia. Due to the remarkable relationship between cataract extraction and a reduced incidence of dementia, the enhancement in quality of life for the afflicted patients and their households is anticipated to be significant. There is a need for more research into the mechanisms via which cataract removal may influence the probability of dementia.

Declaration of Interest

None.

Conflict of Interest

The authors confirm that they have no conflicts of interest with respect to the work described in this manuscript.

References

Ackland, P., Resnikoff, S., & Bourne, R. (2017). World blindness and visual impairment: despite many successes, the problem is growing. *Community eye health,* 30(100), 71.

Anstey, K. J., Lord, S. R., Hennessy, M., Mitchell, P., Mill, K., & von Sanden, C. (2006). The effect of cataract surgery on neuropsychological test performance: a randomized controlled trial. *Journal of the international neuropsychological society*, 12(5), 632–639.

Anstey, K. J., von Sanden, C., Salim, A., & O'Kearney, R. (2007). Smoking as a risk factor for dementia and cognitive decline: a meta-analysis of prospective studies. *American journal of epidemiology*, 166(4), 367–378.

Asbell, P. A., Dualan, I., Mindel, J., Brocks, D., Ahmad, M., & Epstein, S. (2005). Age-related cataract. *Lancet,* 365(9459), 599–609.

Ayaki, M., Muramatsu, M., Negishi, K., & Tsubota, K. (2013). Improvements in sleep quality and gait speed after cataract surgery. *Rejuvenation research,* 16(1), 35–42.

Baltes, P. B., & Lindenberger, U. (1997). Emergence of a powerful connection between sensory and cognitive functions across the adult life span: a new window to the study of cognitive aging?. *Psychology and aging,* 12(1), 12–21.

Benedek, G. B. (1971). Theory of transparency of the eye. *Applied optics,* 10(3), 459–473.

Boucard, C. C., Hernowo, A. T., Maguire, R. P., Jansonius, N. M., Roerdink, J. B., Hooymans, J. M., & Cornelissen, F. W. (2009). Changes in cortical grey matter density associated with long-standing retinal visual field defects. *Brain,* 132(Pt 7), 1898–1906.

Brenner, D. E., Kukull, W. A., van Belle, G., Bowen, J. D., McCormick, W. C., Teri, L., & Larson, E. B. (1993). Relationship between cigarette smoking and Alzheimer's disease in a population-based case-control study. *Neurology,* 43(2), 293–300.

Chapman, F. M., Dickinson, J., McKeith, I., & Ballard, C. (1999). Association among visual hallucinations, visual acuity, and specific eye pathologies in Alzheimer's disease: treatment implications. *The American journal of psychiatry,* 156(12), 1983–1985.

Chen, S. P., Bhattacharya, J., & Pershing, S. (2017). Association of vision loss with cognition in older adults. *JAMA ophthalmology,* 135(9), 963–970.

Congdon, N., Vingerling, J. R., Klein, B. E., West, S., Friedman, D. S., Kempen, J., O'Colmain, B., Wu, S. Y., Taylor, H. R., & Eye diseases prevalence research group (2004). Prevalence of cataract and pseudophakia/aphakia among adults in the United States. *Archives of ophthalmology,* 122(4), 487–494.

Coogan, A. N., Schutová, B., Husung, S., Furczyk, K., Baune, B. T., Kropp, P., Häßler, F., & Thome, J. (2013). The circadian system in Alzheimer's disease: disturbances, mechanisms, and opportunities. *Biological psychiatry,* 74(5), 333–339.

Crabtree, H. L., Hildreth, A. J., O'Connell, J. E., Phelan, P. S., Allen, D., & Gray, C. S. (1999). Measuring visual symptoms in British cataract patients: the cataract symptom scale. *The British journal of ophthalmology*, 83(5), 519–523.

Delaye, M., & Tardieu, A. (1983). Short-range order of crystallin proteins accounts for eye lens transparency. *Nature,* 302(5907), 415–417.

Drobny, J. V., Anstey, K. J., & Andrews, S. (2005). Visual memory testing in older adults with age-related visual decline: a measure of memory performance or visual functioning?. *Journal of clinical and experimental neuropsychology,* 27(4), 425–435.

Ferri, C. P., Prince, M., Brayne, C., Brodaty, H., Fratiglioni, L., Ganguli, M., Hall, K., Hasegawa, K., Hendrie, H., Huang, Y., Jorm, A., Mathers, C., Menezes, P. R., Rimmer, E., Scazufca, M., & Alzheimer's disease international (2005). Global prevalence of dementia: a Delphi consensus study. *Lancet* (London, England), 366(9503), 2112–2117.

Fillit, H., Nash, D. T., Rundek, T., & Zuckerman, A. (2008). Cardiovascular risk factors and dementia. *The American journal of geriatric pharmacotherapy*, 6(2), 100–118.

Fischer, M. E., Cruickshanks, K. J., Schubert, C. R., Pinto, A. A., Carlsson, C. M., Klein, B. E., Klein, R., & Tweed, T. S. (2016). Age-related sensory impairments and risk of cognitive impairment. *Journal of the American geriatrics society,* 64(10), 1981–1987.

Flaxman, S. R., Bourne, R. R. A., Resnikoff, S., Ackland, P., Braithwaite, T., Cicinelli, M. V., Das, A., Jonas, J. B., Keeffe, J., Kempen, J. H., Leasher, J., Limburg, H., Naidoo, K., Pesudovs, K., Silvester, A., Stevens, G. A., Tahhan, N., Wong, T. Y., Taylor, H. R., & Vision loss expert group of the global burden of disease study (2017). Global causes of blindness and distance vision impairment 1990-2020: a systematic review and meta-analysis. *The Lancet. Global health,* 5(12), e1221–e1234.

François, J. (1982). Genetics of cataract. Ophthalmologica. Journal international d'ophtalmologie. *International journal of ophthalmology. Zeitschrift fur Augenheilkunde*, 184(2), 61–71.

Goldstein, L. E., Muffat, J. A., Cherny, R. A., Moir, R. D., Ericsson, M. H., Huang, X., Mavros, C., Coccia, J. A., Faget, K. Y., Fitch, K. A., Masters, C. L., Tanzi, R. E., Chylack, L. T., Jr, & Bush, A. I. (2003). Cytosolic beta-amyloid deposition and supranuclear cataracts in lenses from people with Alzheimer's disease. *Lancet,* 361(9365), 1258–1265.

Gray, C. S., Karimova, G., Hildreth, A. J., Crabtree, L., Allen, D., & O'connell, J. E. (2006). Recovery of visual and functional disability following cataract surgery in older people: Sunderland Cataract Study. *Journal of cataract and refractive surgery,* 32(1), 60–66.

Grodstein, F., Chen, J., & Hankinson, S. E. (2003). Cataract extraction and cognitive function in older women. *Epidemiology,* 14(4), 493–497.

Haargaard, B., Wohlfahrt, J., Rosenberg, T., Fledelius, H. C., & Melbye, M. (2005). Risk factors for idiopathic congenital/infantile cataract. *Investigative ophthalmology & visual science,* 46(9), 3067–3073.

Hall, T. A., McGwin, G., Jr, & Owsley, C. (2005). Effect of cataract surgery on cognitive function in older adults. *Journal of the American geriatrics society,* 53(12), 2140–2144.

Hanson, R. L. W., Gale, R. P., Gouws, A. D., Airody, A., Scott, M. T. W., Akthar, F., Waterson, S., Wells, M. T., Wright, A. J., Bell, K., Silson, E., Baseler, H. A., & Morland, A. B. (2019). Following the status of visual cortex over time in patients with macular degeneration reveals atrophy of visually deprived brain regions. *Investigative ophthalmology & visual science*, 60(15), 5045–5051.

Harada, C. N., Natelson Love, M. C., & Triebel, K. L. (2013). Normal cognitive aging. *Clinics in geriatric medicine,* 29(4), 737–752.

Harding, J. J. (1998). Cataract, Alzheimer's disease, and other conformational diseases. *Current opinion in ophthalmology*, 9(1), 10–13.

Hurd, M. D., Martorell, P., Delavande, A., Mullen, K. J., & Langa, K. M. (2013). Monetary costs of dementia in the United States. *The New England journal of medicine,* 368(14), 1326–1334.

Ishii, K., Kabata, T., & Oshika, T. (2008). The impact of cataract surgery on cognitive impairment and depressive mental status in elderly patients. *American journal of ophthalmology*, 146(3), 404–409.

Jay, J. L., Mammo, R. B., & Allan, D. (1987). Effect of age on visual acuity after cataract extraction. *The British journal of ophthalmology,* 71(2), 112–115.

Jefferis, J. M., Mosimann, U. P., & Clarke, M. P. (2011). Cataract and cognitive impairment: a review of the literature. *The British journal of ophthalmology,* 95(1), 17–23.

Jefferis, J. M., Taylor, J. P., & Clarke, M. P. (2015). Does cognitive impairment influence outcomes from cataract surgery? Results from a 1-year follow-up cohort study. *The British journal of ophthalmology,* 99(3), 412–417.

Kheirkhah, F., Roustaei, G., Mohebbi Abivardi, E., Hamidia, A., & Javadian Kutenai, S. (2018). Improvement in cognitive status and depressive symptoms three months after cataract surgery. *Caspian journal of internal medicine,* 9(4), 386–392.

Kiyosawa, M., Bosley, T. M., Chawluk, J., Jamieson, D., Schatz, N. J., Savino, P. J., Sergott, R. C., Reivich, M., & Alavi, A. (1989). Alzheimer's disease with prominent visual symptoms. Clinical and metabolic evaluation. *Ophthalmology*, 96(7), 1077–1086.

Kondratova, A. A., & Kondratov, R. V. (2012). The circadian clock and pathology of the ageing brain. Nature reviews. *Neuroscience,* 13(5), 325–335.

Kovacs, G. G., Alafuzoff, I., Al-Sarraj, S., Arzberger, T., Bogdanovic, N., Capellari, S., Ferrer, I., Gelpi, E., Kövari, V., Kretzschmar, H., Nagy, Z., Parchi, P., Seilhean, D., Soininen, H., Troakes, C., & Budka, H. (2008). Mixed brain pathologies in dementia: the Brain Net Europe consortium experience. *Dementia and geriatric cognitive disorders*, 26(4), 343–350.

Lee, A. G., & Martin, C. O. (2004). Neuro-ophthalmic findings in the visual variant of Alzheimer's disease. *Ophthalmology*, 111(2), 376–381.

Lee, A. G., Beaver, H. A., Jogerst, G., & Daly, J. M. (2003). Screening elderly patients in an outpatient ophthalmology clinic for dementia, depression, and functional impairment. *Ophthalmology*, 110(4), 651–657.

Lee, C. M., & Afshari, N. A. (2017). The global state of cataract blindness. *Current opinion in ophthalmology,* 28(1), 98–103.

Lee, C. S., Gibbons, L. E., Lee, A. Y., Yanagihara, R. T., Blazes, M. S., Lee, M. L., McCurry, S. M., Bowen, J. D., McCormick, W. C., Crane, P. K., & Larson, E. B. (2022). Association between cataract extraction and development of dementia. *JAMA internal medicine,* 182(2), 134–141.

Leske, M. C., Chylack, L. T., Jr, & Wu, S. Y. (1991). The lens opacities case-control study. risk factors for cataract. *Archives of ophthalmology,* 109(2), 244–251.

Lin, H., Zhang, L., Lin, D., Chen, W., Zhu, Y., Chen, C., Chan, K. C., Liu, Y., & Chen, W. (2018). Visual restoration after cataract surgery promotes functional and structural brain recovery. *EBioMedicine,* 30, 52–61.

Lin, M. Y., Gutierrez, P. R., Stone, K. L., Yaffe, K., Ensrud, K. E., Fink, H. A., Sarkisian, C. A., Coleman, A. L., Mangione, C. M., & Study of osteoporotic fractures research group (2004). Vision impairment and combined vision and hearing impairment predict cognitive and functional decline in older women. *Journal of the American geriatrics society,* 52(12), 1996–2002.

Lindenberger, U., & Baltes, P. B. (1994). Sensory functioning and intelligence in old age: a strong connection. *Psychology and aging,* 9(3), 339–355.

Liu, Y. C., Wilkins, M., Kim, T., Malyugin, B., & Mehta, J. S. (2017). Cataracts. *Lancet,* 390(10094), 600–612.

Livingston, G., Huntley, J., Sommerlad, A., Ames, D., Ballard, C., Banerjee, S., Brayne, C., Burns, A., Cohen-Mansfield, J., Cooper, C., Costafreda, S. G., Dias, A., Fox, N., Gitlin, L. N., Howard, R., Kales, H. C., Kivimäki, M., Larson, E. B., Ogunniyi, A., Orgeta, V., Ritchie, K., Rockwood, K., Sampson, E. L., Samus, Q., Schneider, L. S., Selbæk, G., Teri, L., Mukadam, N. (2020). Dementia prevention, intervention, and care: 2020 report of the Lancet Commission. *Lancet,* 396(10248), 413–446.

Maharani, A., Dawes, P., Nazroo, J., Tampubolon, G., Pendleton, N., & SENSE-Cog WP1 group (2018). Cataract surgery and age-related cognitive decline: A 13-year follow-up of the English longitudinal study of ageing. *PloS one,* 13(10), e0204833.

McCarty, C. A., & Taylor, H. R. (2001). The genetics of cataract. *Investigative ophthalmology & visual science,* 42(8), 1677–1678.

McGwin, G., Jr, Li, J., McNeal, S., & Owsley, C. (2003). The impact of cataract surgery on depression among older adults. *Ophthalmic epidemiology,* 10(5), 303–313.

Merin, S. (2005). *Inherited eye diseases: diagnosis and management* (2nd ed.). CRC Press.

Mitchell, S. L., Teno, J. M., Miller, S. C., & Mor, V. (2005). A national study of the location of death for older persons with dementia. *Journal of the American geriatrics society,* 53(2), 299–305.

Miyata, K., Yoshikawa, T., Morikawa, M., Mine, M., Okamoto, N., Kurumatani, N., & Ogata, N. (2018). Effect of cataract surgery on cognitive function in elderly: Results of Fujiwara-kyo Eye Study. *PloS one,* 13(2), e0192677.

Monge, Z. A., & Madden, D. J. (2016). Linking cognitive and visual perceptual decline in healthy aging: The information degradation hypothesis. *Neuroscience and biobehavioral reviews,* 69, 166–173.

Norouzpour Deilami, K., Ali Heidari Gorji M, Hamzeh Hoseini S and Farookhfar A. The impact of cataract surgery on depression in elderly Iranian patients: a case–control study. *Sudan journal of medical sciences* (2021) 16(4):439–449.

Ockleford E. *The Handbook of Aging and Cognition* (3rd Ed.). Craik, F. I. M., Timothy, A., Salthouse, T. A. (Eds.). Psychology Press, Taylor and Francis Group, New York and Hove, 2008. No. of Pages 672. ISBN 978-0-8058-5990-4.

Pellegrini, M., Bernabei, F., Schiavi, C., & Giannaccare, G. (2020). Impact of cataract surgery on depression and cognitive function: Systematic review and meta-analysis. *Clinical & experimental ophthalmology,* 48(5), 593–601.

Prince, M., Bryce, R., Albanese, E., Wimo, A., Ribeiro, W., & Ferri, C. P. (2013). The global prevalence of dementia: a systematic review and metaanalysis. *Alzheimer's & dementia: the journal of the Alzheimer's Association*, 9(1), 63–75.e2.

Qiu, C., Kivipelto, M., & von Strauss, E. (2009). Epidemiology of Alzheimer's disease: occurrence, determinants, and strategies toward intervention. *Dialogues in clinical neuroscience*, 11(2), 111–128.

Reichman, W. E., Fiocco, A. J., & Rose, N. S. (2010). Exercising the brain to avoid cognitive decline: examining the evidence. *Aging health,* 6(5), 565–584.

Sadun, A. A., Borchert, M., DeVita, E., Hinton, D. R., & Bassi, C. J. (1987). Assessment of visual impairment in patients with Alzheimer's disease. *American journal of ophthalmology*, 104(2), 113–120.

Salthouse, T. (2012). Consequences of age-related cognitive declines. *Annual review of psychology,* 63, 201–226.

Savica, R., Grossardt, B. R., Bower, J. H., Boeve, B. F., Ahlskog, J. E., & Rocca, W. A. (2013). Incidence of dementia with Lewy bodies and Parkinson disease dementia. *JAMA neurology,* 70(11), 1396–1402.

Schaumberg, D. A., Glynn, R. J., Christen, W. G., Hankinson, S. E., & Hennekens, C. H. (2000). Relations of body fat distribution and height with cataract in men. *The American journal of clinical nutrition*, 72(6), 1495–1502.

Schmidt, W., Klopp, N., Illig, T., & Graw, J. (2008). A novel GJA8 mutation causing a recessive triangular cataract. *Molecular vision*, 14, 851–856.

Schmoll, C., Tendo, C., Aspinall, P., & Dhillon, B. (2011). Reaction time as a measure of enhanced blue-light mediated cognitive function following cataract surgery. *The British journal of ophthalmology*, 95(12), 1656–1659.

Shiels, A., & Hejtmancik, J. F. (2013). Genetics of human cataract. *Clinical genetics*, 84(2), 120–127.

Sperduto, R. D., Milton R. C., Lindblad A. S., Klein B. E. K., Ferris F. L. and Clemons T. E. Risk factors associated with age-related nuclear and cortical cataract. *Ophthalmology* (2001) 108(8):1400–1408.

Swenor, B. K., Wang, J., Varadaraj, V., Rosano, C., Yaffe, K., Albert, M., & Simonsick, E. M. (2019). Vision impairment and cognitive outcomes in older adults: the health ABC study. *The journals of gerontology. Series A, Biological sciences and medical sciences*, 74(9), 1454–1460.

Tamura, H., Tsukamoto, H., Mukai, S., Kato, T., Minamoto, A., Ohno, Y., Yamashita, H., & Mishima, H. K. (2004). Improvement in cognitive impairment after cataract surgery in elderly patients. *Journal of cataract and refractive surgery*, 30(3), 598–602.

Tan, J. S., Wang, J. J., & Mitchell, P. (2008). Influence of diabetes and cardiovascular disease on the long-term incidence of cataract: the Blue Mountains eye study. *Ophthalmic epidemiology*, 15(5), 317–327.

Verdina, T., Stiro, F., Bruni, F., Spedicato, G. A., Mastropasqua, R., & Cavallini, G. M. (2022). Evaluation of the impact of cataract surgery on cognitive function in very elderly patients: a prospective, observational study. *Aging clinical and experimental research*, 34(3), 661–669.

von dem Hagen, E. A., Houston, G. C., Hoffmann, M. B., Jeffery, G., & Morland, A. B. (2005). Retinal abnormalities in human albinism translate into a reduction of grey matter in the occipital cortex. *The European journal of neuroscience*, 22(10), 2475–2480.

West, S. K., & Valmadrid, C. T. (1995). Epidemiology of risk factors for age-related cataract. *Survey of ophthalmology*, 39(4), 323–334.

Westcott, M. C., Tuft, S. J., & Minassian, D. C. (2000). Effect of age on visual outcome following cataract extraction. *The British journal of ophthalmology*, 84(12), 1380–1382.

Williams, A., Sloan, F. A., & Lee, P. P. (2006). Longitudinal rates of cataract surgery. *Archives of ophthalmology*, 124(9), 1308–1314.

Wong T. Y. (2001). Effect of increasing age on cataract surgery outcomes in very elderly patients. *BMJ (Clinical research ed.)*, 322(7294), 1104–1106.

Zhang, Q., Guo, X., Xiao, X., Yi, J., Jia, X., & Hejtmancik, J. F. (2004). Clinical description and genome wide linkage study of Y-sutural cataract and myopia in a Chinese family. *Molecular vision*, 10, 890–900.

Zheng, D. D., Swenor, B. K., Christ, S. L., West, S. K., Lam, B. L., & Lee, D. J. (2018). Longitudinal Associations between visual impairment and cognitive functioning: The salisbury eye evaluation study. *JAMA ophthalmology*, 136(9), 989–995.

Chapter 2

Advances in Neurodegenerative Disorder Diagnoses

Sailee Chowdhury[1,*],
Koyel Kar[1],
Priyanka Chakraborty[1],
Dipanjana Ash[1],
Ayon Dutta[2]
and Rana Mazumder[3]
[1]Department of Pharmaceutical Technology, BCDA College of Pharmacy & Technology, Hridaypur, Kolkata, West Bengal, India
[2]Department of Pharmaceutical Technology, Brainware University, Barasat, Kolkata, West Bengal, India
[3]Department of Pharmaceutics, Gitanjali College of Pharmacy, Lohapur, Birbhum, West Bengal, India

Abstract

Neurodegenerative disorders are progressive neurological degenerative conditions that have a big socioeconomic impact everywhere. For the purpose of offering suitable therapeutic interventions, their early detection is required. One of the tools of the next generation for seeing and keeping track of physiochemical variations linked to neurological illnesses is the development of biomarkers. Beta-amyloid, neurofilament light chain, tau protein, glial fibrillary protein, and alpha-synuclein are a few recent developments in fluid biomarkers. A brief discussion of imaging biomarkers is also included. Developments made in the

* Corresponding Author's Email: me_sailee@yahoo.com.

In: Neurogenerative Disorders
Editors: Mohit Agrawal, Manmohan Singhal, Amit Kumar Nayak et al.
ISBN: 979-8-89530-143-2

treatment plan different diseases like Parkinson, Huntington, Alzheimer, Amyotrophic lateral sclerosis and therefore offer a perception on the imminent projections to offer an outline for additional advancements and improvement of molecular diagnostics to combat neurodegenerative disorders is explored.

Keywords: neurodegenerative disorder, biomarkers, amyotrophic lateral sclerosis

Abbreviations

8OH2′dG	8-Hydroxy-2′-Deoxyguanosine
AI	Artificial Intelligence
ANXA3	Annexin A3
AQP9	Aquaporin 9
BBB	Blood-Brain-Barrier
C9orf72	Chromosome 9 Open Reader Frame 72
CBD	Corticobasal Degeneration
CNS	Central Nervous System
CYSTM	Cysteine-rich, Transmembrane Module
EEG	Electron Rncephalography
EMG	Electromyography
FFPET	Formalin-Fixed, Paraffin-Embedded Tissues
fMRI	Functional Magnetic Resonance Imaging
FTD	Frontotemporal Disorders
FUS	Fused in Sarcoma
H&Y	Hoehn and Yahr
IF	Interferon-γ
IL-6	Interleukin-6
LBD	Lewy Body Dementia
LRRK2	Leucine-Rich Repeat Kinase 2
MCP	Monocyte Chemoattractant Protein
mHTT protein	Mutant Huntingtin Protein
MRI	Magnetic Resonance Imaging
MRS	Magnetic Resonance Spectroscopy
MS	Multiple Sclerosis
MSA	Multisystem Atrophy
MUNE	Motor Unit Number Estimation

NDDs	Neurodegenerative Disorders
Nogo	Neurite Outgrowth Inhibitor
PARK2	Parkin
PET	Positron Emission Tomography
PINK1	PTEN-induced Putative Kinase 1
PROK2	Prokineticin 2
PS1	Presenilin 1
PSP	Progressive Supranuclear Palsy
SCOPA	Scales for Outcomes in Parkinson's Diseases
SMC	Single Molecule Counting
SPECT	Single Photon Emission Tomography
TARDBP	Transactive Response DNA Binding Protein
TLS	Translocated in Liposarcoma
TNF	Tumor Necrosis Factor
UCH-L1	Ubiquitincarboxy-Terminal Hydrolase L1
UPDRS	Unified Parkinson's Disease Rating Scale
wrCRP	Wide-Range C-Reactive Protein
ZNF238	Zinc Finger Protein 238
α-SNCA	α-Synuclein

Introduction

The hallmarks of NDDs are gradual disruption with subsequent structure or function loss of CNS manifesting cognitive deterioration and dementia (Lamptey et al., 2022). The most prevalent forms of NDDs include multiple sclerosis, Parkinson's disease, Huntington's disease, Alzheimer's disease and others (Peng et al., 2020).

Clinical medicine is always in need of objective evaluations of physical as well as cognitive roles as the foundation for diagnosis and health monitoring. In the future decades, there will likely be a sharp rise in the prevalence of NDDs, particularly those that afflict the elderly. Degenerative diseases' range widens to encompass an increasing number of recognised disorders, but it also narrows as usual patterns in chronic degeneration appear. To keep up with these quick changes, a variety of diagnostic tests have emerged, marrying cutting-edge imaging and neuro-physiological modalities with quantifiable phenotypic features employing neuropsychological methodologies and approaches (Henriques et al., 2018). Early neurodegeneration discovery is crucial since it can offer an opportunity for an early treatment that might be useful to stop the disease's future progression. The early diagnosis of NDD has seen a rise in the use of cutting-edge brain imaging methods like MRI, fMRI, PET and EEG. But some of the major drawbacks of cerebral imaging are the expensive expense of the equipment, the lack of initial scanning slots, and ineligibility for patients with pacemaker like metallic implants (Schwarz, 2021).

However, to emphasis more carefully on the biochemical anomalies in NDD, biochemical tests involve detecting changes of various proteins, metabolites, Ribonucleic acid and different molecules in the blood and CSF. Electrochemical sensors have paid attention recently due to their ability to detect biomarker amount in CSF and blood as well as their lower price, improved stability, increased precision, ease in downsizing (Agrawal and Biswas, 2015; Cohen et al., 2019).

Necessity for Biomarkers as a Diagnostic Tool

The issue of inter-individual variation in clinical aspects and progression of NDDs is what's driving the growing demand for precise and specific biomarker diagnostic techniques (Dorsey et al., 2018; Johansson et al., 2023). Additionally, a patient may have numerous NDDs simultaneously, such as Alzheimer's disease, Lewy Body Dementia and cerebral amyloid angiopathy, that result in fatal intra-cerebral haemorrhage (Robinson et al., 2018). Along with imaging and clinical histories, biomarkers can be used to detect concurrent disease processes. Different neurodegenerative disorders can currently be distinguished by a number of fluid biomarkers. However, CSF assays for Aβ42 orpTau-181 are the only assays that the FDA has approved demonstrating90% agreement with the results of PET scans (Shaw et al., 2019). Another use for biomarkers is to screen for NDDs because they can distinguish between pathological cognitive decline and normal ageing therefore can show up in CSF or plasma years before symptoms start to manifest. Definitely, some of these people have a higher-than-average hereditary risk of developing dementia. Through the use of biomarkers, patients may be given disease-specific or disease-preventive medications earlier or be able to take part in relevant studies when pathological alterations are still in an early stage. Access to clinical trials can be accelerated by incorporating biomarkers into clinical practise (Mattsson et al., 2015).

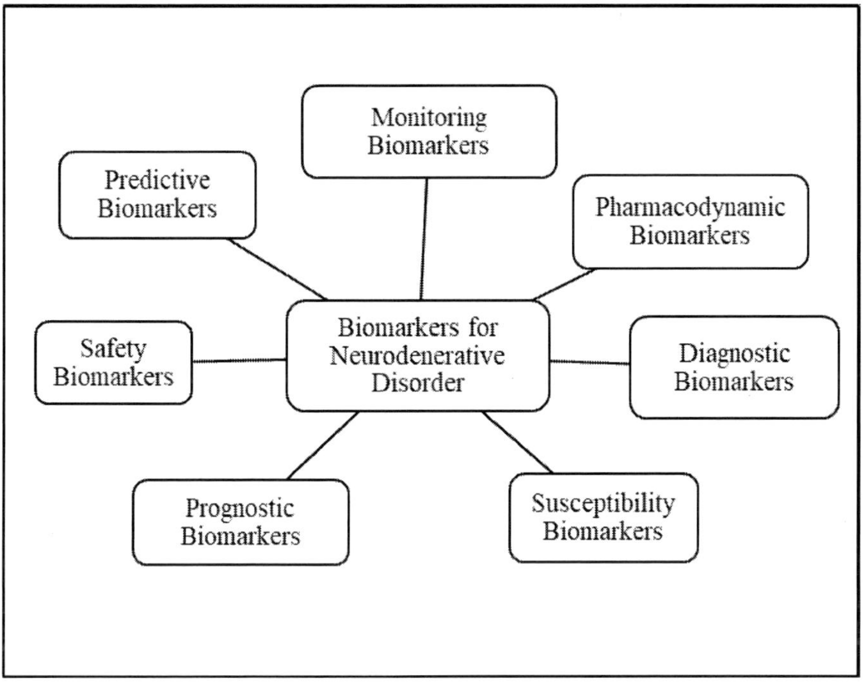

Figure 1. Different types of biomarkers for neurodegenerative disorder.

Common Biomarkers as Diagnostics for Neurodegenerative Disorders

A recent hot subject in neurodegenerative illnesses is the identification of biomarkers. Biomarkers, measurable and evaluable indicators, can be used to define diseased processes, usual biological processes and the pharmacological interactions to medications. The different categories of biomarkers used in neuro-degenerative disorders are represented in Figure 1.

Tau Protein Biomarkers

Neuronal microtubule stability is aided by the intracellular Tau protein. Increased A appears to cause tau and kinases to interact negatively, phosphorylate tau proteins inside of cells, and promote the creation of neuro-fibrillary tangles (NFTs), which disrupt cell communication (Tiwari et al., 2019). Increases in p-Tau (mainly phosphorylated form of Tau on threonine) at sites 181, 217, and 231 can act as a biomarker for AD (Palmqvist et al., 2019; Suárez-Calvet et al., 2020; Ossenkoppele et al., 2022). It may also help to distinguish between AD and FTD because levels of pTau 217 and 181 are raised in AD without unchanging in FTD (Thijssen et al., 2021). CSF pTau 231 may be 1sttau biomarker to be seen in early-onset AD (Ashton et al., 2022). Plasma pTau 181 can forecast the onset of AD. The ideal practice is to use combination of pTau and other biomarkers in clinical situation. The right cutoff for pTau positive needs to be defined by more research (Dubois et al., 2021).

Amyloid-β Biomarkers

Extra-neuronal and entwined peptides, Plaques, are aggregated as neurodegenerative disorder (LBD, AD) progresses resulting in altered protein synthesis showing oxidative stress and the disruption of synaptic signaling and ion transport in neurons (Tiwari et al., 2019). The two main A-peptides (A-40, A-42) in CSF and serum, are distinguished on the basis of length peptide chains via PET (Olsson et al., 2016). In CNS, more neurotoxicity and cellular disruptsionabilityofA-42 is observed than A-40 (Lee et al., 2017). The expense, availability, and invasiveness of CSF collection are drawbacks (Hansson et al., 2019). Recently, biomarker plasma levels (A42/40) have shown better predictive value in precise manner. Although CSF and plasma A biomarkers for AD are equally accurate, this is not currently for amnestic MCI (Chen et al., 2021).

A-Synuclein Biomarkers

A possible biomarker for detection of PD and LBD in CSF and plasma is α-syn. At presynaptic terminals, α-syn is packed in vesicles packaging (Rocha et al., 2018). In CSF both α-syn (oligomeric and phosphorylated) are elevated. Moreover, CSF α-syn (oligomeric) distinguishes between the healthy controls and PD more effectively than CSF or plasmaα-syn levels. Between AD and PD, CSF oligomeric α-syn may be distinguished (Hansson et al., 2014). The evidence for α-syn as a biomarker is clouded for inconsistent sample numbers, study designs and PD heterogeneity (Eusebi et al., 2017).

Glial Biomarkers

Astrocytes grow larger and produce more intermediate filaments, including GFAP, under stressful conditions, such as those associated with neurodegenerative diseases. Elevated systemic GFAP specifically as well as accurately can detect decreased myelin and axonal density than CSF levels (Walker et al., 2023; Benedet et al., 2021; Pereira et al., 2021). It has been suggested that GFAP can be used to distinguish between different NDDs because levels were elevated in AD and LBD but not PD and FTD. Studies found that GFAP was linked with the severity of FTD but not PD or AD. For neurodegenerative conditions other than AD, stronger proof is required (Abdelhak et al., 2022). When dementia occurs with other neurological circumstances, elevated levels of GFAP may be challenging to interpret as it is also raised with several brain injuries (Wang et al., 2018). Combining plasma GFAP with additional biomarkers, such as A and pTau, may be beneficial.

Neurofilament (NfL) Biomarkers

Acytoplasmic protein called Nf, a non-specific, reliable biomarker for axonal damage and non- symptomatic of Charcot-Marie-Tooth disease, AD, atypical PD, FTD, MS and FTD pathology, serves as an intermediate filament in the formation of axons (Khalil et al., 2018; Gaetani et al., 2019; Milà-Alomà et al., 2020). Although greater NfL levels are linked to cognitive deterioration, there is disagreement due to methodological discrepancies between studies (Ramani et al., 2021). Rises in NfL in AD were comparable to age-induced healthy individuals' NfL progression. NfL should be utilized along with A and pTau in older persons who may have neurological diseases.

Electroencephalogram as a Diagnostic Tool

Typically, researchers and physicians can easily collect objective data to capture quantitative electro encephalography utilizing an array of dense grid of scalp electrodes (250 electrodes arranged at predetermined manner) for measuring electrical activity in brain to understand pathogenesis of neurodegenerative disorders (Seiss et al., 2003). Other neuro-physiological methods, such as electromyography, evoked potentials, nerve conduction part, have a place in the diagnosis of neurodegenerative diseases like ALS and MND, but improving EEG yield has made the most progress in this area (Pezard et al., 2001). Activity at certain brain areas may be recorded with particular electrodes using this standard technique of electrode placement, making it simple to compare activity across people and neurodegenerative illnesses. When EEG data is recorded, the electrical conduction sensed by scalp electrodes is thought to be produced by the AP of cortical neurons, most frequently by excitatory postsynaptic potentials, even if the mechanism generating EEG is not entirely known. EEG analysis may therefore shed light on how information is processed in the cortex (Thakor et al., 2004). A patient's physical activity, such as blinking, yawning, or head movement while recording, can potentially cause artefacts, such as interfering from power lines and additional external electrical sources as well as electromyogram (EMG) artefacts. There has been a rise in interest in creating accurate indicators of memory impairment brought on by aging and illness in recent years. The National Institute on Ageing has promoted the development of inexpensive, easily accessible biomarkers from non-invasive EEG for age and disease-induced neurodegeneration to identify subtle functional alterations associated with either normal aging or structural or metabolic deficits attributing to recent advancements in signal processing and acquisition technology (Jeong, 2004).

Neurodegenerative Disease-Based Diagnostic Tools and Current Advancements

Alzheimer's Disease

Alzheimer's disease (AD), most predominant neurodegenerative disorder, is gradual, degenerative illness affecting the cerebral neurons via deteriorating acetylcholine and altering butyryl cholinesterase and acetyl cholinesterase resulting memory loss, loss of cognitive and linguistic abilities, and behavioural problems (Rachakonda et al., 2004). Extracellular senile plaques comprising of tau protein, are the aberrant lesions accumulating in brains of Alzheimer's patients (Hardy et al., 2002; EI-Agnaf et al., 2002). Clinical examinations and cognitive assessments, such as neuropsychological testing, are frequently used to make the diagnosis of AD (Harvey, 2012).

Genetic Biomarkers for the Diagnosis of Alzheimer's Disease

The following three gene mutations account for less than 5% of all instances of AD. The majority of known familial AD cases are caused by mutations in the two homologous presenilin genes, PS1 and PS2, located on chromosomes 14 and 1, respectively. In contrast, mutations in APP gene, located on chromosome 21, are relatively uncommon (Gasser et al., 2001). The presenilin genes produce presenilin proteins, which regulate the breakdown of the APP into smaller peptides (Goodall et al., 2013). Any mutation of missense in one of these presenilin genes results in the making of additional Aβ peptides causing an aberrant increase in APP activity (Berezovska et al., 2003). The βAPP gene was the site of the initial genetic variation connected to AD. The E4 allele of the ApoE is linked to the genetic AD in addition to the mutations previously discussed that can cause AD. (Bekris et al., 2010) Moreover, the E4 allele was found in all AD patients (approximately 40–50%) and could not recognise as a diagnostic marker.

Biochemical Markers for the Diagnosis of Alzheimer's Disease

Tau protein and Aβ concentrations in CSF are two most potential biochemical indicators. Aβ42, a significant indication (sensitivity80-90%) of AD, is secreted extracellular lyin biological fluids (CSF) and considered as great biomarker coupling with other AD biomarkers (Sunderland et al., 2003). A peptide from the CSF forms plaques in cerebral as AD worsens, reducing the amount of Aβ in the CSF.CSF-tau, a sensitive biomarker for AD, however, is unclear why it abnormally rises in AD patients. CSF-Aβ-42 and CSF-tau combination may enhance specificity and sensitivity becomes an ideal pair of biomarkers for AD (Sjögren et al., 2003). 2-[[18F] Fluoro ethyl] (methyl)amino] 1-(1-6Due to its capacity to pass BBB, 2-naphthyl-ethylidenemalononitrile ([18F] FDDNP)-PET, a novel method for early diagnosis of AD, can identify amount of neuro fibrillary tangles and senile amyloid plaques in cerebral with location. 18-FDG-PET (91 ± 3% sensitive) is used to estimate synapse number and assess the energy consumption of the brain (Bokde et al., 2011; Wurtman, 2015). FDDNP binding results in the identification of a novel binding site to A40 fibrils, opening up new possibilities for the treatment of AD in its early stages. Both sensitive tracers, SPECT and PET were employed in the diagnosis of AD (Bokde et al., 2011). Most tracers show the condition's neuronal death causing localized minimization of glucose uptake and investigated by 18F-FDG PET imaging (Young, 2009). MicroRNAs (miRNAs), acting as crucial regulators of several biological processes (synaptic plasticity and neurogenesis), have been used to identify AD early (Grasso et al., 2014; Goodall et al., 2013). The researchers then discovered two sets of bio-molecular diagnostic marker pairs consisting of miR134/miR370, miR3233p/miR370, and miR382/miR370, with relatively high sensitivity (79-100%) and specificity (79-95%). In long-term investigation the discovered miRNA diagnostic biomarker pairs diagnosed MCI in most of patients at asymptomatic stage (1-5 years before clinical conditions) successfully (Sheinerman et al., 2012). Recent findings about changes in plasma phospholipid concentrations can be used to create novel bimolecular diagnostic markers for AD. The drop in phospholipid levels will make it possible to predict with accuracy whether a person with cognitively normal abilities will experience MCI or AD over the next 2 years (Wurtman, 2015). Additionally blood-based biomarker panel (>90% accurate) was used to identify preclinical AD (Mapstone et al., 2014).

Parkinson's Disease

The marked symptoms of Parkinson's disease, an age-inducing disorder, include stiffness, unstable posture, bradykinesia, rest shaking, and a wide range of additional kinetic and non-motor manifestations (Obeso et al., 2017; Armstrong and Okun, 2020). In Parkinson's disease, dopaminergic neurons located between substantia nigra and inner striatum experience deterioration resulting in major loss of dopamine-expressing cells. Based on the worldwide disease burden study (2016), there will be approximately 13 million cases of Parkinson's disease within 2040, highlighting the possible outbreak of Parkinson's disease (Joseph and Tan, 2020; Dorsey et al., 2018). Therefore, finding of initial stages molecular biological markers for Parkinson's disease is essential since it enables for an assessment of the efficacy of neurologically beneficial treatments for the condition. Based on clinical criteria (condition and progression) Parkinson's disease is assessed employing several organised scales including H&Y staging, SCOPA and UPDRS (Molochnikov et al., 2012).

Genetic Biomarkers for the Diagnosis of Parkinson's Disease

In only a small percentage of families, Parkinson's disease develops in a Mendelian dominant autosomal or autosomal regressive manner. For late-onset and early-stage of symptoms alterations have been identified in the genes encoding α-SNCA, LRRK2 and PARK2, UCH-L1, PINK1, oncogene DJ1 respectively (Grasso et al., 2014). A distinctive feature of this neurodegenerative disease, particularly the uncommon early onset familial variant, is the presence of pointed mutations, replications, and triplications in α-SNCA gene on the 4th chromosome. The monogenetic autosomal recessive variants of PD have been studied to identify genes and variants of gene expression. Numerous genetic products of the dominantly inherited autosomal genes have been associated with lack of mitochondrial function and improper functioning of the genetic resultant products in defective or anomalous forms such as oligometric α-SNCA (Miller and O'Callaghan, 2015). The early-stage variant of Parkinson's illness has been linked to greater than 70 alterations on the most prevalent parkin gene that are potentially responsible for hereditary instances of autosomal dominant adolescent Parkinsonism (maximum 50%) (Pankratz et al., 2003). A gene on the 4th chromosome (UCH-L1) encoding a protein (belonging to family, deubiquitinating enzyme), comprised 1% of brain proteins, have been hypothesized to act to reprocess ubiquitin via hydrolysis of ubiquitinated peptides. This deubiquitinating enzyme contributes to the modification of damaged proteins that would otherwise build up in the cell to hazardous levels (Leroy et al., 1998). Furthermore, two identical PINK1 genetic variants (correlated with PD) in families from Spain and Italy were discovered offering additional confirmation to establish a relationship between PINK1 mutations and PARK6, PARK7 (in DJ1 oncogene) (Bonifati et al., 2003; Valente et al., 2004). The DJ-1 proteins, significance in neurotoxicity and cellular oxidative stress, caused slow development of signs and endure response to levodopa therapy (Dekker et al., 2003). Understanding the function of the mentioned genes might help us better comprehend how brain neuronal maintenance mechanisms perform.

Biochemical Markers for the Diagnosis of Parkinson's Disease

For recognizing the initialization of PD, the following bio-molecular screening markers have been used namely α -synuclein protein (existence detected in the Lewy body injuries) and dopamine transporter "DAT" (disappearance identified via PET scanning). Dopamine is taken up by dopaminergic neurons through electrogenic, Na^+ and Cl^- transport-coupled process controlled by DAT. Both the united and distinct regions on the transporter, which is seen to be significantly impacted by the existence of cations, are bound to uptake blockers (Dopamine and cocaine). Additionally, Parkinson's illness causing chemicals are taken up by DAT. As a result, the concentration of DAT in the striatum (putamen) is thought to be the greatest biochemical screening symbol for the onset of PD (Marek et al., 2000; Rachakonda et al., 2004; Shinto et al., 2014). Two variants in the α-synuclein gene (present in multiple synucleinopathies) have been accountable for finding of both Lewy bodies and neuritis, the distinctive pathologies in cerebrum of people suffering PD and dementia. The usage of α-synuclein should be coupled with other diagnostic techniques (such as PET with [^{18}F]-Dopa tracer and SPECT with [123I]-β-CIT) in order to improve its accuracy and efficacy for PD (Tissingh et al., 1997; Duyckaerts et al., 2003; Loane and Politis, 2011). By observing the discharge of positrons from the cerebral cortex following a modest dose of radioactive elements or markers administered into the circulatory system, PET is thought to be the most effective method for diagnosing PD. Studies revealed average 40% decrease in striatal 18F-Dopa consumption in PD patients in comparison to controls (Bokde et al., 2011). PD Patients consuming medication often show an average profile of 18F-Dopa. Ioflupane Iodine-123, a widely available and more clinically accessible SPECT tracer than [18F]-Dopa, stimulates the structure of the presynaptic dopamine receptor system. The SPECT is distinct from PET is via using isotopes having longer half-lives retaining on site (Rachakonda et al., 2004; Young, 2009). Shinto et al., (2014) revealed progressive decline in particular striatal uptake of 99mTc-TRODAT-1 (after 3h of injecting) in Stage I, II and III 16 PD individuals (9 men, 7 women) compared to 6 identical aged healthy ones via SPECT imaging (Shinto et al., 2014). 99mTc-TRODAT-1 is a reliable and frequently used in Parkinsonism differential diagnostic tool for quantifying DAT activity however the cost-effectiveness is still an issue (Jankovic et al., 2000; Molochnikov et al., 2012). Body fluids are suitable platforms for biomarkers representing the biological status of the cells and are easy to access and inexpensive (Shinde et al., 2015). The potential for developing circulatory biomarkers for PD is enormous considering the rising significance of miRNAs in biologicals (Soreq et al., 2013; Grasso et al., 2014). Parkinson's disease has no standardised diagnostic procedure. An accurate biomarker including blood test or scanning is currently being developed by researchers to detect the dopamine and its metabolism in the brain. However, these examinations are pricey and are only carried out in specialised imaging facilities (Torrent et al., 2015).

Amyotrophic Lateral Sclerosis

Amyotrophic lateral sclerosis (ALS), a form of NDDs, mostly impacts on both motor neurons (motor neurons in motor cortex, cerebral nuclei and anterior part of the spinal cord) and extra-motor regions resulting in gradual fatigue of muscles, fasciculation and atrophy. Oxidative damage, ER stress, impaired mitochondrial function, malfunctioning endosomal slavery, gene transcription, and RNA degradation, excito-toxicity, sudden cellular death, swelling, and genetic predisposition are just a few of the many factors that contribute to ALS (Masrori and Philip, 2020; Srinivasan et al., 2020). The manifestations, clinical assessment, and multiple rounds of testing (such as MUNE and EMG) govern the diagnosis of ALS (Joyce and Gregory, 2013).

Genetic Biomarkers for the Diagnosis of Amyotrophic Lateral Sclerosis

Genetic ALS is thought to be caused by alterations in over a dozen varieties of genes. A malfunction in a gene, C9orf72 accounts for about 1/3rd of all genetic instances (and a tiny proportion of random cases). Genetic (gene superoxide dismutase 1 producing copper-zinc superoxide dismutase 1) alteration is also responsible for another 20% of heredity cases (Agrawal and Biswas, 2015). The purpose of genes is still a mystery. The hereditary instances (3%) occur from abnormalities in the TARDBP gene encoding for TAR DNA binding protein-43 and another 5% of familial and <1% of occasional instances result from alterations in the FUS gene encoding FUS/TLS (Robelin et al., 2014). Chromosomal structure can be reversibly and inheritably altered through epigenetic processes (for example DNA methylation and acetylation of histone) however non-heritable alterations affect the layout of chromatin or DNA but not DNA sequence (Martin et al., 2013). Studies reported that DNA samples from post-mortem spinal cord tissue from occasional ALS individuals were characterised using the micro array technique (Figueroa-Romero et al., 2012).

Bio-Chemical Markers for the Diagnosis of Amyotrophic Lateral Sclerosis

Studies revealed that mGLUR2, belonging to metabotropic glutamate receptor category, provided safe-guardian contradiction of excitotoxicity and diminished in ALS T lymphocytes (Poulopoulou et al., 2005). Additionally, the levels of glutathione peroxidase and SOD1 enzyme expression were shown to be reduced in erythrocytes of ALS patients (Cova et al., 2010). Another helpful indicator for ALS is increased levels of 8OH2′dG, a byproduct of oxidative damage to DNA (Bogdanov et al., 2000). Microglial cells and other immune cells proliferate unregulated in CNS, causing ALS neuronal deterioration (Philips and Robberecht, 2011). In the peripheral of ALS patients the concentration of IF-γ, IL-6, TNF, MCP and wrCRP was found to be increased attributing to cytokines, novel biomarkers (Robelin and Gonzalez,

2014). Nogo, a potential biochemical marker, exhibits synaptic expansion suppressive function and is essential to the disease (Fergani et al., 2005).

Table 1. Genetic/molecular and bio-chemical markers of different neurodegenerative disorders

Neurodegenerative disorders	Diagnostic tools		
	Genetic/molecular	Bio-chemical	References
AD	PS1, PS2 mutations, APP, ApoEisoforms	Cerebro-spinal fluid tau protein, Phospho-tau	Gasser et al., 2001; Sunderland et al., 2003; Bekris et al., 2010
PD	α-SNCA, LRRK2 and PARK2, UCH-L1, PINK1, oncogene DJ1 mutations	Disappearance of DAT, Injuries in Lewy body	Grasso et al., 2014; Agawal and Biswas, 2015
ALS	C9orf72, TARDBP gene, FUS gene mutations	mGLUR2, IF-γ, IL-6, TNF, MCP and wrCRP	Cova et al., 2010; Philips and Robberecht, 2011; Robelin et al., 2014; Agrawaland Biswas, 2015
HD	H2AFY, PROK2, ZNF238, AQP9, ANXA3, CYSTM gene mutations	8OHdG, lactic acid, 4-hydroxynoneal, malondialdehyde, Interleukins, TNF-α, clusterin, glutathione peroxidase, copper-zinc superoxide dismutase	Agrawaland Biswas, 2015

Huntington's Disease

Huntington's disease (HD), a completely infiltrating neurodegenerative disorder, is triggered via rapid and significant rising of hereditary CAG trinucleotide in the Huntington's gene on 4th chromosome (Andhale and Shrivastava, 2022). Recently SMC mHTT immunoassay and microarray technology were adapted to determine mHTT levels and alteration of mRNA in blood in HD patient respectively (Lovrecic et al., 2009; Wild et al., 2015). The evaluation of HD biomarkers has always been difficult because the disease manifests itself via a range of characteristics and progresses at different speeds.

Molecular Biomarkers for the Diagnosis of Huntington's Disease

Clinical study reported the overexpression (1.6-times) of gene H2AFY in both blood and brain of HD patients (Hu et al., 2011). Next-generation DNA sequencing and Fluidigm methodologies demonstrated an analysis of gene expression and identified a group of five genes (PROK2, ZNF238, AQP9, ANXA3 and CYSTM as expected HD biomarkers that are considerably detected in HD blood (Borovecki et al., 2005; Zhai et al., 2005; Aziz et al., 2010; Mesko et al., 2010; Venancio and Aravind, 2010; Mastrokolias et al., 2015). PROK2 and ZNF238 plays aemerging role in modifications of circadian rhythms and brain progression respectively associated with HD (Zhai et al., 2005; Aziz et al., 2010). Inflammatory mechanisms was found to be raised for the overexpression of AQP9 in blood (Mesko et al., 2010).

Biochemical Markers for the Diagnosis of Huntington's Disease

The recognition of impaired homoeostasis in this disease has led to the identification of numerous feasible biomarkers. Recent investigation via cross-sectional MRS putaminal metabolic products in pre-manifest and previously detected HD people were differentiated from healthy controls using (Sturrock et al., 2015). In a recent investigation employing cross-sectional MRS differentiate putaminal metabolic products as potential bio-chemical marker for example elevation and reduction of myo-inositol and N-acetyl Aspartate in pre-clinical and initial stage HD patient from controls (Sturrock et al., 2015). A higher serum concentration of vasopressin (assists in homoeostasis) in HD individual was established vasopressin as influential biomarker (Wood et al., 2008). Elevated levels of 8OHdG, Interleukins, TNF-α, clusterin (in plasma and brain) and lowering of copper-zinc superoxide dismutase (in plasma) and glutathione peroxidase of HD patients were found to be significant biomarkers (Chen et al., 2007; Dalrymple et al., 2007; Weir et al., 2011).

All of these biomarkers (listed in Table 1) would make it easier to assess therapeutic efficacy accurately and would enhance the security and effectiveness of clinical studies.

Recent Challenges

Undoubtedly, these advanced biosensors have facilitated the diagnosis and management of neurodegenerative disorders offering a number of advantages over traditional methods for diagnosing different neurological diseases (Hyodoet al., 2022). The continual modernization and modification of the electrodes used in production of transducer have also lately increased the benefits of the biosensors. Despite all these advantages, there are still difficulties when using biosensors for NDD control and detection in practical settings. Biosensor performance, production costs, disposal costs, and sensitivity are all influenced by the electrode's physical and chemical composition, which in turn depends on how the material is manufactured and how it is designed. Furthermore, the cost of gold and platinum metals may be high due to their application in the manufacture of electrodes. The process of making metal electrodes often involves chopping off pieces of larger metal components, which drives up production costs (Tao et al., 2021). In order for wearables and other IoT-connected devices to operate fast in real-time, they need a strong connection and extremely low latency. The materials or nanomaterials used to make electrodes may have neuro-toxic effects; therefore, this must be taken into account as well. Due to the multiple *in vitro* research involved, biocompatibility assessment occasionally needs a lot of labour. Therefore, when utilising diverse biosensors for the detection of NDD, a basic understanding of physiological condition, cognitive dysfunctions, and epidemiological part is required. There are presently few blood signs that can be used to precisely detect NDD (Hansson, 2021). Neuroscientists are forced to employ an invasive procedure to gather samples and implant electrodes as a result of these barriers (Terstappen et al., 2021).

Future Projections

Nanotechnology can be used in the production of electrodes to address the numerous problems with employing biosensors for NDD. In order to identify and monitor a range of brain alterations, NDD bio-sensing techniques have been improved with the aid of nanotechnological tools (Liang and Jeong-Yeol, 2021). Current years have observed an increase in the use of nanoparticles, which has resulted in advancements, particularly in sensitivity, detection range, and response time (Rohilla et al., 2021). The ability of carbon nanoparticles to interact with, detect, and remove amyloid plaques have been demonstrated in a recent study on its use in the diagnosis of AD. Similar to this, graphene's carbon nanotubes can improve sensor conductivity. Nanoscale modifications have also been observed in antibodies, receptors, enzymes, and other elements involved in analyte recognition. Access to the 5

G communication network is projected to increase the output of AI biosensors by delivering faster wireless connectivity and speed. Data collection, better detection accuracy, more effective treatment, monitoring of symptoms, analysis of NDD progression, forecasting of symptom incidence, and the creation of NDD-related government policies can all benefit from this (Gopinath et al., 2022).

Conclusion

Applications for biosensors span a wide range of fields, such as forensics, ecological monitoring, food protection, medication improvement, and illness (especially in NDDs) detection. A measurable and quantifiable signal is generated via magnetic, optical, electrochemical, and mechanical biosensors when bio-molecular analytes interact with a useful biosensor electrode. Recent research points to nanomaterial-based biosensors as a potential replacement for the traditional, labor-intensive methods of finding biomarkers. However, there are immobile barriers standing in the way of improved biosensors realizing their full potential. Therefore, future research must focus on creating reliable and accurate electrochemical sensors that can recognise biomarkers as well as finding novel composite materials with potent anti-interference properties that can improve the analytical process's sensitivity and specificity.

Disclaimer

None.

References

Abdelhak, A., Foschi, M., Abu-Rumeileh, S., Yue, J. K., D'Anna, L., Huss, A., Oeckl, P., Ludolph, A. C., Kuhle, J., Petzold, A., & Manley, G. T. (2022). Blood GFAP as an emerging biomarker in brain and spinal cord disorders. *Nature Reviews Neurology,* 18(3), 158-172. https://doi.org/10.1038/s41582-021-00609-8.

Agrawal, M., & Abhijit, B. (2015). Molecular diagnostics of neurodegenerative disorders. *Frontiers in Molecular Biosciences,* 2, 54. https://doi.org/10.3389/fmolb.2015.00054.

Andhale, R., & Deepti, S. (2022). Huntington's disease: A clinical review. *Cureus,* 14(8), e28484. https://doi.org/10.7759/cureus.28484.

Ariyurek, A., Y., Goeman, J. J., Van Duijn, E., Roos, R. A., Van Der Mast, R. C., Van Ommen, G. B., Den Dunnen, J. T., t Hoen, P. A., & van Roon-Mom, W. (2015). Huntington's disease biomarker progression profile identified by transcriptome sequencing in peripheral blood. *European Journal of Human Genetics,* 23(10), 1349-1356. https://doi.org/10.1038/ejhg.2014.292.

Armstrong, M. J., & Michael, S. O. (2020). Diagnosis and treatment of Parkinson disease: A review. *JAMA,* 323(6), 548-560. https://doi.org/10.1001/jama.2020.0710.

Ashton, N. J., L. B. Andrea, T. K. Tharick, K. K. Thomas, R. J. Juan, S. B. Wagner, M. Sulantha, et al., (2022). Cerebrospinal fluid p-tau231 as an early indicator of emerging pathology in Alzheimer's disease. *EBioMedicine,* 76, 103836. https://doi.org/10.1016/j.ebiom.2022.103836.

Aziz, N. A., V. A. Galia, M. Johan, J. L. Gert, & A. C. Raymund. (2010). Sleep and circadian rhythm alterations correlate with depression and cognitive impairment in Huntington's disease. *Parkinsonism & Related Disorders,* 16(5), 345-350. https://doi.org/10.1016/j.parkreldis.2009.12.007.

Bekris, L. M., Chang-En, Y., Thomas, D. B., & Debby, W. T. (2010). Genetics of Alzheimer disease. *Journal of Geriatric Psychiatry and Neurology*, 23(4), 213-227. https://doi.org/10.1177/0891988710383554.

Benedet, A. L., Marta, M. A., Agathe, V., Nicholas, J. A., Tharick, P., Firoza, L., Thomas, K. K., et al., (2021). Differences between plasma and cerebrospinal fluid glial fibrillary acidic protein levels across the Alzheimer disease continuum. *JAMA Neurology*, 78(12), 1471-1483. https://doi.org/10.1001/jamaneurol.2021.3350.

Berezovska, O., Pavan, R., Jesse, S., Michael, S. W., Brian, J. B., & Bradley, T. H. (2003). Amyloid precursor protein associates with a nicastrin-dependent docking site on the presenilin 1–γ-secretase complex in cells demonstrated by fluorescence lifetime imaging. *Journal of Neuroscience*, 23(11), 4560-4566. https://doi.org/10.1523/JNEUROSCI.23-11-04560.2003.

Bogdanov, M., Robert, H. B. J., Wayne, M., Ryan, S., Doug, H., Heather, O. D., Mflint, B., & Merit, C. (2000). Increased oxidative damage to DNA in ALS patients. *Free Radical Biology and Medicine,* 29(7), 652-658. https://doi.org/10.1016/S0891-5849(00)00440-1.

Bokde, A. L. W., James, F. M. M., Niall, P. S., Richard, B. R., Sharon, A., & Colin, P. D. (2011). Advances in diagnostics for neurodegenerative disorders. In *Neurodegenerative Disorders: A Clinical Guide* (pp. 17-42).

Bonifati, V., Patrizia, R., Marijke, J. V. B., Onno, S., Guido, J. B., Elmar, K., Marieke, C. J. D., et al., (2003). Mutations in the DJ-1 gene associated with autosomal recessive early-onset parkinsonism. Science, 299(5604), 256-259. https://doi.org/10.1126/science.1077205.

Borovecki, F. L., Lovrecic, J. Z., Hyun, J., Florian, T., H. D. Rosas, S. M. Hersch, et al., (2005). Genome-wide expression profiling of human blood reveals biomarkers for Huntington's disease. *Proceedings of the National Academy of Sciences,* 102(31), 11023-11028. https://doi.org/10.1073/pnas.0502824102.

Chen, C. M., Yih-RW, Mei-LC, Jun-LL, Yu-ML, Po-WL, Bing-WS, & Daniel, T. Y. C. (2007). Increased oxidative damage and mitochondrial abnormalities in the peripheral blood of Huntington's disease patients. *Biochemical and Biophysical Research Communications,* 359(2), 335-340. https://doi.org/10.1016/j.bbrc.2007.05.066.

Chen, Y. R., Chih, S. L., Hsin, C., Joachim, V., Xiao, L. K., Grant, O. C., Hsiu, J. J., Doresses, L., Shu, T. S. H., & Kuei, R. C. (2021). Diagnostic accuracy of blood biomarkers for Alzheimer's disease and amnestic mild cognitive impairment: A meta-analysis. *Ageing Research Reviews*, 71, 101446. https://doi.org/10.1016/j.arr.2021.101446.

Cohen, A. D., Susan, M. L., Beth, E. S., William, E. K., Kaj, B., & Henrik, Z. (2019). Fluid and PET biomarkers for amyloid pathology in Alzheimer's disease. *Molecular and Cellular Neuroscience*, 97, 3-17. https://doi.org/10.1016/j.mcn.2019.01.003.

Cova, E., Paolo, B., Cristina, C., Maria, R. M., Laura, S., Stefano, B., Stefania Guareschi, Bruno, R., & Mauro, C. (2010). Time course of oxidant markers and antioxidant defenses in subgroups of amyotrophic lateral sclerosis patients. *Neurochemistry International,* 56(5), 687-693. https://doi.org/10.1016/j.neuint.2009.12.002.

Dalrymple, A., Edward, J. W., Richard, J., Kirupa, S., Maria, B., Åsa, P., Graham, S. J., et al., (2007). Proteomic profiling of plasma in Huntington's disease reveals neuroinflammatory activation and biomarker candidates. *Journal of Proteome Research,* 6(7), 2833-2840. https://doi.org/10.1021/pr0701250.

Dekker, M., Vincenzo, B., John, V. S., Nico, L., Robert, J. G., Pieter, S., Marten, H., Peter, H., Ben, O., & Cornelia, V. D. (2003). Clinical features and neuroimaging of PARK7-linked parkinsonism. *Movement Disorders*, 18(7), 751-757. https://doi.org/10.1002/mds.11660.

Dorsey, E. R., Alexis, E., Emma, N., Nooshin, A., Foad, A. A., Ahmed, A., José, C. A., et al., (2018). Global, regional, and national burden of Parkinson's disease, 1990–2016: A systematic analysis for the Global Burden of Disease Study 2016. *The Lancet Neurology*, 17(11), 939-953. https://doi.org/10.1016/S1474-4422(18)30295-3.

Dorsey, E. R., Alistair, M. G., Melissa, R. H., Gretchen, L. B., & Lee, H. (2018). Teleneurology and mobile technologies: The future of neurological care. *Nature Reviews Neurology*, 14(5), 285-297. https://doi.org/10.1038/s41582-018-0001-7.

Dubois, B., Nicolas, V., Giovanni, B. F., Gil, D. R., Marwan, S., Stefano, C., Alexandre, B., et al., (2021). Clinical diagnosis of Alzheimer's disease: Recommendations of the International Working Group. *The Lancet Neurology,* 20(6), 484-496. https://doi.org/10.1016/S1474-4422(21)00045-2.

Duyckaerts, C., & Jean-Jacques, H. (2003). Lewy bodies, a misleading marker for Parkinson's disease? *Bulletin de l'Academie Nationale de Medecine*, 187(2), 277-292. https://doi.org/10.1016/S0007-5509(03)00051-0.

EI-Agnaf, O. M. A., & Irvine, G. B. (2002). Aggregation and neurotoxicity of α-synuclein and related peptides. *Biochemical Society Transactions*, 30(4), 559-565. https://doi.org/10.1042/bst0300559.

Eusebi, P., David, G., Leonardo, B., Iosief, A., Davide, C., Massimiliano, O., Paolo, C., & Lucilla, P. (2017). Diagnostic utility of cerebrospinal fluid α-synuclein in Parkinson's disease: A systematic review and meta-analysis. *Movement Disorders*, 32(10), 1389-1400. https://doi.org/10.1002/mds.27007.

Fergani, A., Luc, D., Natasa, J., Yves, L., Marc, D. T., Frederique, R., Jean-Philippe, L., & Jose-Luis, G. A. (2005). Reticulons as markers of neurological diseases: Focus on amyotrophic lateral sclerosis. Neurodegenerative *Diseases,* 2(3-4), 185-194. https://doi.org/10.1159/000087219.

Figueroa, R., C. J. H., Diane, E. B., Colin, E. D., Michael, D. C., Andrea, L. S., Raymond, Y., Douglas, M. R., Brian, C. C., & Eva, L. F. (2012). Identification of epigenetically altered genes in sporadic amyotrophic lateral sclerosis. *PLoS ONE*, 7(12), e52672. https://doi.org/10.1371/journal.pone.0052672.

Gaetani, L., Kaj, B., Paolo, C., Massimiliano, D. F., Lucilla, P., & Henrik, Z. (2019). Neurofilament light chain as a biomarker in neurological disorders. *Journal of Neurology, Neurosurgery & Psychiatry,* 90(8), 870-881. https://doi.org/10.1136/jnnp-2018-320804.

Gasser, T. M., Dichgans, J. F. I., Hausmanowa-Petrusewicz, K., Jurkat-Rott, T., Klopstock, E. L., et al., (2001). EFNS task force on molecular diagnosis of neurologic disorders: Guidelines for the molecular diagnosis of inherited neurologic diseases. First of two parts. *European Journal of Neurology,* 8(4), 299-314. https://doi.org/10.1046/j.1468-1331.2001.00109.x.

Goodall, E. F., Paul, R. H., Oliver, B., Janine, K., & Pamela, J. S. (2013). Neuronal dark matter: The emerging role of microRNAs in neurodegeneration. *Frontiers in Cellular Neuroscience*, 7, 178. https://doi.org/10.3389/fncel.2013.00178.

Gopinath, S. C. B., Zool, H. I., Mohd, I. S., & Mohd, N. M. Y. (2022). Advancement in biosensor: Telediagnosis and remote digital imaging. *Biotechnology and Applied Biochemistry*, 69(3), 1199-1208. https://doi.org/10.1002/bab.2262.

Grasso, M., Paola, P., Annamaria, C., & Michela, A. D. (2014). Circulating miRNAs as biomarkers for neurodegenerative disorders. *Molecules,* 19(5), 6891-6910. https://doi.org/10.3390/molecules19056891.

Hansson, O. (2021). Biomarkers for neurodegenerative diseases. *Nature Medicine*, 27(6), 954-963. https://doi.org/10.1038/s41591-021-01368-0.

Hansson, O., Sara, H., Annika, Ö., Henrik, Z., Kaj, B., Lennart, M., & Katarina, N. (2014). Levels of cerebrospinal fluid α-synuclein oligomers are increased in Parkinson's disease with dementia and dementia with Lewy bodies compared to Alzheimer's disease. *Alzheimer's Research & Therapy,* 6(3), 1-6. https://doi.org/10.1186/alzrt268.

Hansson, O., Sylvain, L., Markus, O., Henrik, Z., & Piotr, L. (2019). Advantages and disadvantages of the use of the CSF Amyloid β (Aβ) 42/40 ratio in the diagnosis of Alzheimer's Disease. *Alzheimer's Research & Therapy*, 11(1), 1-15. https://doi.org/10.1186/s13195-019-0467-7.

Hardy, J., & Dennis, J. S. (2002). The amyloid hypothesis of Alzheimer's disease: Progress and problems on the road to therapeutics. *Science*, 297(5580), 353-356. https://doi.org/10.1126/science.1077779.

Harvey, P. D. (2012). Clinical applications of neuropsychological assessment. *Dialogues in Clinical Neuroscience,* 14(1), 91-99. https://doi.org/10.31887/DCNS.2012.14.1/pharvey.

Henriques, A. D., Andrea, L. B., Einstein, F. C., Pedro, R., & Otávio, T. N. (2018). Fluid and imaging biomarkers for Alzheimer's disease: Where we stand and where to head to. *Experimental Gerontology,* 107, 169-177. https://doi.org/10.1016/j.exger.2018.03.013

Hu, Y., Vanita, C., Raman, C., Joseph, J. L., Zhixiang, L., Hongliu, D., Bin, Z., et al., (2011). Transcriptional modulator H2A histone family, member Y (H2AFY) marks Huntington disease activity in man and mouse. *Proceedings of the National Academy of Sciences,* 108(41), 17141-17146. https://doi.org/10.1073/pnas.1107187108.

Hyodo, T., Wataru, S., Taro, U., & Yasuhiro, S. (2022). Effects of surface modification of platinum electrodes with gold on hydrogen-sensing properties of diode-type sensors. *ECS Sensors Plus,* 1(1), 013602. https://doi.org/10.1149/ecsensorsplus.1.013602.

Jankovic, J., & Tan, E. K. (2020). Parkinson's disease: Etiopathogenesis and treatment. *Journal of Neurology, Neurosurgery & Psychiatry,* 91(8), 795-808. https://doi.org/10.1136/jnnp-2020-323940.

Jankovic, J., Ali, H. R., Michael, M., Daniel, P., & Parkinson Study Group. (2000). The evolution of diagnosis in early Parkinson disease. *Archives of Neurology,* 57(3), 369-372. https://doi.org/10.1001/archneur.57.3.369.

Jeong, J. (2004). EEG dynamics in patients with Alzheimer's disease. *Clinical Neurophysiology*, 115(7), 1490-1505. https://doi.org/10.1016/j.clinph.2004.01.015.

Johansson, C., Thordardottir, S., Laffita-Mesa, J., Rodriguez-Vieitez, E., Zetterberg, H., Blennow, K., & Graff, C. (2023). Plasma biomarker profiles in autosomal dominant Alzheimer's disease. *Brain,* 146(3), 1132-1140. https://doi.org/10.1093/brain/awad026.

Joyce, N. C., & Carter, G. T. (2013). Electrodiagnosis in persons with amyotrophic lateral sclerosis. *PM&R,* 5(5), S89-S95. https://doi.org/10.1016/j.pmrj.2013.01.012.

Khalil, M., Teunissen, C. E., Otto, M., Piehl, F., Sormani, M. P., Gattringer, T., Barro, C., Kappos, L., Comabella, M., Fazekas, F., & Petzold, A. (2018). Neurofilaments as biomarkers in neurological disorders. *Nature Reviews Neurology*, 14(10), 577-589. https://doi.org/10.1038/s41582-018-0070-3.

Lamptey, R. N., Chaulagain, B., Trivedi, R., Gothwal, A., Layek, B., & Singh, J. (2022). A review of the common neurodegenerative disorders: Current therapeutic approaches and the potential role of nanotherapeutics. *International Journal of Molecular Sciences,* 23(3), 1851. https://doi.org/10.3390/ijms23031851.

Lee, S. J., Nam, E., Lee, H. J., Savelieff, M. G., & Lim, M. H. (2017). Towards an understanding of amyloid-β oligomers: Characterization, toxicity mechanisms, and inhibitors. *Chemical Society Reviews*, 46(2), 310-323. https://doi.org/10.1039/C6CS00319A.

Leroy, E., Boyer, R., Auburger, G., Leube, B., Ulm, G., Mezey, E., Harta, G., Brownstein, M. J., Jonnalagada, S., Chernova, T., & Dehejia, A. (1998). The ubiquitin pathway in Parkinson's disease. *Nature,* 395(6701), 451-452. https://doi.org/10.1038/26752.

Liang, Y., & Yoon, J. Y. (2021). *In situ* sensors for blood-brain barrier (BBB) on a chip. *Sensors and Actuators Reports,* 3, 100031. https://doi.org/10.1016/j.snr.2021.100031.

Lovrecic, L., Kastrin, A., Kobal, J., Pirtosek, Z., Krainc, D., & Peterlin, B. (2009). Gene expression changes in blood as a putative biomarker for Huntington's disease. *Movement Disorders,* 24(15), 2277-2281. https://doi.org/10.1002/mds.22509.

Mapstone, M., Cheema, A. K., Fiandaca, M. S., Zhong, X., Mhyre, T. R., MacArthur, L. H., Hall, W. J., Fisher, S. G., Peterson, D. R., Haley, J. M., & Nazar, M. D. (2014). Plasma phospholipids identify antecedent memory impairment in older adults. *Nature Medicine,* 20(4), 415-418. https://doi.org/10.1038/nm.3490.

Marek, K., Seibyl, J., & Holloway, R. A. (2000). Multicenter assessment of dopamine transporter imaging with DOPASCAN/SPECT in parkinsonism. *Neurology,* 55(10), 1540-1547. https://doi.org/10.1212/WNL.55.10.1540.

Martin, L. J., & Wong, M. (2013). Aberrant regulation of DNA methylation in amyotrophic lateral sclerosis: A new target of disease mechanisms. *Neurotherapeutics,* 10, 722-733. https://doi.org/10.1007/s13311-013-0175-1.

Masrori, P., & Van Damme, P. (2020). Amyotrophic lateral sclerosis: A clinical review. European *Journal of Neurology,* 27(10), 1918-1929. https://doi.org/10.1111/ene.14208Mastrokolias.

Mattsson, N., Carrillo, M. C., Dean, R. A., Devous, M. D. Sr, Nikolcheva, T., Pesini, P., Salter, H., Potter, W. Z., Sperling, R. S., Bateman, R. J., & Bain, L. J. (2015). Revolutionizing Alzheimer's disease and clinical trials through biomarkers. *Alzheimer's & Dementia: Diagnosis, Assessment & Disease Monitoring,* 1(4), 412-419. https://doi.org/10.1016/j.dadm.2015.10.001.

Mesko, B., Poliskal, S., Szegedi, A., Szekanecz, Z., Palatka, K., Papp, M., & Nagy, L. (2010). Peripheral blood gene expression patterns discriminate among chronic inflammatory diseases and healthy controls and identify novel targets. *BMC Medical Genomics*, 3, 1-3. https://doi.org/10.1186/1755-8794-3-16.

Meyer, G. C., A. H., Bell, R. D., & Zhang, W. (2021). Strategies for delivering therapeutics across the blood-brain barrier. *Nature Reviews Drug Discovery,* 20(5), 362-383. https://doi.org/10.1038/s41573-021-00272-0.

Milà-Alomà, M., Salvadó, G., Gispert, J. D., Vilor-Tejedor, N., Grau-Rivera, O., Sala-Vila, A., Sánchez-Benavides, G., Arenaza-Urquijo, E. M., Crous-Bou, M., González-de-Echávarri, J. M., & Minguillon, C. (2020). Amyloid beta, tau, synaptic, neurodegeneration, and glial biomarkers in the preclinical stage of the Alzheimer's continuum. *Alzheimer's & Dementia,* 16(10), 1358-1371. https://doi.org/10.1002/alz.12176.

Miller, D. B., & O'Callaghan, J. P. (2015). Biomarkers of Parkinson's disease: Present and future. *Metabolism,* 64(3), S40-S46. https://doi.org/10.1016/j.metabol.2014.07.026.

Molochnikov, L., Rabey, J. M., Dobronevsky, E., Bonuccelli, U., Ceravolo, R., Frosini, D., Grünblatt, E., Riederer, P., Jacob, C., Aharon-Peretz, J., & Bashenko, Y. (2012). A molecular signature in blood identifies early Parkinson's disease. *Molecular Neurodegeneration,* 7(1), 1-0. https://doi.org/10.1186/1750-1326-7-26.

Obeso, J. A., Stamelou, M., Goetz, C. G., Poewe, W., Lang, A. E., Weintraub, D., Burn, D., Halliday, G. M., Bezard, E., Przedborski, S. J., & Lehericy, S. (2017). Past, present, and future of Parkinson's disease: A special essay on the 200th Anniversary of the Shaking Palsy. *Movement Disorders,* 32(9), 1264-1310. https://doi.org/10.1002/mds.27035.

Olsson, B., Lautner, R., Andreasson, U., Öhrfelt, A., Portelius, E., Bjerke, M., Hölttä, M., Rosén, C., Olsson, C., Strobel, G., & Wu, E. (2016). CSF and blood biomarkers for the diagnosis of Alzheimer's disease: A systematic review and meta-analysis. *The Lancet Neurology,* 15(7), 673-684. https://doi.org/10.1016/S1474-4422(16)00070-3.

Ossenkoppele, R., van der Kant, R., & Hansson, O. (2022). Tau biomarkers in Alzheimer's disease: Towards implementation in clinical practice and trials. *The Lancet Neurology*, 21(8), 726-734. https://doi.org/10.1016/S1474-4422(22)00160-1.

Palmqvist, S., Insel, P. S., Stomrud, E., Janelidze, S., Zetterberg, H., Brix, B., Eichenlaub, U., Dage, J. L., Chai, X., Blennow, K., & Mattsson, N. (2019). Cerebrospinal fluid and plasma biomarker trajectories with increasing amyloid deposition in Alzheimer's disease. *EMBO Molecular Medicine*, 11(12), e11170. https://doi.org/10.15252/emmm.201911170.

Palmqvist, S., Janelidze, S., Quiroz, Y. T., Zetterberg, H., Lopera, F., Stomrud, E., Su, Y. I., Chen, Y., Serrano, G. E., Leuzy, A., & Mattsson-Carlgren, N. (2020). Discriminative accuracy of plasma phospho-tau217 for Alzheimer disease vs other neurodegenerative disorders. *JAMA,* 324(8), 772-781. https://doi.org/10.1001/jama.2020.11358.

Pankratz, N., Nichols, W. C., Uniacke, S. K., Halter, C., Rudolph, A., Shults, C., Conneally, P. M., & Foroud, T. (2003). Significant linkage of Parkinson disease to chromosome 2q36-37. *The American Journal of Human Genetics,* 72(4), 1053-1057. https://doi.org/10.1086/374172.

Peng, C., Trojanowski, J. Q., & Lee, V. M. (2020). Protein transmission in neurodegenerative disease. *Nature Reviews Neurology*, 16(4), 199-212. https://doi.org/10.1038/s41582-019-0316-7.

Pereira, J. B., Janelidze, S., Smith, R., Mattsson-Carlgren, N., Palmqvist, S., Teunissen, C. E., Zetterberg, H., Stomrud, E., Ashton, N. J., Blennow, K., & Hansson, O. (2021). Plasma GFAP is an early marker of amyloid-β but not tau pathology in Alzheimer's disease. *Brain,* 144(11), 3505-3516. https://doi.org/10.1093/brain/awab232.

Pezard, L., Jech, R., & Růžička, E. (2001). Investigation of non-linear properties of multichannel EEG in the early stages of Parkinson's disease. *Clinical Neurophysiology*, 112(1), 38-45. https://doi.org/10.1016/S1388-2457(00)00588-0.

Philips, T., & Robberecht, W. (2011). Neuroinflammation in amyotrophic lateral sclerosis: Role of glial activation in motor neuron disease. *The Lancet Neurology*, 10(3), 253-263. https://doi.org/10.1016/S1474-4422(10)70250-2.

Poulopoulou, C., Davaki, P., Koliaraki, V., Kolovou, D., Markakis, I., & Vassilopoulos, D. (2005). Reduced expression of metabotropic glutamate receptor 2 mRNA in T cells of ALS patients. *Annals of Neurology: Official Journal of the American Neurological Association and the Child Neurology Society*, 58(6), 946-949. https://doi.org/10.1002/ana.20604.

Rachakonda, V., Pan, T. H., & Le, W. D. (2004). Biomarkers of neurodegenerative disorders: How good are they? *Cell Research,* 14(5), 349-358. https://doi.org/10.1038/sj.cr.7290214.

Ramani, S., Berard, J. A., & Walker, L. A. (2021). The relationship between neurofilament light chain and cognition in neurological disorders: A scoping review. *Journal of the Neurological Sciences,* 420, 117229. https://doi.org/10.1016/j.jns.2020.117229.

Robelin, L., & Gonzalez De Aguilar, J. L. (2014). Blood biomarkers for amyotrophic lateral sclerosis: Myth or reality? *BioMed Research International,* 2014. https://doi.org/10.1155/2014/286213.

Robinson, J. L., Lee, E. B., Xie, S. X., Rennert, L., Suh, E., Bredenberg, C., Caswell, C., Van Deerlin, V. M., Yan, N., Yousef, A., & Hurtig, H. I. (2018). Neurodegenerative disease concomitant proteinopathies are prevalent, age-related and APOE4-associated. *Brain,* 141(7), 2181-2193. https://doi.org/10.1093/brain/awy138.

Rocha, E. M., De Miranda, B., & Sanders, L. H. (2018). Alpha-synuclein: Pathology, mitochondrial dysfunction and neuroinflammation in Parkinson's disease. *Neurobiology of Disease,* 109, 249-257. https://doi.org/10.1016/j.nbd.2017.10.014.

Rohilla, D., Chaudhary, S., & Umar, A. (2021). An overview of advanced nanomaterials for sensor applications. *Engineered Science,* 16, 47-70. https://doi.org/10.30919/es21001641.

Schwarz, A. J. (2021). The use, standardization, and interpretation of brain imaging data in clinical trials of neurodegenerative disorders. *Neurotherapeutics,* 18(2), 686-708. https://doi.org/10.1007/s13311-021-01056-4.

Seiss, E., Praamstra, P., Hesse, C., & Rickards, H. (2003). Proprioceptive sensory function in Parkinson's disease and Huntington's disease: Evidence from proprioception-related EEG potentials. *Experimental Brain Research,* 148, 308-319. https://doi.org/10.1007/s00221-002-1265-8.

Shaw, L. M., Hansson, O., Manuilova, E., Masters, C. L., Doecke, J. D., Li, Q. X., Rutz, S., Widmann, M., Leinenbach, A., & Blennow, K. (2019). Method comparison study of the Elecsys® β-amyloid (1–42) CSF assay versus comparator assays and LC-MS/MS. *Clinical Biochemistry,* 72, 7-14. https://doi.org/10.1016/j.clinbiochem.2019.06.008.

Sheinerman, K. S., Tsivinsky, V. G., Crawford, F., Mullan, M. J., Abdullah, L., & Umansky, S. R. (2012). Plasma microRNA biomarkers for detection of mild cognitive impairment. *Aging (Albany NY),* 4(9), 590-600. https://doi.org/10.18632/aging.100510.

Shinde, S., Mukhopadhyay, S., Mohsen, G., & Khoo, S. K. (2015). Biofluid-based microRNA biomarkers for Parkinson's disease: An overview and update. *Journal of Parkinson's Disease,* 5(4), 827-844. https://doi.org/10.3233/JPD-151759.

Shinto, A., Antony, J., Kamaleshwaran, K., Vijayan, K., Selvan, A., Korde, A., Kameshwaran, M., & Samuel, G. (2014). Correlative 99mTc-labeled tropane derivative single photon emission computed tomography and clinical assessment in the staging of Parkinson disease. *World Journal of Nuclear Medicine,* 13(03), 178-183. https://doi.org/10.4103/1450-1147.142365.

Sjögren, M., Andreasen, N., & Blennow, K. (2003). Advances in the detection of Alzheimer's disease - Use of cerebrospinal fluid biomarkers. *Clinica Chimica Acta,* 332(1-2), 1-10. https://doi.org/10.1016/S0009-8981(03)00204-0.

Soreq, L., Salomonis, N., Bronstein, M., Greenberg, D. S., Israel, Z., Bergman, H., & Soreq, H. (2013). Small RNA sequencing-microarray analyses in Parkinson leukocytes reveal deep brain stimulation-induced splicing changes that classify brain region transcriptomes. *Frontiers in Molecular Neuroscience,* 6, 10. https://doi.org/10.3389/fnmol.2013.00010.

Srinivasan, E., & Rajasekaran, R. (2020). A systematic and comprehensive review on disease-causing genes in amyotrophic lateral sclerosis. *Journal of Molecular Neuroscience,* 70(11), 1742-1770. https://doi.org/10.1007/s12031-020-01467-3.

Sturrock, A., Laule, C., Wyper, K., Milner, R. A., Decolongon, J., Santos, R. D., Coleman, A. J., Carter, K., Creighton, S., Bechtel, N., & Bohlen, S. (2015). A longitudinal study of magnetic resonance spectroscopy Huntington's disease biomarkers. *Movement Disorders,* 30(3), 393-401. https://doi.org/10.1002/mds.25962.

Suárez-Calvet, M., Karikari, T. K., Ashton, N. J., Lantero Rodriguez, J., Milà-Alomà, M., Gispert, J. D., Salvadó, G., Minguillon, C., Fauria, K., Shekari, M., & Grau-Rivera, O. (2020). Novel tau biomarkers phosphorylated at T181, T217 or T231 rise in the initial stages of the preclinical Alzheimer's continuum when only subtle changes in Aβ pathology are detected. *EMBO Molecular Medicine*, 12(12), e12921. https://doi.org/10.15252/emmm.202012921.

Sunderland, T., Linker, G., Mirza, N., Putnam, K. T., Friedman, D. L., Kimmel, L. H., Bergeson, J., Manetti, G. J., Zimmermann, M., Tang, B., & Bartko, J. J. (2003). Decreased β-amyloid1-42 and increased tau levels in cerebrospinal fluid of patients with Alzheimer disease. *JAMA,* 289(16), 2094-2103. https://doi.org/10.1001/jama.289.16.2094.

Tao, Y., Chen, L., Pan, M., Zhu, F., & Zhu, D. (2021). Tailored biosensors for drug screening, efficacy assessment, and toxicity evaluation. *ACS Sensors,* 6(9), 3146-3162. https://doi.org/10.1021/acssensors.1c00757Terstappen.

Thakor, N. V., & Tong, S. (2004). Advances in quantitative electroencephalogram analysis methods. *Annual Review of Biomedical Engineering,* 6, 453-495. https://doi.org/10.1146/annurev.bioeng.6.040803.140216.

Thijssen, E. H., La Joie, R., Strom, A., Fonseca, C., Iaccarino, L., Wolf, A., Spina, S., Allen, I. E., Cobigo, Y., Heuer, H., & VandeVrede, L. (2021). Plasma phosphorylated tau 217 and phosphorylated tau 181 as biomarkers in Alzheimer's disease and frontotemporal lobar degeneration: A retrospective diagnostic performance study. *The Lancet Neurology,* 20(9), 739-752. https://doi.org/10.1016/S1474-4422(21)00232-3.

Tiwari, S., Atluri, V., Kaushik, A., Yndart, A., & Nair, M. (2019). Alzheimer's disease: Pathogenesis, diagnostics, and therapeutics. *International Journal of Nanomedicine*, 14, 5541-5564. https://doi.org/10.2147/IJN.S206867.

Torrent, R., De Angelis Rigotti, F., Dell'Era, P., Memo, M., Raya, A., & Consiglio, A. (2015). Using iPS cells toward the understanding of Parkinson's disease. *Journal of Clinical Medicine*, 4(4), 548-566. https://doi.org/10.3390/jcm4040548.

Valente, E. M., Abou-Sleiman, P. M., Caputo, V., Muqit, M. M. K., Harvey, K., Gispert, S., Ali, Z., Del Turco, D., Bentivoglio, A. R., Healy, D. G., & Albanese, A. (2004). Hereditary early-onset Parkinson's disease caused by mutations in PINK1. *Science,* 304(5674), 1158-1160. https://doi.org/10.1126/science.1096284.

Venancio, T. M., & Aravind, L. (2010). CYSTM, a novel cysteine-rich transmembrane module with a role in stress tolerance across eukaryotes. *Bioinformatics,* 26(2), 149-152. https://doi.org/10.1093/bioinformatics/btp620.

Walker, K. A., Duggan, M. R., Gong, Z., Dark, H. E., Laporte, J. P., Faulkner, M. E., An, Y., Lewis, A., Moghekar, A. R., Resnick, S. M., & Bouhrara, M. (2023). MRI and fluid biomarkers reveal determinants of myelin and axonal loss with aging. *Annals of Clinical and Translational Neurology*, 10(3), 397-407. https://doi.org/10.1002/acn3.17714.

Wang, K. K., Yang, Z., Zhu, T., Shi, Y., Rubenstein, R., Tyndall, J. A., & Manley, G. T. (2018). An update on diagnostic and prognostic biomarkers for traumatic brain injury. *Expert Review of Molecular Diagnostics,* 18(2), 165-180. https://doi.org/10.1080/14737159.2018.1422748.

Weir, D. W., Sturrock, A., & Leavitt, B. R. (2011). Development of biomarkers for Huntington's disease. *The Lancet Neurology,* 10(6), 573-590. https://doi.org/10.1016/S1474-4422(11)70072-2.

Wild, E. J., Boggio, R., Langbehn, D., Robertson, N., Haider, S., Miller, J. R., Zetterberg, H., Leavitt, B. R., Kuhn, R., Tabrizi, S. J., & Macdonald, D. (2015). Quantification of mutant huntingtin protein in cerebrospinal fluid from Huntington's disease patients. *The Journal of Clinical Investigation,* 125(5), 1979-1986. https://doi.org/10.1172/JCI78712.

Wood, N. I., Goodman, A. O., van der Burg, J. M., Gazeau, V., Brundin, P., Björkqvist, M., Petersén, Å., Tabrizi, S. J., Barker, R. A., & Morton, A. J. (2008). Increased thirst and drinking in Huntington's disease and the R6/2 mouse. *Brain Research Bulletin,* 76(1-2), 70-79. https://doi.org/10.1016/j.brainresbull.2008.02.013

Wurtman, R. (2015). Biomarkers in the diagnosis and management of Alzheimer's disease. *Metabolism,* 64(3), S47-S50. https://doi.org/10.1016/j.metabol.2015.01.003.

Young, A. B. (2009). Four decades of neurodegenerative disease research: How far we have come! *Journal of Neuroscience,* 29(41), 12722-12728. https://doi.org/10.1523/JNEUROSCI.3684-09.2009.

Zhai, W., Jeong, H., Cui, L., Krainc, D., & Tjian, R. (2005). *In vitro* analysis of huntingtin-mediated transcriptional repression reveals multiple transcription factor targets. *Cell,* 123(7), 1241-1253. https://doi.org/10.1016/j.cell.2005.11.038.

Chapter 3

Alzheimer's Disease: An Overview

Himanshu Sharma,
Siddhant Jai Tyagi,
Phool Chandra, PhD,
and Anurag Verma, PhD
Teerthanker Mahaveer College of Pharmacy, Teerthanker Mahaveer University, Moradabad (UP), India

Abstract

A serious brain ailment that affects millions of people worldwide, Alzheimer's disease (AD) is covered in detail in this book chapter. The chapter starts with an explanation of the intricate pathophysiology of AD before focusing on the functions of amyloid-beta (Aβ) and tau protein in the formation of identifiable neurofibrillary tangles and senile plaques. Mutations in the genes encoding for APP, PSEN1, and PSEN2 are one of the genetic and environmental factors being looked into as probable disease-causing causes. The right steps are taken to address the sluggish cognitive decline, aberrant behavior, and memory loss that are clinical indications of AD. The book chapter emphasizes the importance of early diagnosis, the use of biomarkers, and neuroimaging techniques to more precisely differentiate AD from other dementias. Additionally included in this chapter are contemporary medication therapy, behavioral strategies, and caregiver support programs. Discussion topics include the challenges of creating novel medications, the potential for treating diseases in several methods, and the value of non-pharmacological treatments like mental stimulation and exercise. It is vital to employ a holistic and compassionate approach that includes interdisciplinary teamwork, public awareness initiatives, and legislative action to improve

In: Neurogenerative Disorders
Editors: Mohit Agrawal, Manmohan Singhal, Amit Kumar Nayak et al.
ISBN: 979-8-89530-143-2

the overall quality of life for AD patients. Readers should leave this book chapter with a good understanding of AD, including its pathophysiology, clinical signs, and potential therapies. By supporting continuing research and collaborative efforts, there is potential for progress toward new therapies and, ultimately, a reduction in the burden of this crippling neurological disorder.

Keywords: Alzheimer's disease, neurodegenerative disorder, amyloid-beta, tau protein, pathogenesis, clinical manifestations, early diagnosis, biomarkers

Introduction

Memory, thinking, and reasoning are the three main cognitive processes impacted by AD, a chronic neurological condition. One of the most prevalent types of dementia, AD results in a steady deterioration in cognitive ability, seriously impairing everyday functioning and behavior. This disorder, which has a significant impact on millions of people worldwide, is characterized by the slow and irreversible loss of nerve cells (neurons) and brain connections. Memory loss struggles with problem-solving, confusion, and communication difficulties are frequently early signs of AD (Mudar et al., 2019). As the illness worsens, people may experience personality changes, mood fluctuations, and challenges doing everyday activities like dressing, eating, and maintaining personal cleanliness (Sharma et al., 2023a). AD progresses relentlessly, causing a progressive loss of independence and a significant dependency on carers. The origins of AD may be traced to the early 20th century when a young German psychiatrist and neurologist named Dr. Alois Alzheimer made a revolutionary discovery that would permanently change the field of neuroscience. A fascinating case involving Auguste Deter, a 51-year-old woman who had been displaying acute memory loss, paranoia, and bewilderment, was reported to Dr. Alzheimer in 1906. Dr. Alzheimer watched Auguste Deter's health intently, fascinated by the patient's symptoms and eager to comprehend the pathology at play (Ribas et al., 2023). He thoroughly examined the tissue under a microscope after her death, including a postmortem analysis of her brain (Sharma et al., 2024c). To his surprise, he discovered strange protein plaque deposits outside the nerve cells and twisted fibers inside the cells. Amyloid plaques and neurofibrillary tangles, which have come to be recognized as the distinguishing markers of AD, were identified in this groundbreaking study. Though his findings and subsequent case studies helped establish our understanding of this new neurological disorder, it was long later that the term "AD" was developed to recognize Dr. Alzheimer's great contribution. Despite continuing to be a relatively unexplored area of study, AD's scientific and medical interest rose considerably over the coming decades. In the middle of the 20th century, there was a greater emphasis on dementia and age-related cognitive decline, with AD coming to be recognized as a serious public health issue. Medical experts may now more accurately diagnose AD and discriminate between different types of dementia because of improvements in diagnostic methods like brain imaging and cognitive tests (Sharma et al., 2024a). As public understanding of dementia increased, the stigma associated with it started to disappear, enabling more sympathetic and knowledgeable treatment for people who were affected. Late 20th century genetic research revealed specific genetic alterations linked to familial early-onset Alzheimer's disease. (Modir et al., 2023).

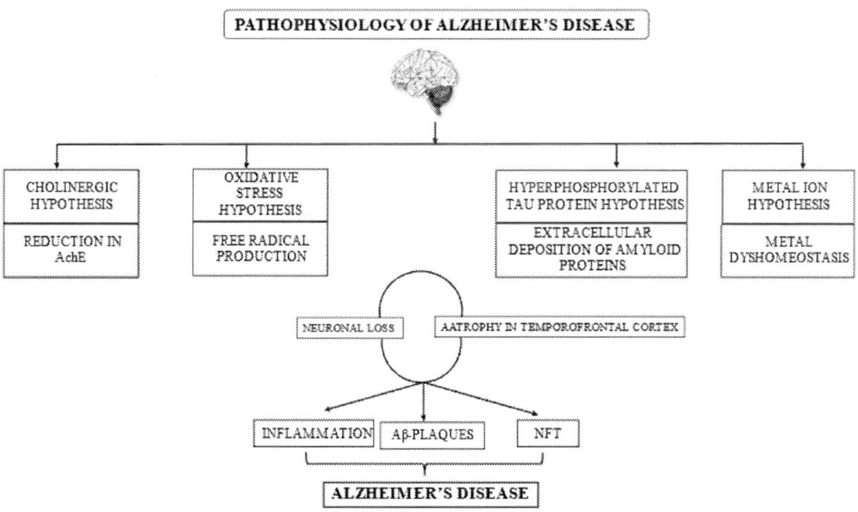

Figure 1. Speculation regarding the pathophysiology of Alzheimer's disease.

Causes and Risk Factors of Alzheimer's Disease

Genetics and Familial Alzheimer's Disease

A small percentage of Alzheimer's patients, ranging from 1 to 5 percent, are classified as familial AD (FAD). FAD is distinguished by a significant genetic component, as opposed to sporadic Alzheimer's, which usually manifests in late adulthood and has no obvious familial pattern (Sharma et al., 2024b). It is brought on by mutations in particular genes that are crucial for the synthesis and processing of amyloid-beta, a protein that builds up in the brain and causes amyloid plaques, the pathology that distinguishes AD, and these mutations are the origin of the disease. The three main genes that contribute to FAD (Kirkeby et al., 2023).

Brain Injury

Alzheimer's disease may be more likely to manifest later in life if a person has a history of severe head trauma or TBI (Ashique et al., 2024). Figure 1 illustrates the importance of taking the right precautions to avoid head injuries and obtaining medical assistance when they do occur (Cook and Polgar, 2015).

Pathophysiology of Alzheimer's Disease

Amyloid Plaques and Tau Tangles

Two pathological characteristics that characterize AD are amyloid plaques and tau tangles. It is thought that these aberrant protein aggregates have a substantial impact on the neurodegenerative process, which results in cognitive decline and memory impairment in those who are affected (Hoque et al., 2023).

Amyloid Plaques

Amyloid plaques, which are sticky collections of amyloid-beta protein, develop between neurons in the brain. Amyloid-beta protein, a larger APP involved in brain cellular processes, is produced in a healthy brain due to neuronal activity and eliminated through various enzymes and clearance mechanisms. The imbalance in the production and clearance of Aβ is observed in Alzheimer's disease. Amyloid plaques start to form when there are too many Aβ molecules accumulating. These plaques harm neurons and impair their ability to operate normally (Kumar et al., 2024). They interfere with synaptic transmission between neurons, affecting the brain's ability to transmit impulses (Sharma et al., 2024c). Amyloid plaques have the potential to cause inflammation, harm to synapses, and degeneration of neurons over time (Dominko et al., 2022).

Tau Tangles

Neuronal tau tangles, also known as NFTs or aberrant tau protein accumulations, are found within neurons. Tau is a microtubule-associated protein that is critical for maintaining the internal organization of neurons and for facilitating the passage of nutrients and other vital materials inside the cell. In AD, tau proteins experience excessively high levels of phosphorylation, which leads to their misfolding and tangle formation inside the neurons. Tau tangle buildup impairs neurons' ability to function normally, interferes with cellular transport processes, and ultimately results in neuronal malfunction and cell death. Tau tangles are especially harmful to parts of the brain that are involved in memory, cognition, and learning, like the cerebral cortex and hippocampus. Their existence is directly correlated with the degree of cognitive deterioration in AD (Colom-Cadena et al., 2023).

Relationship Between Amyloid Plaques and Tau Tangles

Research on the connection between tau tangles and amyloid plaques is ongoing since it is not yet fully understood. However, it is thought that the two illnesses are related and may have an impact on one another's development of the disease. According to the "amyloid cascade hypothesis," the buildup of amyloid plaques sets off a series of incidents that finally result in tau tangles and neurodegeneration. This model postulates that the aggregation of Aβ in amyloid plaques results in a cascade of neurotoxic processes, including inflammation and oxidative stress, which in turn cause tau proteins to be hyperphosphorylated and misfolded, ultimately leading to the formation of tau tangles (Yang et al., 2023). According to this hypothesis, amyloid plaques are the first sign of the disease, and tau pathology develops as a result. Recent findings, however, cast doubt on the amyloid cascade hypothesis's assumption that tau pathology necessarily follows amyloid accumulation in particular brain regions. While amyloid plaques and tau tangles are characteristic of AD, it is crucial to remember that they are not specific to this disease and can also be detected, to a lesser extent, in the brains of some older persons who are cognitively well. In the effort to comprehend and successfully treat AD, research is still being done to determine the link between these diseases and their precise role in the disease's development and cognitive decline (Lin et al., 2023).

Neurotransmitter Changes

Neurotransmitters are chemical messengers that are essential for communication between the brain's neurons. They enable information to be transmitted and control numerous brain activities by sending impulses across synapses, the connectors between neurons. The levels and functioning of a few neurotransmitters are significantly altered in AD, which contributes to the cognitive and behavioral symptoms seen in affected people (Kumar and Kumar, 2014). Key neurotransmitter alterations in AD include, among others:

Acetylcholine

Acetylcholine, a neurotransmitter, plays a crucial role in memory, learning, and cognitive processes. Acetylcholine-producing neurons gradually disappear in AD, especially in areas of the brain that are important for memory and cognitive processing, such as the basal forebrain and hippocampus. Memory loss and cognitive decline in Alzheimer's patients are a result of the decreased production of acetylcholine, which also affects cholinergic signaling. As acetylcholine becomes more readily available in the brain, some people with Alzheimer's may experience a temporary improvement in their cognitive symptoms. These medications are referred to as cholinesterase inhibitors (Van der Zee and Luiten, 1999).

Glutamate

Glutamate, the primary excitatory neurotransmitter in the brain, is also involved in synaptic plasticity and transmission. Glutamate signaling appears to be dysregulated in AD, which results in excessive glutamate release and poor clearance. Glutamate overexposure can damage neurons by causing excitotoxicity, which exacerbates synaptic dysfunction and neuronal damage. According to current theories, the progressive loss of synapses and neuronal death seen in the affected brain regions are caused by elevated glutamate levels in Alzheimer's (Ahmad et al., 2023).

GABA

GABA, the primary inhibitory neurotransmitter in the brain, plays a crucial role in regulating neuronal excitability. Changes in GABAergic transmission have been linked to changes in the balance between excitation and inhibition in some brain circuits in AD. GABAergic neuron dysfunction can upset the harmony of neuronal activity and exacerbate cognitive decline in Alzheimer's patients (Wu et al., 2023).

Serotonin and Norepinephrine

Neurotransmitters that help regulate mood and process emotions include serotonin and norepinephrine. Changes in these neurotransmitter systems have been seen in AD and may be a factor in mood disorders, including anxiety and depression, that afflicted people typically suffer. Changes in the serotonin and norepinephrine pathways can have an impact on a patient's overall quality of life and emotional well-being (Marino and Williams, 2007).

Brain Atrophy and Neurodegeneration

Fundamental traits of AD include brain atrophy and neurodegeneration. The cognitive and functional decline seen in affected individuals is caused by these processes, which include the progressive loss and degeneration of brain tissue. Alzheimer's disease predominantly affects the parts of the brain responsible for memory, learning, and cognitive skills. This causes brain atrophy and neurodegeneration (Martins-Macedo et al., 2021).

Brain Atrophy

Brain atrophy is the term used to describe the thinning or loss of brain volume, especially in particular brain regions. One of the brain areas most impacted by atrophy in AD is the cerebral cortex, which is involved in cognitive processing, and the hippocampus, which is essential for memory storage. These brain regions are thought to have atrophy due to the loss of synaptic connections between nerve cells (neurons) and their progressive demise. The brain networks that control memory and cognitive function are made up of connections that are disturbed as neurons die. Memory loss and cognitive decline are linked to the diminished size and integrity of these brain areas. MRI (Magnetic Resonance Imaging) is a brain imaging technique used to detect and quantify brain atrophy in Alzheimer's Disease (AD). (Khalil et al., 2022).

Neurodegeneration

The progressive loss and degeneration of neurons in the brain is referred to as neurodegeneration. Neurodegeneration in AD is primarily caused by aberrant amyloid-beta protein buildup and the development of neurofibrillary tangles made of hyperphosphorylated tau protein. Neurotoxic amyloid plaques and neurofibrillary tangles limit neurons' ability to function normally. Inflammation, oxidative stress, and compromised cellular functions are just a few of the neurotoxic events that are brought on by the buildup of these protein aggregates. As dementia progresses, the brain areas affected experience a significant loss of neurons and synaptic connections. The extensive death of neurons is a factor in AD's cognitive decline and functional limitations (Dewanjee et al., 2022).

Disconnection Syndrome

Disconnection syndrome is a condition characterized by severe neuronal loss and synaptic disruption in Alzheimer's disease (AD). This phrase describes how the loss of neuronal connections causes communication between various brain regions to become disconnected and disrupted. The condition worsens as the brain's networks become disconnected, making it more difficult for the brain to coordinate complex cognitive tasks including memory, attention, and problem-solving (Savage et al., 2007).

Impacts on Brain Function

In AD, brain atrophy and neurodegeneration have a significant impact on cognitive performance. Memory deficits, thought, and reasoning are brought on by the steady loss of neurons and synaptic connections. Alzheimer's patients could struggle with short-term memory, learning new material, finding the proper words, spatial orientation, and executive functions (including planning and organizing tasks). Daily tasks become more difficult as the condition worsens, impairing functionality and necessitating the assistance of others for care (Lacava et al., 2014).

Diagnostic Methods for Alzheimer's Disease

Clinical Assessment

Clinical assessment for AD involves a thorough and multidimensional evaluation of an individual's cognitive, functional, and behavioral abilities. Healthcare professionals conduct a comprehensive examination to assess memory, attention, language, executive functions, and visuospatial abilities through standardized cognitive tests. They also take a thorough medical history, perform a physical exam, and look at any existing illnesses, medications, and family dementia history. Information from close family members or caregivers is gathered through informant interviews, offering valuable insights into changes in behavior, memory, and daily functioning (Lista et al., 2023). ADLs are assessed to gauge the individual's ability to independently manage personal care, prepare meals, handle finances, and navigate familiar environments. In some cases, neuropsychological testing may provide further insight into specific cognitive functions. Brain imaging, such as MRI or PET scans, helps detect brain atrophy and rule out other structural abnormalities. Blood tests aid in identifying underlying medical conditions that may contribute to cognitive decline. Psychological and behavioral assessments assess mood, behavior, and psychological well-being. A crucial aspect of the clinical assessment is to rule out other potential causes of cognitive impairment through a differential diagnosis approach. The collective information obtained guides healthcare professionals in making an accurate diagnosis, determining the stage of AD, and devising an appropriate treatment plan, ensuring optimal care and support for individuals and their caregivers. Early diagnosis facilitates timely intervention and access to resources and services, ultimately improving the individual's quality of life throughout the disease (Hasan et al., 2020).

Cognitive Tests and Scoring Systems

The clinical evaluation of AD requires the use of cognitive tests and scoring methods. These standardized tests are made to analyze many facets of cognitive function, offering insightful information about the subject's cognitive capabilities and spotting early indications of cognitive decline. The assessment of AD frequently involves the use of several cognitive tests. The MMSE is a widely-used cognitive assessment tool that evaluates various aspects of cognitive function, including orientation, registration, attention, calculation, recollection, and language. Lower scores indicate more severe cognitive impairment. The test gives a total score out of 30. The MoCA is another frequently used cognitive exam that assesses a wider range of cognitive areas, including executive skills and visuospatial ability (Manning, 2004). Additionally, the MoCA provides a 30-point overall score, with lower values indicating a cognitive decline. The Clock Drawing Test evaluates visual-spatial and executive ability. People are requested to design a clock face with a certain time on it. The test is graded based on the drawing's many elements, including the arrangement of the numerals and clock hands. The Trail Making Test, among others, measures cognitive flexibility, visual scanning, and attention. Participants must swiftly connect ascending numbers or letters to pass the test. Clinicians can quantify and monitor cognitive changes over time with the help of scoring systems for these exams. Furthermore, neuropsychological testing may encompass more thorough evaluations of particular cognitive areas, delivering a comprehensive profile of cognitive strengths and deficits (Lewis and Trempe, 2017). Making an accurate diagnosis of AD and separating it from other cognitive illnesses depends on the outcomes of cognitive tests and scoring methodologies. They assist in guiding treatment choices, monitoring the illness' progression, and assessing the efficacy of therapy. Early detection of cognitive impairment through tests allows for prompt intervention, support services, and improved quality of life, enhancing management techniques' efficiency. Since AD is a progressive disorder, routine re-evaluation utilizing cognitive tests and scoring systems is essential to customize care and support as the illness progresses and to provide the best results for afflicted people and their caregivers ("Parkinson's Disease, Movement Disorders, and Dementia," 2012).

Imaging Techniques

AD is difficult to diagnose and must be closely monitored, which requires the use of imaging techniques like MRI and PET scans. With the aid of these imaging techniques, doctors and scientists can see and evaluate disease-related alterations to the brain (Alberdi et al., 2016). An overview of MRI and PET scan applications in AD is provided below.

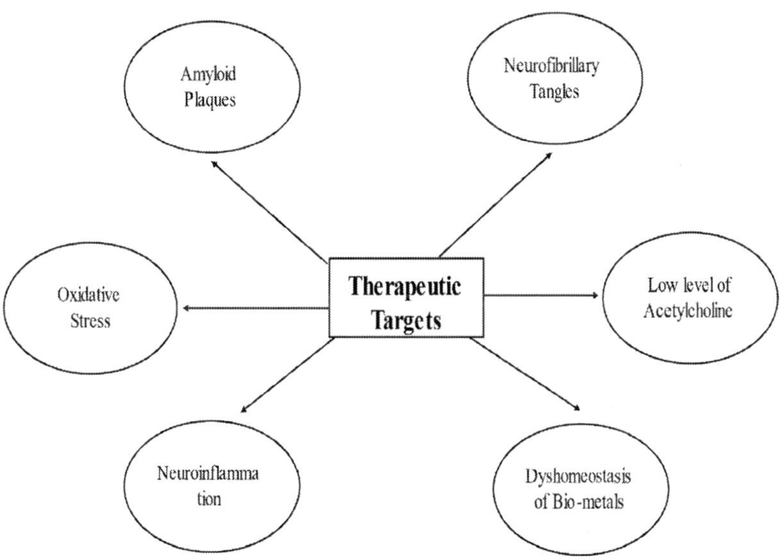

Figure 2. Targets to manage Alzheimer's disease.

Magnetic Resonance Imaging

With the help of strong magnets and radio waves, the non-invasive imaging method known as MRI.

Biomarker Analysis for Alzheimer's Disease

CSF analysis can identify specific biomarkers linked to Alzheimer's disease. Biomarkers are biological indicators that can signal the presence of a disease or its progression. In the context of AD, two essential biomarkers originate in CSF see Figure 2 (Rossini et al., 2020).

Amyloid-Beta Protein

Amyloid-beta plaques building up in the brain are one of AD's hallmarks. Reduced levels of A-β42, a particular type of amyloid-beta, and elevated levels of A-β40 in the CSF can signify amyloid-beta buildup in the brain, respectively (Bensalem et al., 2023).

Tau Protein

In nerve cells, the protein tau keeps microtubules in place. Inside the brain cells, aberrant tau protein tangles form in AD (Sharma et al., 2023b). Increased concentrations of total tau and phosphorylated tau (p-tau) in CSF are linked to neurodegeneration and may be an early sign of Alzheimer's disease (Dewanjee et al., 2022).

Differential Diagnoses

CSF testing can help distinguish AD from other neurological disorders such as frontotemporal dementia, Lewy body dementia, or normal pressure hydrocephalus that share some of the same symptoms as AD. Making a more precise diagnosis may be aided by the unique biomarker patterns found in CSF (Gifford et al., 2023).

Treatment Approaches for Alzheimer's Disease

Pharmacological Interventions (Cholinesterase Inhibitors, Memantine)

Drug treatments for Alzheimer's disease aim to manage symptoms and prevent its progression. At the moment, memantine and cholinesterase inhibitors are the two primary pharmacological groups that have been licensed for the treatment of Alzheimer's. Depending on the stage and severity of the ailment, these drugs, which each target a different component of the disease's pathology, may be administered singly or in combination (Sharma et al., 2023c). It's important to understand that these medications only treat symptoms and cannot cure AD. This is a summary of these pharmaceutical therapies (Akbari et al., 2020).

Cholinesterase Inhibitors

Cholinesterase inhibitors enhance the production of acetylcholine, a crucial neurotransmitter for memory and cognitive function. The progressive degeneration of cholinergic neurons in AD leads to decreased levels of acetylcholine. Acetylcholine is prevented from being degraded by cholinesterase inhibitors, which improve cholinergic neurotransmission. The three main cholinesterase inhibitors that have been approved for the treatment of AD are donepezil (Aricept), rivastigmine (Exelon), and galantamine (Razadyne, Reminyl). These medications can help with daily living tasks, behavior, and cognitive function and are frequently used in mild to moderate AD. Although they differ from person to person, their effects are often moderate (Iversen, 1998).

Memantine

Memantine is a drug used to treat Alzheimer's disease, especially in milder to more advanced stages. Memantine functions differently from cholinesterase inhibitors because it prevents glutamate, a neurotransmitter that can be harmful when present in high concentrations, from being overactive. Although glutamate plays a role in many mental processes, including memory and learning, an excessive amount of it can harm neurons and cause excitotoxicity. Memantine helps control glutamate activity, guarding against overstimulation and consequent damage to nerve cells. In those with mild to moderate Alzheimer's disease, it can help stabilize cognitive and functional abilities (Thakral et al., 2023).

Dementia and Alzheimer's-Related Disorders

Dementia and Alzheimer's-related illnesses often lead to a decline in daily tasks due to their impact on memory and cognitive function. (Prajjwal et al., 2023). Although many symptoms of cognitive decline fall under the general term "dementia," Alzheimer's disease (AD) is the leading cause of dementia see Table 1.

Prevention of Alzheimer's Disease

Since the etiology of AD is yet unknown, preventing the disease is a difficult objective. However, there is evidence to support the idea that some lifestyle choices and risk-reduction measures may help lower the likelihood of acquiring Alzheimer's or postpone the disease (Sharma and Chandra, 2023). These steps can help improve overall well-being and brain health, even though they might not completely avoid the disease. Here are several preventative actions and lifestyle choices that have been linked to a lower risk of AD (Rogers et al., 2023). There are many services and support alternatives available to assist you in navigating this difficult journey if AD or associated disorders affect you or someone you love. See Table 2 for more information (Çakmak et al., 2020).

Discussion

Alzheimer's disease is a progressive neurodegenerative disorder that primarily affects older adults, causing a decline in cognitive function and memory. It is characterized by the accumulation of abnormal protein deposits, such as beta-amyloid plaques and tau tangles, in the brain. Early symptoms include forgetfulness and confusion, which worsen over time, leading to severe impairment in daily life activities. The exact cause remains unclear, but genetics, age, and lifestyle factors may play a role. Currently, there is no cure for Alzheimer's, and available treatments aim to alleviate symptoms temporarily. Research continues to explore potential therapies and early detection methods to address this global health challenge.

Table 1. Frontotemporal dementia, vascular dementia, Lewy body dementia, and illnesses connected to dementia and Alzheimer's

Vascular dementia	Lewy body dementia	Frontotemporal dementia	References
Vascular dementia ranks behind Alzheimer's disease as the second most common cause of dementia. Blood flow to the brain is reduced, which causes damage to brain tissue. The illnesses that may be responsible for this decreased blood flow include small vessel disease, strokes, and other vascular-related problems	Lewy body dementia is a typical form of progressive dementia. The telltale signs include Lewy bodies, and abnormal protein deposits in the brain. These deposits interfere with normal brain function, causing cognitive impairment and other symptoms	Frontotemporal dementia is a dangerous condition despite being a less common type of dementia. This causes slow damage to the frontal and temporal lobes of the brain, affecting behavior, and personality, and leading to linguistic problems	(Ordóñez and Ordóñez, 2021)
Vascular dementia symptoms include memory loss, confusion, and disorientation	Lewy body symptoms Visual hallucinations, fluctuating alertness, and attention	Frontotemporal dementia signs issues with language, such as difficulty speaking or interpreting speech, and issues with judgment and decision-making	(Ordóñez and Ordóñez, 2021)

Table 2. Alzheimer's disease support services and resources

Support organizations	Caregiver resources	Clinical trial registries	References
The Alzheimer's Association is one of the leading organizations battling dementia and AD. They offer a wealth of services, including study materials, support groups, and a round-the-clock helpline	The NIA features a comprehensive caregiving area that contains dementia caregiving information, resources, and guidance for managing caregiving responsibilities	ClinicalTrials.gov is a database of international clinical studies, including those investigating dementia and Alzheimer's disease. People can look for clinical trials using this site that might be suitable for their condition	(Jicha et al., 2010)
Website: www.alz.org	Website: www.nia.nih.gov/health/caregiving	Website: www.clinicaltrials.gov	(Jicha et al., 2010)

Future Prospects

Continuous research and breakthroughs in various areas are enhancing the future prospects for Alzheimer's Disease (AD), thereby enhancing prevention, detection, and treatment (Levine and Lawlor, 1991). More sensitive and precise biomarkers for AD are being sought after through research. Early disease discovery can result in earlier therapies, which may help to halt the trajectory of cognitive deterioration (E et al., 2021). The use of precision medicine techniques may increase as our knowledge of the genetic and molecular causes of Alzheimer's disease expands. More individualized and successful therapies might result from treating patients according to their genetic profile (E et al., 2021). The amyloid-beta and tau proteins are the targets of some disease-modifying treatments and immunotherapies. These therapies seek to slow or stop the progression of Alzheimer's, opening the door to more potent therapeutic approaches (Marsool et al., 2023). Researchers are investigating therapy combinations that target various AD-related pathways. Combining various therapy modalities may increase their effectiveness and offer a more thorough approach to disease care (Mauskopf et al., 2004). Additional methods for enhancing brain health and lowering the risk of Alzheimer's may emerge from ongoing research into lifestyle interventions such as exercise, diet, cognitive training, and social involvement (Etherton-Beer, 2014). Monitoring cognitive health, supplying caregivers with remote help, and enhancing access to care are all made possible by technology, which includes wearables, digital health apps, and telemedicine (Alberts, 2013). Complex datasets connected to AD may be more thoroughly analyzed because of developments in big data analytics and artificial intelligence (AI). This might lead to new understandings of the mechanisms behind the disease and possible targets for treatment (De Silva et al., 2021). To develop Alzheimer's research and exchange information and resources, cooperation between scientists, medical professionals, and organizations globally is essential (Broyd et al., 2009).

Conclusion

Alzheimer's disease (AD) is a severe neurological condition causing significant consequences for affected individuals, families, caregivers, and society, with increasing cases expected as the population ages. Despite the difficulties of Alzheimer's, recent research and advancements provide cause for hope. Instruments for earlier detection and more accurate diagnosis may be developed as a result of progress in biomarker research. Targeted therapy and precision medicine techniques are being studied to develop tailored treatments for persons with Alzheimer's. Immunotherapies and disease-modifying drugs are being studied to slow or stop the course of illness. Changes in lifestyle and technologically based solutions are also promising for promoting brain health and improving treatment. To treat those with Alzheimer's disease with decency, respect, and compassion, ethics must always come first. Comprehensive support networks that include resources, assistance for caregivers, and public awareness initiatives greatly enhance the quality of life for those with Alzheimer's. While there is presently no cure for AD, the dedication of researchers, medical professionals, advocates, and carers inspires hope that the disease's symptoms will one day be decreased. Continuous collaboration, financial support, and public acceptance are necessary for the advancement of Alzheimer's research and care. The fight against AD ultimately requires cooperation from all parties. Together, we can design a future with effective therapies, prevention measures, and assistance services, offering a more optimistic outlook to people with Alzheimer's and the people who care about them.

Acknowledgments

The authors express their gratitude to the Honorable Chancellor of Teerthanker Mahaveer University, Moradabad for providing the necessary facilities.

Disclaimer

None.

References

Ahmad, F., Javed, M., Athar, M., & Shahzadi, S. (2023). Determination of affected brain regions at various stages of Alzheimer's disease. *Neuroscience Research, 192*, 77–82. https://doi.org/https://doi.org/10.1016/j.neures.2023.01.010.

Akbari, V., Ghobadi, S., Mohammadi, S., & Khodarahmi, R. (2020). The antidepressant drug; trazodone inhibits Tau amyloidogenesis: Prospects for prophylaxis and treatment of AD. *Archives of Biochemistry and Biophysics, 679*, 108218. https://doi.org/https://doi.org/10.1016/j.abb.2019.108218.

Alberdi, A., Aztiria, A., & Basarab, A. (2016). On the early diagnosis of Alzheimer's Disease from multimodal signals: A survey. *Artificial Intelligence in Medicine, 71*, 1–29. https://doi.org/https://doi.org/10.1016/j.artmed.2016.06.003.

Alberts, M. J. (2013). Chapter 30 - *Clinical Presentation and Diagnosis of Cerebrovascular Disease* (M. A. Creager, J. A. Beckman, & J. B. T.-V. M. A. C. to B. H. D. (Second E. Loscalzo (eds.); pp. 361–371). W. B. Saunders. https://doi.org/10.1016/B978-1-4377-2930-6.00030-6.

Ashique, S., Pal, R., Sharma, H., Mishra, N., & Garg, A. (2024). Unraveling the Emerging Niche Role of Extracellular Vesicles (EVs) in Traumatic Brain Injury (TBI). *CNS & Neurological Disorders Drug Targets.*

Bensalem, J., Hein, L. K., Hassiotis, S., Trim, P. J., Proud, C. G., Heilbronn, L. K., & Sargeant, T. J. (2023). Modifying Dietary Protein Impacts mTOR Signaling and Brain Deposition of Amyloid β in a Knock-In Mouse Model of Alzheimer Disease. *The Journal of Nutrition, 153*(5), 1407–1419. https://doi.org/https://doi.org/10.1016/j.tjnut.2023.02.035.

Broyd, S. J., Demanuele, C., Debener, S., Helps, S. K., James, C. J., & Sonuga-Barke, E. J. S. (2009). Default-mode brain dysfunction in mental disorders: A systematic review. *Neuroscience & Biobehavioral Reviews, 33*(3), 279–296. https://doi.org/https://doi.org/10.1016/j.neubiorev.2008.09.002.

Çakmak, O., Ökten, S., Alımlı, D., Ersanlı, C. C., Taslimi, P., & Koçyiğit, Ü. M. (2020). Novel piperazine and morpholine substituted quinolines: Selective synthesis through activation of 3,6,8-tribromoquinoline, characterization and their some metabolic enzymes inhibition potentials. *Journal of Molecular Structure, 1220*, 128666. https://doi.org/https://doi.org/10.1016/j.molstruc.2020.128666.

Colom-Cadena, M., Davies, C., Sirisi, S., Lee, J.-E., Simzer, E. M., Tzioras, M., Querol-Vilaseca, M., Sánchez-Aced, É., Chang, Y. Y., Holt, K., McGeachan, R. I., Rose, J., Tulloch, J., Wilkins, L., Smith, C., Andrian, T., Belbin, O., Pujals, S., Horrocks, M. H., … Spires-Jones, T. L. (2023). Synaptic oligomeric tau in Alzheimer's disease — A potential culprit in the spread of tau pathology through the brain. Neuron, *111*(14), 2170-2183.e6. https://doi.org/https://doi.org/10.1016/j.neuron.2023.04.020.

Cook, A. M., & Polgar, J. M. (2015). Chapter 15 - *Assistive Technologies for Cognitive Augmentation 11* In the previous edition of this book this chapter was co-written by Kim Adams, Roger Calixto, Lui Shi Gan, Andrew Ganton, Andrew Rees, Tyler Simpson, and Rebecca Watchorn. (A. M. Cook & J. M. B. T. A. T. (Fourth E. Polgar (eds.); pp. 375–410). Mosby. https://doi.org/https://doi.org/10.1016/B978-0-323-09631-7.00015-6.

De Silva, K., Mathews, N., Teede, H., Forbes, A., Jönsson, D., Demmer, R. T., & Enticott, J. (2021). Clinical notes as prognostic markers of mortality associated with diabetes mellitus following critical care: A retrospective cohort analysis using machine learning and unstructured big data. *Computers in Biology and Medicine, 132*, 104305. https://doi.org/https://doi.org/10.1016/j.compbiomed.2021.104305.

Dewanjee, S., Chakraborty, P., Bhattacharya, H., Chacko, L., Singh, B., Chaudhary, A., Javvaji, K., Pradhan, S. R., Vallamkondu, J., Dey, A., Kalra, R. S., Jha, N. K., Jha, S. K., Reddy, P. H., & Kandimalla, R. (2022). Altered glucose metabolism in Alzheimer's disease: Role of mitochondrial dysfunction and oxidative stress. *Free Radical Biology and Medicine, 193*, 134–157. https://doi.org/https://doi.org/10.1016/j.freeradbiomed.2022.09.032.

Dominko, K., Rastija, A., Smiljanic, K., Mladenovic, A., Lešnjaković, L., Kanazir, S., Milanovic, D., & Hecimovic, S. (2022). Amyloid-ß plaque formation and BACE1 accumulation in the brains of a 5xFAD Alzheimer's disease mouse model is associated with altered distribution and not proteolysis of BACE1 substrates Sez6 and Sez6L. *Mechanisms of Ageing and Development, 207*, 111726. https://doi.org/https://doi.org/10.1016/j.mad.2022.111726.

E, B., D, B., Elumalai, V. K., & K, U. (2021). Data-driven gait analysis for diagnosis and severity rating of Parkinson's disease. *Medical Engineering & Physics*, *91*, 54–64. https://doi.org/https://doi.org/10.1016/j.medengphy.2021.03.005.

Etherton-Beer, C. D. (2014). Vascular cognitive impairment in dementia. *Maturitas, 79*(2), 220–226. https://doi.org/https://doi.org/10.1016/j.maturitas.2014.06.004.

Gifford, A., Praschan, N., Newhouse, A., & Chemali, Z. (2023). Biomarkers in frontotemporal dementia: Current landscape and future directions. *Biomarkers in Neuropsychiatry, 8*, 100065. https://doi.org/https://doi.org/10.1016/j.bionps.2023.100065.

Hasan, T. F., Kelley, R. E., Cornett, E. M., Urman, R. D., & Kaye, A. D. (2020). Cognitive impairment assessment and interventions to optimize surgical patient outcomes. *Best Practice & Research Clinical Anaesthesiology, 34*(2), 225–253. https://doi.org/https://doi.org/10.1016/j.bpa.2020.05.005.

Hoque, M., Samanta, A., Alam, S. S. M., Zughaibi, T. A., Kamal, M. A., & Tabrez, S. (2023). Nanomedicine-based immunotherapy for Alzheimer's disease. *Neuroscience & Biobehavioral Reviews, 144*, 104973. https://doi.org/https://doi.org/10.1016/j.neubiorev.2022.104973.

Iversen, S. D. (1998). The pharmacology of memory. Comptes Rendus de l'Académie Des Sciences - Series III - *Sciences de La Vie, 321*(2), 209–215. https://doi.org/https://doi.org/10.1016/S0764-4469(97)89824-1.

Jicha, G. A., Schmitt, F. A., Abner, E., Nelson, P. T., Cooper, G. E., Smith, C. D., & Markesbery, W. R. (2010). Prodromal clinical manifestations of neuropathologically confirmed Lewy body disease. *Neurobiology of Aging, 31*(10), 1805–1813. https://doi.org/https://doi.org/10.1016/j.neurobiolaging.2008.09.017.

Khalil, M., Hollander, P., Raucher-Chéné, D., Lepage, M., & Lavigne, K. M. (2022). Structural brain correlates of cognitive function in schizophrenia: A meta-analysis. *Neuroscience & Biobehavioral Reviews, 132*, 37–49. https://doi.org/https://doi.org/10.1016/j.neubiorev.2021.11.034.

Kirkeby, E. K., Chyan, M.-K., Diehl, G., Wilbur, D. S., Li, Y., Roberts, A. G., & Mastren, T. (2023). Design and synthesis of astatinated benzothiazole compounds for their potential use in Targeted Alpha Therapy (TAT) strategies to treat Alzheimer's disease-associated amyloid plaques. *Applied Radiation and Isotopes*, *191*, 110555. https://doi.org/https://doi.org/10.1016/j.apradiso.2022.110555.

Kumar, N., & Kumar, R. (2014). Chapter 3 - *Nanomedicine for Neurological Disorder* (N. Kumar & R. B. T. N. and N. in the T. of L. D. Kumar (eds.); pp. 109–175). William Andrew Publishing. https://doi.org/https://doi.org/10.1016/B978-0-323-26433-4.00003-8.

Kumar, P., Sharma, H., Singh, A., Pandey, S. N., & Chandra, P. (2024). Correlation Between Exosomes and Neuro-inflammation in Various Brain Disorders BT - *Exosomes Based Drug Delivery Strategies for Brain Disorders* (N. Mishra, S. Ashique, A. Garg, V. Chithravel, & K. Anand (eds.); pp. 273–302). Springer Nature Singapore. https://doi.org/10.1007/978-981-99-8373-5_11.

Lacava, R., Gareri, P., Castagna, A., Mazzei, F., Cotroneo, A. M., Ruberto, C., Aversa, A., & Mattace Raso, F. (2014). P049: The importance of electrolyte balance: marine plasma treatment in elderly patients with dementia and psychotic disorders. *European Geriatric Medicine, 5*, S97–S98. https://doi.org/https://doi.org/10.1016/S1878-7649(14)70225-6.

Levine, J., & Lawlor, B. A. (1991). Family Counseling and Legal Issues in Alzheimer's Disease. *Psychiatric Clinics of North America, 14*(2), 385–396. https://doi.org/https://doi.org/10.1016/S0193-953X(18)30314-9.

Lewis, T. J., & Trempe, C. L. (2017). Chapter 3 - *Diagnosis of Alzheimer's - Standard-of-Care* (T. J. Lewis & C. L. B. T. T. E. of A. (Second E. Trempe (eds.); pp. 52–77). Academic Press. https://doi.org/https://doi.org/10.1016/B978-0-12-812112-2.00003-3.

Lin, X., Liu, W., Dong, X., & Sun, Y. (2023). Epigallocatechin gallate-derived carbonized polymer dots: A multifunctional scavenger targeting Alzheimer's β-amyloid plaques. *Acta Biomaterialia, 157*, 524–537. https://doi.org/https://doi.org/10.1016/j.actbio.2022.11.063.

Lista, S., Vergallo, A., Teipel, S. J., Lemercier, P., Giorgi, F. S., Gabelle, A., Garaci, F., Mercuri, N. B., Babiloni, C., Gaire, B. P., Koronyo, Y., Koronyo-Hamaoui, M., Hampel, H., & Nisticò, R. (2023). Determinants of approved acetylcholinesterase inhibitor response outcomes in Alzheimer's disease: relevance for precision medicine in neurodegenerative diseases. *Ageing Research Reviews, 84*, 101819. https://doi.org/https://doi.org/10.1016/j.arr.2022.101819.

Manning, C. (2004). Beyond memory: neuropsychologic features in differential diagnosis of dementia. *Clinics in Geriatric Medicine, 20*(1), 45–58. https://doi.org/https://doi.org/10.1016/j.cger.2003.10.002.

Marino, M. J., & Williams, M. (2007). *Central Nervous System Drugs Overview* (J. B. Taylor & D. J. B. T. C. M. C. I. I. Triggle (eds.); pp. 1–16). Elsevier. https://doi.org/https://doi.org/10.1016/B0-08-045044-X/00161-9.

Marsool, M. D. M., Prajjwal, P., Reddy, Y. B., Marsool, A. D. M., Lam, J. R., & Nandwana, V. (2023). Newer modalities in the management of Alzheimer's dementia along with the role of aducanumab and lecanemab in the treatment of its refractory cases. *Disease-a-Month, 69*(5), 101547. https://doi.org/https://doi.org/10.1016/j.disamonth.2023.101547.

Martins-Macedo, J., Salgado, A. J., Gomes, E. D., & Pinto, L. (2021). Adult brain cytogenesis in the context of mood disorders: From neurogenesis to the emergent role of gliogenesis. *Neuroscience & Biobehavioral Reviews, 131*, 411–428. https://doi.org/https://doi.org/10.1016/j.neubiorev.2021.09.030.

Mauskopf, J., Paramore, C., Chan Lee, W., McBurney, C. R., & Snyder, E. H. (2004). P1-373 Drug persistence is similar with rivastigmine and donepezil in Alzhemier's disease patients. *Neurobiology of Aging, 25*, S204. https://doi.org/https://doi.org/10.1016/S0197-4580(04)80685-7.

Modir, A., Shamekhi, S., & Ghaderyan, P. (2023). A systematic review and methodological analysis of EEG-based biomarkers of Alzheimer's disease. *Measurement, 220*, 113274. https://doi.org/https://doi.org/10.1016/j.measurement.2023.113274.

Mudar, R. A., Nguyen, L. T., Eroh, J., Chiang, H.-S., Rackley, A., & Chapman, S. B. (2019). Event-related neural oscillation changes following reasoning training in individuals with Mild Cognitive Impairment. *Brain Research, 1704*, 229–240. https://doi.org/https://doi.org/10.1016/j.brainres.2018.10.017.

Ordóñez, M. de los Á., & Ordóñez, P. de los Á. (2021). Sleep in Persons Living with Alzheimer's Disease and Related Dementias. *Nursing Clinics of North America, 56*(2), 249–263. https://doi.org/https://doi.org/10.1016/j.cnur.2021.02.004.

Parkinson Disease, Movement Disorders and Dementia. (2012). *Basal Ganglia, 2*(3, Supplement), e1–e87. https://doi.org/https://doi.org/10.1016/j.baga.2012.10.001.

Prajjwal, P., Marsool, M. D. M., Inban, P., Sharma, B., Asharaf, S., Aleti, S., Gadam, S., Al Sakini, A. S., & Hadi, D. D. (2023). Vascular dementia subtypes, pathophysiology, genetics, neuroimaging, biomarkers, and treatment updates along with its association with Alzheimer's dementia and diabetes mellitus. *Disease-a-Month, 69*(5), 101557. https://doi.org/https://doi.org/10.1016/j.disamonth.2023.101557.

Ribas, M. Z., Paticcié, G. F., Noleto, F. M., Ramanzini, L. G., Veras, A. de O., Dall'Oglio, R., Filho, L. B. de A., Martins da Silva, J. G., Lima, M. P. P., Teixeira, B. E., Nunes de Sousa, G., Alves, A. F. C., Vieira Lima, L. M. F., Sallem, C. C., Garcia, T. F. M., Ponte de Oliveira, I. M., Rocha, R. S. de C., Jucá, M. de S., Barroso, S. T., & Claudino dos Santos, J. C. (2023). Impact of dysexecutive syndrome in quality of life in Alzheimer disease: What we know now and where we are headed. *Ageing Research Reviews, 86*, 101866. https://doi.org/https://doi.org/10.1016/j.arr.2023.101866.

Rogers, C. J., Ayuso, J., Hackney, M. E., & Penza, C. (2023). Alzheimer Disease and Related Cognitive Impairment in Older Adults: A Narrative Review of Screening, Prevention, and Management for Manual Therapy Providers. *Journal of Chiropractic Medicine, 22*(2), 148–156. https://doi.org/https://doi.org/10.1016/j.jcm.2023.03.001.

Rossini, P. M., Di Iorio, R., Vecchio, F., Anfossi, M., Babiloni, C., Bozzali, M., Bruni, A. C., Cappa, S. F., Escudero, J., Fraga, F. J., Giannakopoulos, P., Guntekin, B., Logroscino, G., Marra, C., Miraglia, F., Panza, F., Tecchio, F., Pascual-Leone, A., & Dubois, B. (2020). Early diagnosis of Alzheimer's disease: the role of biomarkers including advanced EEG signal analysis. Report from the IFCN-sponsored panel of experts. *Clinical Neurophysiology, 131*(6), 1287–1310. https://doi.org/https://doi.org/10.1016/j.clinph.2020.03.003.

Savage, L. M., Roland, J., & Klintsova, A. (2007). Selective septohippocampal – but not forebrain amygdalar – cholinergic dysfunction in diencephalic amnesia. *Brain Research, 1139*, 210–219. https://doi.org/https://doi.org/10.1016/j.brainres.2006.12.083.

Sharma, H., & Chandra, P. (2023). Challenges and Future Prospects: A Benefaction of Phytoconstituents on Molecular Targets Pertaining to Alzheimer's Disease. *International Journal of Pharmaceutical Investigation, 14*(1), 117–126. https://doi.org/10.5530/ijpi.14.1.15.

Sharma, H., Chandra, P., Verma, A., Pandey, S. N., Kumar, P., & Sigh, A. (2023). Therapeutic approaches of nutraceuticals in the prevention of neurological disorders. *European Chemical Bulletin, 12*(5), 1575 – 1596. https://doi.org/10.48047/ecb/2023.12.si5a.038.

Sharma, H., Kaushik, M., Goswami, P., Sreevani, S., Chakraborty, A., Ashique, S., & Pal, R. (2024). Role of miRNAs in Brain Development. *MicroRNA, 13*. https://doi.org/10.2174/0122115366287127240322054519.

Sharma, H., Pathak, R., Kumar, N., Nogai, L., Mishra, R., Bhandari, M., Koli, M., & Pandey, P. (2023). Endocannabinoid System: Role in Depression, Recompense, And Pain Control. *Journal of Survey in Fisheries Sciences, 10*(4S), 2743–2751.

Sharma, H., Rachamalla, H. K., Mishra, N., Chandra, P., Pathak, R., & Ashique, S. (2024). *Introduction to Exosome and Its Role in Brain Disorders BT - Exosomes Based Drug Delivery Strategies for Brain Disorders* (N. Mishra, S. Ashique, A. Garg, V. Chithravel, & K. Anand (Eds.); pp. 1–35). Springer Nature Singapore. https://doi.org/10.1007/978-981-99-8373-5_1.

Sharma, H., Rani, T., & Khan, S. (2023). An insight into neuropathic pain: a systemic and up-to-date review. *IJPSR, 14*(2), 607–621.

Sharma, H., Tyagi, S. J., Chandra, P., Verma, A., Kumar, P., Ashique, S., & Hussain, A. (2024). *Role of Exosomes in Parkinson's and Alzheimer's Diseases BT - Exosomes Based Drug Delivery Strategies for Brain Disorders* (N. Mishra, S. Ashique, A. Garg, V. Chithravel, & K. Anand (Eds.); pp. 147–182). Springer Nature Singapore. https://doi.org/10.1007/978-981-99-8373-5_6.

Thakral, S., Yadav, A., Singh, V., Kumar, M., Kumar, P., Narang, R., Sudhakar, K., Verma, A., Khalilullah, H., Jaremko, M., & Emwas, A. H. (2023). Alzheimer's disease: Molecular aspects and treatment opportunities using herbal drugs. *Ageing Research Reviews, 88*, 101960. https://doi.org/https://doi.org/10.1016/j.arr.2023.101960.

Van der Zee, E. A., & Luiten, P. G. M. (1999). Muscarinic acetylcholine receptors in the hippocampus, neocortex and amygdala: a review of immunocytochemical localization in relation to learning and memory. *Progress in Neurobiology, 58*(5), 409–471. https://doi.org/https://doi.org/10.1016/S0301-0082(98)00092-6.

Wu, T., Cai, W., & Chen, X. (2023). Epigenetic regulation of neurotransmitter signaling in neurological disorders. *Neurobiology of Disease, 184*, 106232. https://doi.org/https://doi.org/10.1016/j.nbd.2023.106232.

Yang, Y., García-Cruzado, M., Zeng, H., Camprubí-Ferrer, L., Bahatyrevich-Kharitonik, B., Bachiller, S., & Deierborg, T. (2023). LPS priming before plaque deposition impedes microglial activation and restrains Aβ pathology in the 5xFAD mouse model of Alzheimer's disease. *Brain, Behavior, and Immunity, 113*, 228–247. https://doi.org/https://doi.org/10.1016/j.bbi.2023.07.006.

Chapter 4

Parkinson's Disease: Background, Molecular Mechanisms, Diagnosis, and Therapeutic Advancements

Mudit Kumar[1], M.Pharm,
Shweta Jain[2], PhD,
and Ankur Vaidya[1,*], PhD

[1]Faculty of Pharmacy, Uttar Pradesh University of Medical Sciences, Saifai, Etawah (U.P.), India
[2]Sir MadanLal Institute of Pharmacy, Etawah (U.P.), India

Abstract

Parkinson's disease (PD) is a nervous system illness that causes uncontrollable movement. Tremor, loss of smell, and balance issues are early warning indicators. The hallmark of Parkinson's disease is a progressive loss and degeneration of dopaminergic neurons in the substantia nigra and pars compacta, which results in a decrease in dopamine levels in the striatum and motor impairments. Patients with Parkinson's disease also have front striatal-mediated executive dysfunction, which includes deficiencies in focus, short-term memory, processing speed, and impulsivity. Parkinson's disease cannot yet be diagnosed using a diagnostic test. A neurologist, a physician skilled in disorders of the neurological system, makes a diagnosis. Parkinson's disease is identified by reviewing your symptoms, medical history, and the results of a neurological and physical examination. The most effective metabotropic glutamate receptors to target for Parkinson's

* Corresponding Author's Email: ankur_vaidya2000@yahoo.co.in.

In: Neurogenerative Disorders
Editors: Mohit Agrawal, Manmohan Singhal, Amit Kumar Nayak et al.
ISBN: 979-8-89530-143-2

disease treatments are mGluR5 and mGluR4. New non-dopaminergic Parkinson's disease therapies are now being developed; thanks to the recent emergence of new medicines that target these receptors and have good pharmacokinetic profiles and brain permeability. The most popular Parkinson's disease treatments are only partially or momentarily helpful, and only a small percentage of patients can get or use them. Because current treatments neither stop or slow the progression of the disease, nor do they restore lost or degenerated dopaminergic neurons, the search for more effective medications is imperative. The prevailing knowledge of the molecular signalling systems connected to Parkinson's disease. Emerging treatments to stop or slow the progression of this complex disease include pharmaceutical interventions, surgical procedures, stem cell transplants, gene therapy, and complementary, supportive, and rehabilitation therapies.

Keywords: substantia nigra, dopamine, striatum, metabotropic glutamate

Introduction

In addition to sluggish movement, tremor, rigidity, walking, and imbalance, Parkinson's disease (PD) is a degenerative condition of the brain that also produces a few non-motor consequences, such as mental health issues, cognitive impairment, pain, sleep issues, and other sensory disruptions. Speech and mobility difficulties, as well as limitations in many facets of daily living, are caused by motor disorders such dyskinesias (uncontrollable movements) and dystonias (painful uncontrollable muscular contractions). As these symptoms worsen, a substantial percentage of people become disabled and need care. During their illness, dementia strikes a large number of PD patients (Korczyn et al., 2017).

Aside from multiple system atrophy, chorea, progressive supranuclear palsy, dystonia and ataxia, PD is the most frequent movement condition. Tremor, rigidity and slow movement are several movement disorders that have symptoms with PD. All movement disorders have the same difficulties as PD in terms of pharmaceutical access, diagnostic and treatment gaps, and LMICs (low- and middle-income countries) (Korczynet al., 2017). Growing older is a common risk factor for PD, though it can also strike younger people. Women are less affected than men are. Several studies have suggested that exposure to environmental factors, including air pollution, pesticides, and industrial solvents, may raise the risk of PD. Although the precise cause of PD is unidentified, it is thought to be caused by a complex interaction between inherited genes and a lifetime of exposure to environmental factors including pesticides, and air pollution (Jankovicet al., 2020).

Etiology

Several areas of the cortex send inhibitory and excitatory signals to the striatum. The primary disease that causes the symptoms is the loss of dopaminergic neurons (Jankovicet al., 2020). The usage of herbicides, pesticides, and proximity to industrial sites has all been implicated as contributing factors to PD. After receiving an injection of 1-methyl-4-phenyl-1,2,3,6-tetrahydropyridine, some people have been seen to exhibit parkinsonian-like symptoms. This substance was accumulated by the mitochondria. Furthermore, evidence suggests that the thalamic nuclei may be harmed by the oxidation and generation of free radicals. Genes are significant because, if one family member has PD, the chance of PD in siblings increases. Additionally, these situations frequently start considerably earlier in life. Lewy bodies are mostly composed of abnormally high quantities of aggregated α-synuclein, which is discovered during autopsies. Altered α-synuclein function is believed to add to the aetiology of PD. The goal of current research is to stop α-synuclein from spreading and aggregating (Jankovic et al., 2020).

Epidemiology

PD affects 1 to 2 persons out of every 1000 people at any given moment; the prevalence rises with ageing, affecting 1% of people over the age of 60. 5% to 10% of patients are predisposed genetically. Occurrence and frequency of PD do rise with age, and males are more likely than women to have the disorder.

Pathophysiology

When many members of an Italian family in the New Jersey region were diagnosed with PD in 1999, the pursuit of the disease's genetic cause gathered steam. A further development resulted from research on families that had this disease's uncommon autosomal dominant type. The aggregation of α-synuclein in the brain's SN and other regions appears to be the main cause of degeneration and subsequent DA loss in the basal ganglia, which regulate muscle tone and movement. α-synuclein protein buildup may be caused by an unidentified environmental trigger or be subsequent to a hereditary predisposition, as is the case with the PARK-1 mutation found in the Contursi kindred of New Jersey (Adams et al., 2023). As a result, it is no longer sufficient to believe that the primary cause of PD is a deficiency in DA in the SN. The underlying pathophysiology appears to be more profound and intricate, and research on the non-genetic causes of α-synuclein deposition in the brain is currently underway.

Histopathology

According to histology, PD is characterised by α-synuclein neuronal inclusions in both the cell bodies and processes of neurons. Lewy-related pathology is the term used to describe the presence of Lewy bodies and Lewy neurites together. Any neurodegenerative disease is characterised by a selective neuronal loss, and in PD, this loss is most obvious in the SN pars compacta. However, it has long been understood that Lewy bodies in PD go far beyond the SN. A staging system for PD has been proposed by Braak and colleagues based on the spread of α-synuclein pathology (Adams et al., 2023).

According to this model, the dorsal motor nucleus of the vagus in the medulla and the front olfactory nucleus of the olfactory bulb are where neuronal disease initially appears. The central nervous system (CNS) impacts autonomic neurons in the peripheral nervous system, and it is increasingly recognized that Parkinsons's disease (PD) constitutes a multiorgan disease process beyond CNS involvement. Additionally, it has intensified debate over the possibility of vagus nerve-mediated retrograde transmission of unidentified transmissible chemicals from the gut to the brain.

Symptoms

The most well-known signs of PD include loss of muscular control. But as we now know, PD symptoms can include more than just problems with muscle function.

Motor-Related Symptoms

- *Slowed movements* You must experience this symptom in order for PD to be diagnosed. People who experience it describe their muscles as being weak, but there is actually no loss of strength; instead, it is caused by issues with muscle control.
- *Tremor while muscles are at rest* About 80% of people with PD experience this regular shaking of their muscles, even when they are not actively moving. Essential tremors, which rarely occur when muscles are at rest, are distinct from resting tremors.
- *Stiffness or Rigidity* PD illness commonly manifests as cogwheel and lead-pipe rigidity. When moving a bodily part, lead-pipe rigidity refers to a consistent, unchanging stiffness. Tremor and lead-pipe rigidity together result in cogwheel stiffness. The jerky, stop-and-go aspect of the movements gives it its name.
- *Walking gait or Unstable posture* PD causes rigidity and slowness which results in a slumped or stooped posture. This typically manifests as the illness worsens. When walking, a person with it will take shorter, shuffled strides and use their arms less. While moving, turning may require multiple steps.

Other motor symptoms can include:

- *Cramped or small handwriting* Due to muscle control problems.
- *Gagging* The lack of facial muscular control causes yet another symptom.
- *A mask-like expression on the face* This condition, known as hypomimia, occurs when facial expressions barely or never change.
- *Dysphagia* or difficulty swallowing. Reduced throat muscle control results in this. It makes conditions like pneumonia or choking more likely.
- *Atypically quiet speech* Reduced throat and chest muscular control is the cause of this.

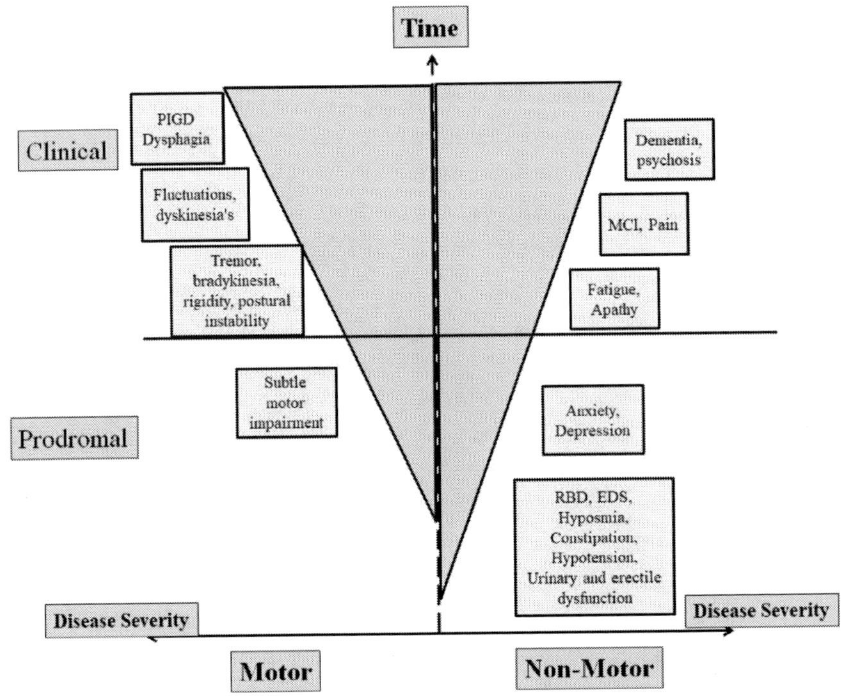

Figure 1. Course of PD from prodromal phase to clinical phase, including levodopa-related complications.

Non-Motor Symptoms

There may be a number of symptoms that are unrelated to movement and muscle control. In the past, medical professionals thought that non-motor symptoms, when present before motor symptoms, were risk factors for this condition as shown in Figure 1 However, there is mounting proof that these signs might emerge even in the early stages of the illness. This means that these symptoms may act as early warning indications for motor issues that appear years or even decades later.

Non-motor symptoms include:

- Orthostatic hypotension, gastrointestinal problems and sexual dysfunctions.
- *Depression.*

- *Anosmia.*
- *Sleep problems*, rapid eye movement, restless legs syndrome and behavior disorder.
- PD related dementia.

Clinical Conditions of PD

PD has been described as a complex neurodegenerative disorder with a range of symptoms brought on by the death of dopaminergic neuronal cells in the SN. Following Alzheimer's disease, PD is the neuropathological ailment with the second-highest prevalence that is linked to severe impairment and a poorer quality of life. It has been discovered that PD incidence rises with aging and is more common in developed nations. PD is extremely uncommon in persons under the age of 40, whereas it affects 1–2% of the global population and 4–5% of those over the age of 85. Men are said to have a higher incidence because estrogen has a protective effect on women, but smokers and coffee drinkers also have lower chances since nicotine is a monoamine-oxidase-B (MAO-B) and caffeine is a receptor antagonist with putative neuroprotective effects (Kalia et al., 2015). Since inpatient treatment at advanced disease stages appears to account for the majority of this cost - which is more expensive than disease medication - early illness identification is imperative. Due to the lack of reliable diagnostic procedures, clinical classification criteria are used to define PD as the presence of both motor and nonmotor symptoms. The monitoring of these essential characteristics, the majority of which are progressive symptoms, serves as one of the present clinical practice's primary decision markers for diagnosing diseases. The fact that a favourable response to dopaminergic medication serves as the primary means of confirming the diagnosis of PD is a clear sign of the diagnosis' ambiguity (Driver et al., 2009).

Pathology

Although various factors are linked to the development of PD, there is little known about how the disease begins. Toxin and methanol exposure, carbon monoxide poisoning, and head trauma are all potential environmental risk factors, but genetic abnormalities can also cause dementia. Together with ageing, these variables can cause mitochondrial malfunction and increased oxidative stress, resulting in neuronal energy failure and neurodegeneration (Prediger et al., 2011). PD is also classified as a synuclein because of aberrant α-synuclein build up and subsequent intracellular aggregation, which results in the creation of Lewy bodies. It is typically found in neuronal cell mitochondria, particularly in the thalamus, olfactory bulb, hippocampus, and striatum. SNCA gene alterations, according to various publications, can influence how intracellular aggregates form. Although -synuclein is the predominant component of LBs, they are made up of more than 90 additional molecules, including mitochondrial, ubiquitin proteasome, and autophagy proteins, as well as PD-related gene products (Thakuret al., 2022).

Cardinal Motor Symptoms in PD Identification

The rigidity, rest tremor, bradykinesia, and loss of postural reflexes are the commonest motor signs of PD. Most motor symptoms respond to dopaminergic medication, which helps differentiate PD from other PD illnesses and aid in disease identification (Jankovic et al., 2008).

Bradykinesia

Bradykinesia is characterized by sluggish movement, declining amplitude, and poor fine motor control because of the decreasing neuronal density in the SN and is the majority recognizable motor sign of PD. Patients with bradykinesia find it difficult to execute quick motions because they are unable to supply the executive muscles with enough energy. Initial signs include difficulty multitasking and poor reaction times, but other symptoms might also include swallowing difficulties, loss of gesticulation, and decreased blinking. Patients with PD who experience bradykinesia may need more external triggers to access their motor programs. Bradykinesia and the extent of DA insufficiency are frequently closely correlated (Obeso et al., 2017).

Tremor

It is a rhythmic muscle relaxation and contraction mostly on the limbs but can stretch to the jaw, lips, and chin, is one of the most instantly recognizable symptoms of PD. Supination and pronation are hallmarks of rest tremors in the hands, which can be reduced by activity or while you sleep. A postural tremor, which is an extended horizontal position against gravity, is frequently mentioned in PD patients. One of the earliest symptoms of Parkinson Diseases, postural tremor, is more noticeable than any other tremor. In contrast to essential tremor, tremors are present in the same frequency range (4-6 Hz) and are susceptible to dopaminergic medication. When there is an essential tremor, the voice and head can be affected more frequently (5-10) and more favourably by alcohol, beta-blockers, and botulinum toxin. Essential tremor at a young age is allegedly a possible risk factor for PD development.

Rigidity

The inflexibility of the limbs, neck, and trunk is referred to as rigidity, which is the second-most prevalent major motor sign of PD. In rigidity, the range of motion is restricted because to muscle stiffness and the inability to relax, while in bradykinesia, the movement is impaired. Shoulder discomfort, which is sometimes mistaken as arthritis, is a typical PD symptom resulting from rigidity. According to reports, dopaminergic agonists can lessen stiffness. as shown in Figure 2.

Postural Instability

The primary sign of diminished postural reflexes usually appears in the late stages of the disease. The majority of falls among PD patients and subsequent hip fractures are caused by this primary symptom. Dopaminergic therapy does not improve postural instability, however deep brain stimulation has been demonstrated to be effective (Armstrong et al., 2020).

There are several different clinical clusters that have been postulated as subtypes of PD, including tremor-dominant and postural-instability-gait disorder subtypes.30-33 According to numerous studies, the tremor-dominant PD phenotype is not as severe in its illness manifestation or its rate of progression as the PIGD phenotype. According to certain theories, the clinical subtypes represent various and diverse disease mechanisms in addition to determining the phenotypic, natural course, and prognosis. This theory has been called into question by the observation that motor subtypes are not fixed, but rather vary with the course of an illness and its treatment.

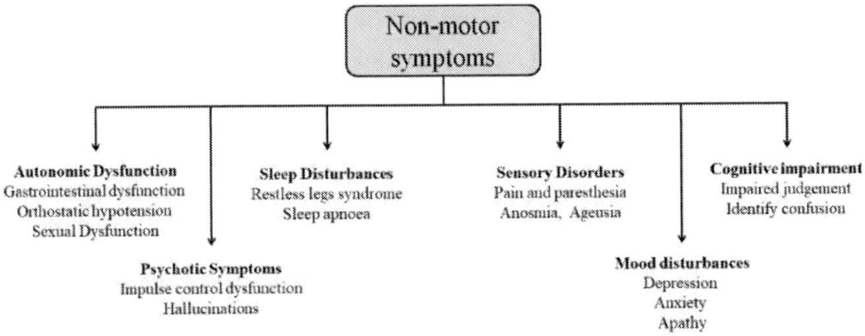

Figure 2. The variety of non-motor symptoms PD sufferers experience.

Environmental Risk Factors

Risk factors for the illness include exposure to pesticides and heavy metals, rural living, agricultural employment, traumatic head injury, melanoma history, use of dairy products, and type 2 diabetes mellitus. A new meta-analysis that included both qualitative and quantitative studies of a variety of environmental exposures reveals that several of these associations - such as rural living, using well water, and pesticide exposure - do not have strong consistency. Some meta-analyses found no evidence to support the beneficial association between pesticide exposure and traumatic brain injury, while others confirmed this association. It is not surprising that such epidemiological research may provide contradictory results due to a number of difficulties and inherent limits (Dorsey et al., 2018).

Neuropathology

Nigrostriatal DA Neuron Vulnerability

The function of α-synuclein in the healthy brain is still not completely understood. Point mutations in α-synuclein, duplications and triplications of genes and polymorphisms that boost the expression of wildtype α -synuclein are all causes of PD. This genetic data and the finding that α -synuclein accumulates in Lewy pathology even in patients of idiopathic PD point to the protein's important role in nearly all cases of the disease. Immunostaining of accumulating α -synuclein, which starts in the caudal brainstem and spreads rostrally to the neocortex over the course of the disease, is used to determine the neuropathological staging of PD progression (Lotharius et al., 2002). Neuronal loss, α-synuclein accumulation, and aggregation are all followed by a neuroinflammatory response that is glial-driven. Glial cells are thought to play a role in the pathophysiology of PD as both a protective reaction to try and save injured neurons and as a source of uncontrolled inflammation that can lead to more neuronal damage. It is still unclear if neuroinflammation is a common cause of PD or only a defence mechanism to lessen existing neuronal damage (Sudhof et al., 2011). Investigating the complex nature of idiopathic PD and the molecular mechanisms that contribute to its genesis is crucial to achieve this goal (Singleton et al., 2003).

DA neurons in the SN are thought to be a particularly vulnerable population of cells in PD, although the nearby DA neurons in the ventral tegmental area are significantly resistant to deterioration. Numerous factors, such as the nigrostriatal neurons' particular morphology, physiology, bioenergetic profile, and neurochemistry, contribute to their sensitivity. First, in rat brain, a single nigrostriatal neuron's axon arbor can be up to 80 cm long; in humans, this length is thought to be 4 m. One nigrostriatal neuron in the rat forms 100000–240000 synapses in the striatum. A nigrostriatal neuron in a human is thought to create 1000000–2400000 synapses. The ventral tegmental area neuron, in comparison, creates roughly 10-fold fewer connections (Deng et al., 2014). There is a lot of proof that PD patients have malfunctioning mitochondria. It is clear that each neuron must sustain at least 10,000,000,000 mitochondria - and must do so over extremely long distances. Nigrostriatal neurons may have "too many mouths to feed," as Paul Bolam has hypothesized. It would stand to reason that the mitochondria that are farthest from the soma would be most susceptible to "wear and tear," and as a result, they could produce less ATP and more ROS. If so, this could explain why the terminals are where nigrostriatal degeneration starts (Tansey et al., 2008). The susceptibility of the dopaminergic nigrostriatal neuron may be influenced by DA itself, primarily in the context of mitochondrial dysfunction. Tyrosine is converted into DA, a catecholamine, through the successive enzymatic operations of amino acid decarboxylase and tyrosine hydroxylase. DA, a redox reactive chemical, is often locked away in synaptic vesicles at levels that are thought to be in the high millimolar range. Therefore, local cytosolic concentrations in the micromolar range might easily be produced even with a little amount of DA leakage from vesicles. Now it is well defined that increased levels of α-synuclein and mitochondrial impairment, which implicated in PD, lead to redistribution of DA from vesicles to cytosol. DA quinone species can be created from cytoplasmic DA through enzymatic oxidation or non-enzymatic auto-oxidation. Covalent cysteinyl-DA adducts are created when the electron-deficient DAQ combines with biological nucleophiles, primarily reduced sulfhydryl groups on free glutathione residues, cysteine, and proteins. (Yokoyama et al., 2020).

Parkinson's Disease-Related Mitochondrial Dysfunction

Reactive oxygen scavenger proteins (such glutathione peroxidase) and other typical compensatory mechanisms, such as antioxidants, will be used by the mitochondria of a healthy neuron to detoxify these ROS. Oxidative stress and mitochondrial dynamics are also significant contributors to the pathophysiology of DA neurons (Martin et al., 2009). The processes of mitochondrial fusion and fission, in which the outer membranes of two mitochondria combine to create a single membrane (fusion) or divide to generate two membranes (fission), are potentially potential causes of neuronal dysfunction (Horowitz et al., 2013). This process regulates synaptic maintenance, mitochondrial synthesis, and neurotransmission, it is not unexpected that genes directing mitochondrial dynamics are required for DA neuron survival (Dias et., al 2013).

Damage to Mitochondrial DNA

Additional support for the association between PD and mutations in genes controlling mitochondrial function comes from the control of mitochondrial DNA. 37 genes, including 13 protein parts for electron transport chain complexes I through V, are encoded by mitochondrial DNA (MT DNA). MT DNA is located in the inner mitochondrial membrane, which is near to the area where oxidative phosphorylation occurs. Additionally, after rotenone therapy in rats, MT DNA basic sites within DA neurons have also been noted; this process takes place before the death of DA cells (Alexeyev et al., 2009).

Since a few years ago, it has become evident that mitochondrial malfunction is a major factor in the development of degeneration (Dauer and Przedborski et al., 2009). After a PD injury, mitochondrial DNA gradually accumulates mutations that hinder efficient mitochondrial activity. ROS levels rise as a result of this process, creating oxidative stress.

Inhibition of Complex I

Rotenone, a traditional complex I inhibitor, is the foundation of PD. Rotenone is a biochemical instrument as well as an organic insecticide that is still used in the US to eradicate invasive aquatic organisms. It differs from 1-methyl-4-phenylpyridinium (MPTP) toxicity in that it doesn't call for astrocyte bioactivation and doesn't have a particular affinity or necessity for the Dopamine transporter (DAT) (Sanders et al., 2014). Rotenone causes neurobehavioral impairments and lesions of the SN and striatum in animal models of PD. It also causes an accumulation of the protein α-synuclein in the cytoplasm of DA neurons. Given that systemic injection of rotenone affects all cells but causes a nigrostriatal lesion, this paradigm is very helpful in demonstrating the specific toxicity of complex I inhibition to DA neurons. The transferrin receptor-2dependent buildup of iron in the SN was accurately predicted by the rotenone model of Parkinson's disease and was later verified in cases of clinical Parkinson's disease. Additionally, it foresaw the development of Mt DNA, a basic lesion in PD's nigrostriatal neurons. Such translational findings highlight the value of neurotoxic models in identifying the pathogenic processes underlying PD. Using any animal model to fully recreate the complicated disease state of PD is obviously difficult, thus it's crucial to be aware of our limits while using these tools (Greenamyre et al., 2003).

Hypertoxic Stress

ROS levels may rise pathologically due to aberrantly elevated production, poor detoxification, or any combination of the two. Despite H2O2's low relative toxicity, it can nonetheless produce highly reactive radicals. Nitric oxide (NO), which is prevalent in the brain, reacts with H2O2 to produce peroxynitrite ($ONOO^-$) and the hydroxyl radical (OH•). It is obvious that oxidative stress is important for this disease's etiology (Roberts et al., 2012). Numerous lines of evidence support the theory that iron metabolism is disrupted in PD, leading to an increase in iron accumulation and oxygen radicals in the SN. Additionally seen to interact with α-synuclein and contribute to the development of Lewy bodies are iron deposits. Iron homeostasis in the brain is mostly regulated by proteins that store iron in an inactive state (such as ferritin and transferrin receptors), and disruption of these proteins may have an impact on neurodegenerative processes (Yoshida et al., 1998).

DA Synthesis

It is not unexpected that DA packaging and storage are tightly controlled cellular processes; sequestering DA into synaptic vesicles offers a storage environment that prevents DA autooxidation by maintaining a low pH and restricting exposure to MAO-B. It has been demonstrated that the vesicular monoamine transporter is essential for the appropriate processing of DA molecules, and knockdown of VMAT2 in mice causes a gradual loss of DA neurons from the SN that is similar to PD. Additionally, there is proof that phospholipase D2 (PLD2) and α-synuclein interact to help create these synaptic vesicles from initial endosomes, and mutations in the α-synuclein gene would probably prevent this from happening. Upsurges in free DA inside the presynaptic cytoplasm are a likely cause of both the observed drop in levels of functional DA neurotransmitter and the magnified amount of oxidative damage seen in PD. This also poses a special problem for the disorder's treatment because DA replacement therapy is crucial for treating motor symptoms but may also increase cellular stress (Jenco et al., 1998).

Neuroinflammation

Numerous downstream proinflammatory mediators, including as inducible nitric oxide synthase, can be upregulated by redox-sensitive transcription factors like NF-κB. This changes citrulline and NO into l-arginine and NADPH (Cho et al., 2011) Anti-inflammatory substances like IL-10, TGF_{β}, and glial-derived neurotrophic factors are expressed during normal inflammation resolution in the brain (Forstermann et al., 2012). Negative feedback processes involving nuclear co-repressors like histone deacetylases (HDAC1-3) and nuclear co-repressor proteins have as a target the suppression of inflammatory transcription. According to studies, p65-NF-B transcription factors attached to inflammatory gene promoters are where the orphan nuclear receptor Nurr1 is recruited. There, it activates the CoREST corepressor complex, which then displaces chromatin-bound NF-B transcription factors. In contrast, adult mice with astrocytic Nurr1 knockdown experienced worsened DA neuron loss after receiving a peripheral injection of bacterial lipopolysaccharide.

Parkinson's Disease - Genetics

The orphan nuclear receptor Nurr1 is recruited to p65-NF-B transcription factors associated with inflammatory gene promoters. There, it activates the REST corepressor complex, which then displaces NF-B transcription factors that are linked to the chromatin. The loss of DA neurons was increased in adult mice with astrocytic Nurr1 knockdown following a peripheral injection of bacterial lipopolysaccharide (Mata et al., 2006). It's interesting to note that Rocha and associates have shown that glucocerebrosidase activity is also decreased in idiopathic PD. The development of small molecule glucocerebrosidase chaperones to improve activity is ongoing. It is not surprising that PD may be linked to mutations that alter proteins involved in antioxidant defence. An early-onset, autosomal recessive variant of PD is brought on by DJ-1 mutations. It's interesting to note that animals with DJ-1 gene deletion have compromised mitochondrial complex I function in the brain. It is significant that postmortem tissue from PD patients has higher levels of astrocytes than neurons in the human brain, where DJ-1 expression is higher in astrocytes. This shows that a primary neuronal phenotype may be caused by a deficiency in the glial protein DJ-1. The DJ-1 expression in astrocytes is being targeted for enhancement (Kim et al., 2005).

Environmental Exposure Risks of Parkinson's Disease

Pesticides

Genetics was assumed to have little to no impact on the pathophysiology of PD and to be secondary to environmental exposures. In contrast, it had been noted that early exposure to a rural setting and well water was linked to an increased incidence of PD. A 'causal agent' that might be hazardous was thought to be transported by well water. The potential impact of pesticides on PD has drawn a lot of attention in this area (Rajput et al., 1987). Both rotenone, a complex I inhibitor, and paraquat, a redox cycling pro-oxidant chemical, have been used in rodents to imitate PD, which is consistent with mechanisms thought to be involved in the disease (Tanner et al., 2011).

Metals

Manganism, a parkinsonian condition brought on by inhalational overexposure to manganese, is the finest example of the close association between occupational metal exposure and neurotoxicity. Although it has long been thought that manganism is clinically distinct from idiopathic PD, some recent investigations indicate that the clinical profile of manganism and PD significantly overlap. Numerous research examining the link between transition-metal exposure and PD have hypothesized that metal buildup in the basal ganglia contributes to mitochondrial dysfunction (Betarbet et al., 2000). The incidence of PD was significantly correlated with occupational exposure to copper, iron, manganese, zinc, mercury, and lead in individuals exposed for more than 20 years (McCormack et al.,2002). Additionally, there is experimental proof that alterations in iron homeostasis may be a factor in the degeneration of nigrostriatal neurons (Lucchini et al., 2014).

Pathogens

The 1918 Spanish influenza postencephalitic cases of parkinsonism best illustrate the historical significance of a pathogenic illness and neurodegeneration. The years after the widespread H1N1 influenza infection saw a significant increase in the prevalence of parkinsonism, even though the clinical signs were obviously different from those of normal PD (Jang et al., 2009). It's interesting that those who were pregnant during the 1918 influenza pandemic, had a higher risk of developing PD. This suggests that immune-based neuroinflammation may be involved, possibly without direct exposure to virus particles. It's interesting to note that modern influenza virus strains, including H5N1, have been discovered to be capable of crossing the CNS and causing neuroinflammation and degeneration of nigrostriatal DA neurons (Rhodes et al., 2014).

The Molecular Mechanism of PD

A complex neurodegenerative disorder, PD manifests both motor and non-motor symptoms. The primary pathogenic change in the parkinsonian brain is the loss of dopaminergic neurons in the SN pars compacta in the ventral midbrain (Dawson et al., 2014). Additionally, elements that are both intracellular and extracellularly found in the SNc are believed to act as damaging pathogenetic components. Intracellular inclusions containing clumps of α-synuclein and neuronal death in the SN, which causes striatal insufficiency of dopamine, are the neuropathological signs of PD (Bloem et al., 2021). The prevalence of PD is more in men as compared to women and rises with age, from 1% of people over 60 to 4% of people over 80, highlighting the negative effects of aging. Although 10% of cases are classified as having youthful onsets, occurring between 20 and 50 years of age, this may represent a separate disease group since the typical age of onset is about 60 years. The most prevalent age-related complicated, idiopathic neurological condition is PD, which is second only to Alzheimer's disease (Lees et al., 2009). PD noted certain typical non-motor symptoms in particular patients, such as autonomies and sleep. There are many nonmotor symptoms. It is uncommon to encounter a patient who does not experience one or more of these. However, the cause of PD is still unknown despite these early descriptions. Novel proteins and pathways that may cause dopaminergic degeneration and a clinical PD illness have been discovered in the last ten years as a result of the discovery of many genes that cause rare familial forms of PD (Armstrong et al., 2020). The greatest contribution to developing novel therapeutics for this prevalent, incurable neurodegenerative ailment will come from knowing the biology of the sporadic form of PD (Dodiya et al., 2020).

Genetics

α-Synuclein (PARK1 and PARK4) Pathway

The α-synuclein family of proteins, which also consists of β synuclein, and includes γ-synuclein. The NAC region primarily distinguishes α-synuclein structurally from the other components. All three members of the family are primarily neuronal proteins that preferentially localize to presynaptic terminals under normal conditions (Shahnawaz et al., 2020). The gene for α-synuclein was discovered to be connected to PD first and A53T, A30P, and E46K mutations in α-synuclein have been linked to familial PD in a number of families See in Table 1. Additionally, α-synuclein protects cysteine-string protein-deficient mice from neurodegeneration. As a result, it is thought to be protective by preserving co-chaperone levels, which safeguard nerve terminal integrity, and it may work partially in place of cysteine-string protein-a, a synaptic co-chaperone. It has been shown that phosphorylation of α-synuclein, particularly at Ser 129, is essential for the formation of fibrils both *in vitro* and *ex* , utilizing a Drosophila model and in the brains of persons with PD and other comparable synucleinopathies. DA leakage from synaptic vesicles as a result of the α-synuclein proto fibrils damaging the vesicular membranes may be a symptom of their toxic effects. The identification of mutations in ATP13A2, which is connected to PARK9, adds to the mounting evidence for the pathogenic role of defective cellular autophagy in PD (Kargbo et al., 2020). There is strong genetic evidence for the following genes' causal involvement in familial Parkinson disease.

LRRK2 (PARK8)

Many PD patients have been shown to have LRRK2 mutations. Particularly, the G2019S mutation was found in 1-2% of sporadic cases and 5-6% of Autosomal dominant familial PD cases. It was discovered that certain populations, such as Ashkenazi Jews and North African Arabs, have an even higher prevalence of this condition.

LRRK2's cellular role is still a mystery. The Golgi apparatus, the outer mitochondrial membrane, and the endoplasmic reticulum are only a few examples of intracellular membranes that it may associate with. Even though LRRK2 is not reported to interact with either protein, the finding of α-synuclein-positive Lewy body pathology or tau-positive neurofibrillary tangle pathology in LRRK2 patients raises the possibility of a shared involvement for LRRK2 in the phosphorylation and processing of these two proteins (Padmanabhan et al., 2020).

Table 1. Parkinson's disease-associated gene

Sr. No.	Gene	Inheritance Base	Causes	Location
1	SNCA (a-synuclein)	Autosomal dominant	Lewy bodies, Lewy neuritis	PARK1/4
2	Parkin	Autosomal recessive	Lewy bodies, Lewy neuritis	PARK2
3	PINK1	Autosomal recessive	Unknown factor	PARK6
4	DJ-1	Autosomal recessive	Unknown factor	PARK7
5	LRRK2 (dardarin)	Autosomal dominant	Lewy body, Lewy neurites, tau inclusion, and amyloid plague	PARK8
6	ATP13A2	Autosomal recessive	Unknown	PARK9

A ubiquitin-like domain and two extremely intriguing novel gene domains are separated by a linker region at the C-terminus of the 465 amino acid E2-dependent E3 ubiquitin ligase known as parkin (Gonzalez-Hunt et al., 2020). To support this claim, however, only a small number of postmortem studies in PD caused by parkin have been carried out. Numerous mis sense and rearrangement-causing homozygous and compound heterozygous mutations in the parkin gene have been discovered.

Missense mutations were primarily discovered in the parkin C-terminal, a highly intriguing novel gene finger domain, of these. This process of loss-of-function is hypothesized to cause neurodegeneration and PD with a deficiency in Lewy bodies. In one instance, however, compound heterozygote mutations that decreased but did not abolish the parkin activity resulted in Lewy bodies being present in a PD brain.

PTEN

PTEN was found to transcriptionally and activate PINK1 in investigations on the expression profiles of cancer cells, giving rise to the moniker PTEN-induced kinase 1 (PINK1) (Jang et al., 2009). PINK1 mutations were later found in three sizable consanguineous families with ARPD, one Spanish and two Italian. A 581 amino acid long protein is encoded by the eight exon PINK1 gene. A mitochondrial serine protease called Omi/HtrA2 prevents apoptosis. It has been shown that Omi/HtrA2's proteolytic activity is regulated by phosphorylation during stress, and that PINK1 is required for this p38 pathway-mediated phosphorylation. This was especially shown when it was shown that patients with PINK1 mutations had less phosphorylated Omi/HtrA2 in their brains than idiopathic PD patients. The direct interaction between PINK1 and Omi/HtrA2 has not been proven, though.

SIRT1 Pathway

Silent information regulator (SIRT) is a term for a group of class III histone deacetylase. There are seven different forms of SIRT, SIRT1 through SIRT7, each of which has unique enzymatic properties, physiological roles, and sub-cellular localisation. SIRT1 has predominantly been identified as a nuclear protein implicated in apoptosis, neuronal differentiation, and the growth of tumours (Kim et al., 2005).

Additionally, SIRT1 induces autophagy by blocking the acetylation process, which is required for its induction. Among the many kinds of SIRT1 activators, L amine A protein, metformin, resveratrol, SRT-1720, and methylene blue are a few examples. The cofactor for SIRT1 activity, AMP-activated protein kinase, is activated directly or indirectly by resveratrol and SRT-1720. In both healthy and diseased cells, the autophagy-lysosomal process is a cellular breakdown mechanism that interacts with various cellular processes. The development of autophagy dysfunction, which results in the build-up of misfolded proteins and DN degeneration, is brought on by genetic variance in PD. Because SIRT1 activates heat shock factor 1 (HSF-1) and the autophagy process, which prevents thc aggregation of α-synuclein, PD neuropathology is less likely to develop and advance. SIRT1 increases autophagy, which lowers the build-up of α-synuclein and mis folded proteins while preserving cellular homeostasis. According to research SIRT1 activators boost the expression of autophagy markers and reduce the deposition of α-synuclein synthesis and aggregation by inhibiting protein hyperphosphorylation. Because of a mitochondrial DNA abnormality, the catalytic component of mitochondrial complex I in the frontal cortex is altered by ROS in PD (Guo et al., 2021). Apoptosis-inducing factors are activated by mitochondrial complex I. SIRT1 and SIRT1 activators have been found to lower the risk of PD in MPTP-model mice by suppressing pro-apoptotic and apoptotic pathways.

NF-κB

The transcription of cytokines and chemokines that support inflammation depends on the DNA-binding protein NF-κB. Extracellular stimuli control NF-κB, and an inhibitor of B (IB) inhibits this regulation by keeping NF-B locked in the cytosol and inhibiting its localization. Extracellular stimuli that activate TLR4 in the presence of CD44 promote NF-κB activation and the release of pro-inflammatory cytokines with the beginning of PD. But the absence of CD44 in PD inhibits the activation of NF-κB and the start of neuroinflammation. Immune dysregulation brought on by aging promotes NF-κB activation with subsequent neuronal damage and neuroinflammation leading to the development of PD (Bian et al., 2020) Results from post-mortem investigations support NF-κB's involvement in the DNs' degeneration in the SN. Notably, SIRT1 regulates oxidative stress and inflammation, whereas NF-κB supports glycolytic energy during inflammation. Inflammation and energy balance are both seriously dysregulated in PD. The SIRT1 factor also prevents NF-κB-mediated immune activation and response.

Pi3/AKT Pathway

According to this pathway AKT contributes to the transmission of PD signalling. AKT and phosphorylated AKT, which are serine/threonine-specific protein kinases, are considerably decreased in the SN pars compacta (SNpc) of PD patients. According to certain studies, PD is characterized by abnormal GSK-3beta expression. The PI3K/AKT/mTOR pathway influences the oxidative stress pathway through additional downstream signalling molecules, such as FOXO3A, in addition to modulating GSK-3beta to affect PD (Mena et al., 2009). When the PI3K/AKT/FOXO3A pathway is disrupted as a result of abnormal Parkin gene expression, oxidative stress becomes imbalanced, resulting in PD. The PI3K/AKT/mTOR pathway inhibitor salidroside (SAL), which can lower GSK-3β and lessen PD symptoms, has been studied as a possible medication for the treatment of PD by researchers.

Mitogen-Activated Protein Kinases (MAPKs)

The minimum of three hierarchically consecutive kinase elements that make up a MAPK signalling cascade are a MAPK kinase 2 and 3(MAP2K, MAP3K). MAP3Ks phosphorylated and activated MAP2Ks, which in turn phosphorylated and activated MAPKs, according to the proposed route. Transcription factors like c-Jun, c-Myc, and ATF2, as well as anti- and pro-apoptotic proteins like Bcl-2 and Bad, are examples of the target proteins that are phosphorylated by active MAPKs. JNK-interacting proteins and p38 MAPK signalling pathways can be activated by various types of cellular stress, including genotoxic, oxidative, and osmotic stress, as well as by microbial substances, like bacterial lipopolysaccharide, and proinflammatory cytokines, like tumour necrosis factor (TNF-α) and IL-1.p38 MAPK signalling pathways may contribute differentially to the dopaminergic neuronal degeneration characteristic of PD (Zhao et al., 2018). Increased levels of phosphorylated (active) versions of JNK and ERK, but not the level of phosphorylated p38 MAPK, were observed to correspond with the confined distribution of neurofibrillary tangles in the brain of a α-synuclein-over expressing mice model of PD (Kaul et al., 2011).

Assessment of Parkinson's Disease Patients

Diagnostic Criteria

The PD tremor often has a unilateral onset, a "pill rolling" quality (with the thumb flexed), and a frequency range of 4-6Hz. Tremor amplitude frequently increases while at rest, while moving, when distracted, when concentrating on a motor or cognitive task (with the contralateral limb), and when under stress. Particularly in early or tremor-predominant disease, tremor variability in PD makes it sometimes difficult to distinguish from a functional (psychogenic) tremor (Deuschl et al., 1998).

The following tests used to distinguish the two:

1. Making ballistic motions with the unaffected limb on the opposite side, which in functional tremor but not in PD results in a momentary tremor stop.
2. To check for entrainment, have the patient tap their fingers at a frequency other than their tremor in order to accomplish a motor activity with the unaffected (or less afflicted) limb.

A functional tremor may be present if the patient experiences severe difficulties doing the task, the tremulous hand adopts the new frequency, or changes dramatically (Bhatia et al., 2017). Even though essential tremor (ET) occasionally resembles PD tremor. This is not perfect, and in a large percentage of instances, there may be overlap in the tremor characteristics, making clinical distinction occasionally challenging (Jankovic et al., 2012).

Differential Diagnoses

There are four different forms of PD: primary (idiopathic), secondary (acquired, symptomatic), heredodegenerative, and multiple system degeneration (parkinsonism plus symptoms). Tremor, early gait abnormalities (such as freezing), pyramidal tract findings, postural instability, and levodopa response are a few characteristics that can be utilized to distinguish PD from other parkinsonian illnesses (Warren et al., 2007). Although the poor response to levodopa medication in patients with PD or other atypical parkinsonian illnesses has been attributed to abnormalities in the density of postsynaptic DA receptors, this may not be the only cause (Parati et al., 1993). Recent positron emission tomography imaging investigations have indicated that DA receptors in PSP are relatively well-preserved, suggesting that downstream alterations may be the cause of the lack of dopamine.

Levodopa improvement is suggestive of PD, but it does not definitely distinguish PD from other Parkinsonian illnesses (Clarke et al., 2007). Only 77% of individuals with pathologically confirmed PD had a "good" or "excellent" initial response to levodopa, according to one study. Apomorphine injection administered subcutaneously has been used to distinguish between PD and other PD illnesses; nevertheless, this test does not outperform levodopa medication and makes little contribution to the diagnostic process (Piccini et al., 2006). These neuroimaging methods show promise, but before their diagnostic potential is completely realized, more resolution and sensitivity enhancement are required (Brooks et al., 1992).

Therapeutic Developments for the Treatment of Parkinson's Disease

Advances in Deep-Brain Stimulation

When levodopa-induced side effects become more troublesome, deep brain stimulation is an additional proven treatment for Parkinson's disease (PD) that is helpful in treating dopamine-dependent motor symptoms. DBS is the surgical implantation of electrodes that stimulate subcortical organs like the globus pallidus internus and the subthalamic nucleus (Spillantini et al., 1997). In some severe PD patients, DBS produces significant reductions in motor symptoms and fluctuations compared to optimal pharmacological therapy, however dopamine-resistant symptoms other than tremor (such as gait disorder and postural instability) do not react well. DBS techniques may result in speech impairment in addition to surgical issues and cognitive and neuropsychiatric side effects. Innovative DBS strategies, including as adaptive DBS that targets various regions and updated intra-operative imaging methods, promise to increase practical applicability and lessen the impact of negative consequences (Polymeropoulos et al., 1997).

Regenerative Treatments

There is a lot of interest in using cell-based and gene therapies in addition to the pharmaceutical methods mentioned above to restore the function of the missing dopaminergic neurons. Clinical trials for two gene treatments using the genes that encode these enzymes are currently being conducted (Kosloski et al., 2013).

Neurotrophic Factors

There has been a lot of interest in creating neuroprotective medicines based on neurotrophic factors since they show positive effects on dopaminergic neurons in pre-clinical models, such as glial cell line-derived neurotrophic factor (GDNF). However, randomised double-blind trials, such as recent research in the UK, have not been able to replicate similar findings. However, there has been substantial debate regarding the reasons why these open and double-blind trials have produced such disparate results. As a result, a workshop was held in 2019 to explore these concerns; the outcomes of which were just recently published. Although GDNF research has so far produced a range of results, this interesting experimental method continues to spark curiosity. Inconsistent outcomes may be somewhat explained by the inclusion of patients with moderately advanced PD, insufficient follow-up, and the significant placebo effect (Hickey et al., 2016).

Targeting Non-Dopaminergic Neurotransmitter Systems

Although DA is responsive to many of the motor symptoms of Parkinson's disease, it has little effect on others, such as freezing of gait and tremor. It is now known that some of these characteristics result from deficits in other neurotransmitter systems. As a result, there is interest in changing how they operate to treat particular PD symptoms that are dopamine resistant. Safinamide, a new medication with multiple potential modes of action, has recently been approved for treatment in PD. It is a powerful reversible monoamine oxidase B inhibitor that is beneficial for treating dopaminergic components of Parkinson's disease. (Stefani et al., 2007). Additionally, it modifies glutamate transmission, which could be related to some non-motor symptoms of PD. Safinamide is now more commonly accessible for clinical usage, while its precise function is still unknown. Right now, it's most likely to be utilized as a supplement to levodopa-based therapies, especially in people who have troublesome dyskinesias and fluctuations (Grabli et al., 2013).

Immunotherapies

The presence of aberrant aggregates of α-synuclein is the main indicator of PD. Although the function of α-synuclein in PD is unclear, it is assumed that it plays a crucial pathogenic role. This is corroborated by multiple independent studies showing the deleterious effects of modifying α-synuclein in cell and animal models, as well as the fact that rare familial forms of the disease are caused by mutations or duplications/triplications of the SNCA gene. Potential pathogenic processes for α-synuclein include disruption of vesicular transport, modifications in the lysosome-autophagy system, mitochondrial malfunction, and oxidative stress. The "strains" supporting the idea that pathogenic forms of α-synuclein can behave in a prion-like manner, allowing pathology to spread from cell to cell, are now being discovered. Approaches for passive and active immunisation against α-synuclein have been shown to have neuroprotective effects in animal models (Stefani A et al., 2007).

Disclaimer

None.

References

Adams, C., Suescun J., Haque A., Block K., Chandra S, Ellmore T. M., Schiess M. C. (2023). Updated Parkinson's disease motor subtypes classification and correlation to cerebrospinal homovanillic acid and 5-hydroxyindoleacetic acid levels. *Clinical Parkinsonism & Related Disorders*, 8, 100187.

Alexeyev, M. F. (2009). Is there more to aging than mitochondrial DNA and reactive oxygen species? *The FEBS Journal*, 276(20), 5768–5787.

Armstrong, M. J., Okun M. S. (2020). Diagnosis and treatment of Parkinson disease: a review. *JAMA*, 323(6), 548-560.

Betarbet, R., Sherer TB, MacKenzie G, Garcia-Osuna M, Panov AV, Greenamyre JT. (2000). Chronic systemic pesticide exposure reproduces features of Parkinson's disease. *Nature Neurosci,* 3(12), 1301–1306.

Bhatia, K. P., Bain P, Bajaj N, Elble RJ, Hallett M, Louis ED. (2018). Consensus statement on the classification of tremors. From the taskforce on the tremor of the international Parkinson and Movement Disorder Society. *Movement Disorders,* 33, 75-87.

Bian, W., Jing X., Yang Z, Shi Z, Chen R, Xu A, Zhang, C. (2020). Downregulation of LncRNA NORAD promotes Ox-LDL-induced vascular endothelial cell injury and atherosclerosis. *Aging* (Albany NY), 12(7), 6385.

Bloem, B. R., Okun MS, Klein C. (2021). Parkinson's disease. *The Lancet,* 397(10291), 2284-2303.

Brooks, D. J., Ibanez V, Sawle GV. (1992). Striatal D2 receptor status in patients with Parkinson's disease, striatonigral degeneration, and progressive supranuclcar palsy, measured with 11C-raclopride and positron emission tomography. *Annals of Neurology*, 31, 184–92.

Cho, B., Kim T., Huh YJ, Lee J, Lee YI. (2019). Amelioration of mitochondrial quality control and proteostasis by natural compounds in Parkinson's disease models. *International Journal of Molecular Sciences*, 20(20), 5208.

Clarke, C. E., Davies P. (2000). Systematic review of acute levodopa and apomorphine challenge tests in the diagnosis of idiopathic Parkinson's disease. *Journal of Neurology and Neurosurgery and Psychiatry*, 69, 590–594.

Dawson, T. M., Dawson VL. (2014). Parkin plays a role in sporadic Parkinson's disease. *Neurodegenerative Diseases,* 13, 69–71.

Deng, H. and Yuan L. (2014). Genetic variants and animal models in SNCA and Parkinson disease. *Ageing Research Review,* 15, 161–176.

Deuschl, G., Bain P, Brin M. (1998). Consensus statement of the movementdisorder society on tremor. Ad Hoc scientific committee. *Movement Disord*, 13, 2–23.

Dias, V., Junn E, Mouradian MM. (2013). The role of oxidative stress in Parkinson's disease. *Journal of Parkinson's Diseases,* 3(4), 461–491.

Dodiya, H. B., Forsyth CB, Voigt RM, Engen PA, Patel J, ShaikhM, Keshavarzian A. (2020). Chronic stress-induced gut dysfunction exacerbates Parkinson's disease phenotype and pathology in a rotenone-induced mouse model of Parkinson's disease. *Neurobiology of Disease,* 135, 104352.

Dorsey, E. R., Bloem BR. (2018). The Parkinson Pandemic - A call to action. *JAMA Neurology*, 75, 9–10.

Driver, J. A., Logroscino G, Gaziano JM, Kurth T. (2009). Incidence and remaining lifetime risk of Parkinson disease in advanced age. *Neurology,* 72, 432–438.

Forstermann, U., Sessa WC. (2012). Nitric oxide synthases: regulation and function. *European Heart Journal*, 33(7), 829–837.

Gonzalez-Hunt, C. P., Thacker EA, Toste CM, Boularand S, Deprets S, Dubois L, Sanders LH. (2020). Mitochondrial DNA damage as a potential biomarker of LRRK2 kinase activity in LRRK2 Parkinson's disease. *Scientific reports* 10(1), 17293.

Grabli, D., Karachi C, Folgoas E. (2013). Gait disorders in parkinsonian monkey with pedunculopontine nucleus lesions: A tale of two systems. *Journal of Neurosciences*, 33(29), 11986–11993.

Greenamyre, J. T., Betarbet R, Sherer TB. (2003). The rotenone model of Parkinson's disease: genes, environment and mitochondria. *Parkinsonism Related Disorders* 9, 59–64.

Guo, K., Zhang Y, Li L, Zhang J, Rong H, Liu D, Zhang X. (2021). Neuroprotective effect of paeoniflorin in the mouse model of Parkinson's disease through α-synuclein/protein kinase C δ subtype signaling pathway. *NeuroReport,* 32(17), 1379-1387.

Hickey, P., Stacy M. (2016). Deep Brain Stimulation: A Paradigm Shifting Approach to Treat Parkinson's Disease. *Frontiers in Neurosciences,* 10, 173.

Jang, H., Boltz D, Sturm-Ramirez K, Shepherd KR, Jiao Y, Webster R. (2009). Highly pathogenic H5N1 influenza virus can enter the central nervous system and induce neuro inflammation and neuro degeneration. *Proceedings of National Academy of Sciences*, 106(33), 14063–14068.

Jankovic, J., Tan EK. (2020). Parkinson's disease: etiopathogenesis and treatment. *Journal of Neurology, Neurosurgery & Psychiatry, 91(8)*, 795-808.

Jankovic, J. (2012). Distinguishing Essential Tremor from Parkinson's Disease. *Practical Neurology*, 2012, 36-38.

Jankovic, J. (2008). Parkinson's disease: Clinical features and diagnosis. *Journal of Neurology Neurosurgery and Psychiatry*, 79, 368–376.

Jenco, J. M., Rawlingson A, Daniels B, Morris AJ. (1998). Regulation of phospholipase D2: selective inhibition of mammalian phospholipase D isoenzymes by alpha- and beta-synucleins. *Biochemistry,* 37(14), 4901–4909.

Kalia, L. V., Lang AE. (2015). Parkinson's disease. *Lancet* 386, 896–912.

Kargbo, R. B. (2020). PROTAC compounds targeting α-synuclein protein for treating neurogenerative disorders: Alzheimer's and Parkinson's diseases. *ACS Medicinal Chemistry Letters,* 11(6), 1086-1087.

Kaul, T., Credle J, Haggerty T, Oaks AW, Masliah E, Sidhu A. (2011). Region-specific tauopathy and synucleinopathy in brain of the alpha-synuclein overexpressing mouse model of Parkinson's disease. *BMC Neurosciences*, 12, 79.

Kim, R. H., Smith PD, Aleyasin H, Hayley S, Mount MP, Pownall S. (2005). Hypersensitivity of DJ-1-deficient mice to 1-methyl- 4-phenyl-1,2,3,6-tetrahydropyrindine (MPTP) and oxidative stress. *Proceedings of National Academy of Sciences*, 102(14), 5215–5220.

Kosloski, L. M., Kosmacek EA, Olson KE. (2013). GM-CSF induces neuroprotective and anti-inflammatory responses in 1-methyl-4-phenyl-1,2,3,6- tetrahydropyridine intoxicated mice. *Journal of Neuroimmunology,* 265(1–2), 1–10.

Lees, A. J., Hardy J, Revesz T. (2009). Parkinson's disease. *The Lancet*, 373(9680), 2055-2066.

Lotharius, J. and Brundin P. (2002). Pathogenesis of parkinson's disease: dopamine, vesicles and α-synuclein. *Nature Review Neurosciences*, 3(12), 932–942.

Lucchini, R. G., Guazzetti S, Zoni S, Benedetti C, Fedrighi C, Peli M. (2014). Neuro Toxicology Neuro functional dopaminergic impairment in elderly after lifetime exposure to manganese. *Neurotoxicology,* 45, 309–317.

Magan, S. K., Mupparthi SD, Gollapalli BP, Shukla D, Tiwari AK, Gorantala J, Tantravahi S. (2020). Salidroside-can it be a multifunctional drug?. *Current Drug Metabolism,* 21(7), 512-524.

Martin, H. L., Teismann P. (2009). Glutathione–a review on its role and significance in Parkinson's disease. *FASEB Journal,* 23(10), 3263–3272.

Mata, I. F., Wedemeyer WJ, Farrer MJ, Taylor JP, Gallo KA. (2006). LRRK2 in Parkinson's disease: protein domains and functional insights. *Trends in Neurosciences,* 29(5), 286–293.

McCormack, A. L., Thiruchelvam M, Manning-Bog AB, Thiffault C, Langston JW, Cory-Slechta DA. (2002). Environmental risk factors and Parkinson's disease: selective degeneration of nigral dopaminergic neurons caused by the herbicide paraquat. *Neurobiology Diseases,* 10(2), 119–127.

Mena, M. A., Casarejos MJ, Solano R, Rodríguez-Navarro JA, Gómez A, Rodal I, De Yebenes JG. (2009). NP7 protects from cell death induced by oxidative stress in neuronal and glial midbrain cultures from parkin null mice. *FEBS Letters,* 583(1), 168-174.

Obeso, J. A., Stamelou M, Goetz CG. (2017). Past, present, and future of Parkinson's disease: a special essay on the 200th anniversary of the shaking palsy. *Movement Disorders* 32, 1264–310.

Ozelius, L. J., Senthil G, Saunders-Pullman R, Ohmann E, Deligtisch A, Tagliati M. (2006). LRRK2G2019S as a Cause of Parkinson's Disease in Ashkenazi Jews. *The New England Journal of Medicine,* 354(4), 424–425.

Padmanabhan, S., Lanz TA, Gorman D, Wolfe M, Joyce A, Cabrera C, Merchant K. (2020). An assessment of LRRK2 serine 935 phosphorylation in human peripheral blood mononuclear cells in idiopathic Parkinson's disease and G2019S LRRK2 cohorts. *Journal of Parkinson's Disease,* 10(2), 623-629.

Parati, E. A., Fetoni V, Geminiani GC. (1993). Response to L-DOPA in multiple system atrophy. *Clinical Neuropharmacology,* 16, 139–44.

Piccini, P., Brooks DJ. (2006). New developments of brain imaging for Parkinson's disease and related disorders. *Movement Disorders,* 21, 2035–41.

Polymeropoulos, M. H., Lavedan C, Leroy E. (1997). Mutation in the -Synuclein Gene Identified in Families with Parkinson's Disease. *Science,* 276(5321), 2045–2047.

Rajput, A. H., Uitti RJ, Stern W, Laverty W, O'Donnell K, O'Donnell D. (1987). Geography, drinking water chemistry, pesticides and herbicides and the etiology of Parkinson's disease. *Canadian Journal of Neurology Sciences,* 14(3), 414–418.

Rhodes, S. L., Buchanan DD, Ahmed I, Taylor KD, Loriot MA , Sinsheimer JS. (2014). Pooled analysis of iron-related genes in Parkinson's disease: association with transferring. *Neurobiology Diseases,* 62, 172–178.

Sanders, L. H., McCoy J, Hu X, Mastroberardino PG, Dickinson DC, Chang CJ. (2014). Mitochondrial DNA damage: Molecular marker of vulnerable nigral neurons in Parkinson's disease. *Neurobiology Diseases,* 70(C), 214–223.

Shahnawaz, M., Mukherjee A, Pritzkow S, Mendez N, Rabadia P, Liu X, Soto C. (2020). Discriminating α-synuclein strains in Parkinson's disease and multiple system atrophy. *Nature,* 578(7794), 273-277.

Singleton, A. B, Farrer M, Johnson J, Singleton A, Hague S, Kachergus J. (2003). alpha-Synuclein locus triplication causes Parkinson's disease. *Science,* 302(5646), 841.

Song, S., Jang S, Park J, Bang S, Choi S, Kwon KY, Chung J. (2013). Characterization of PINK1 (PTEN-induced putative kinase 1) mutations associated with Parkinson disease in mammalian cells and Drosophila. *Journal of Biological Chemistry,* 288(8), 5660-5672.

Spillantini, M. G., Schmidt ML, Lee VM. (1997). Alpha-Synuclein in Lewy bodies. *Nature,* 388(6645), 839–40.

Stefani, A., Lozano AM, Peppe A. (2007). Bilateral deep brain stimulation of the pedunculopontine and subthalamic nuclei in severe Parkinson's disease. *Brain.* 130(6), 1596–607.

Sudhof, T. C., Rizo J. (2011). Synaptic Vesicle Exocytosis, Cold Spring HarborPerspect. *Biology,* 3(12), a005637.

Tanner C. M., Kamel F, Ross GW, Hoppin JA, Goldman SM, Korell M. (2011). Rotenone, Paraquat, and Parkinson's Disease. *Environmental Health Perception,* 119(6), 866–872.

Thakur, S., Singh Y, Goyal P, Kumar M. (2022). Current therapy and protective potential of medicinal mushroom cordycepsmilitaris against alzheimer's disease. *Journal of Positive School Psychology,* 6(8), 2100-2108.

Warren, N. M., Piggott MA, Greally E. (2007). Basal ganglia cholinergic and dopaminergic function in progressive supranuclear palsy. *Movement Disorder,* 22, 1594–1600.

Yoshida, T., Tanaka M, Sotomatsu A, Hirai S , Okamoto K. (1998). Activated microglia cause iron-dependent lipid peroxidation in the presence of ferritin. *NeuroReport,* 9(9), 1929–1933.

Zhao, H. M., Zhang XY, Lu XY, Yu SR, Wang X, Zou Y, Zhou BG. (2018). Erzhi pill® protected experimental liver injury against apoptosis via the PI3K/Akt/Raptor/Rictor pathway. *Frontiers in Pharmacology*, 9, 283.

Chapter 5

Huntington's Disease: Neuropharmacology and Clinical Approaches

Ankit[1],
Jyoti[1],
Shivani[2],
and Shiv Kant Sharma[1,*]
[1]Department of Pharmaceutical Sciences, Gurugram University, Gurugram, India
[2]ICAR-Central Institute for Research on Buffaloes, Hisar, Haryana, India

Abstract

Huntington's disease (HD) is a rare neurodegenerative disorder characterized *via* the progressive loss of neurons in specific regions of the brain. It is brought on by a mutation in the huntingtin gene, which results in the creation of mutant huntingtin, a dangerous protein. This protein interferes with typical cellular functions, which ultimately results in the malfunction and death of neurons. Cognitive, motor and mental disturbances all contribute to the condition's symptoms. Issues with memory, executive function, attention, and language skills are among these cognitive impairments. On the other hand, motor abnormalities include bradykinesia (slow movement), muscle rigidity, and involuntary motions (chorea). Extensive study in this field over the last few decades has shed light on HD's current incidence and prevalence rate, which is expected to be 3.92 per 100,000 people between 1985 and 2022 according to the Medline database. Geographically, the incidence varies, with Venezuela and other nations reporting the greatest prevalence rates. Utilizing neuroprotective drugs and modifying glutamate and dopamine

* Corresponding Author's Email: sksharma@gurugramuniversity.ac.in.

In: Neurogenerative Disorders
Editors: Mohit Agrawal, Manmohan Singhal, Amit Kumar Nayak et al.
ISBN: 979-8-89530-143-2

levels are all part of the clinical care of Huntington's disease. Gene silencing therapies, DNA and RNA-based therapies, tools for genetic manipulation, etc. are some of the most recent therapeutic modalities. The standard and recently approved medicines for the management of Huntington's disease are covered in detail in this chapter.

Keywords: Huntington's disease, glutamate modulation, gene silencing therapies, genetic manipulations

Introduction

Huntington's disease (HD) is a fatal hereditary ailment that affects both affected individuals and their families severely. George Huntington, an American physician, provided the first description of it in 1872. HD is fundamentally brought on by a mutation in the Huntingtin gene (HTT), which results in the synthesis of a toxic huntingtin protein. The disease will manifest in a person who inherits one copy of the mutant gene from either parent due to the autosomal dominant inheritance pattern of this mutation (Eje et al., 2023). Every affected person's child has a 50% chance of inheriting the gene due to this genetic component. Although, the age of start can vary, the hallmark of HD is its progressive nature, which commonly manifests symptoms around mid-adulthood. Mood swings, cognitive deterioration, problems with motor skills and coordination, uncontrollable movements known as chorea, and many other symptoms are included in this list. These symptoms worsen as the illness progresses, frequently robbing patients of their ability to walk, talk, and carry out even the most fundamental daily tasks (Ross and Tabrizi 2011). In order to treat Huntington's Disease (HD), a crippling neurodegenerative condition, neuropharmacology is crucial. This sector focuses on creating drugs to treat the disease's various symptoms, including chorea and mood swings. Overall, neuropharmacology is essential for treating HD symptoms and searching for disease-modifying therapies, providing some hope in the fight against this debilitating disease (Jimenez-Sanchez et al., 2017).

Clinical evaluations based on these distinctive symptoms and genetic tests to validate the existence of the mutant HTT gene are used to make the diagnosis. For those who have a family history of HD, genetic counseling is typically advised to assist them comprehend the risks and implications. While there is currently no cure for HD, there are therapy alternatives to control its symptoms and improve the quality of life for those who are affected. Physical and speech therapy can help with motor and communication difficulties, while medications can be provided to help manage motions and psychological concerns. Living with HD can be physically and emotionally taxing for those who have it as well as their families. Therefore, thorough support systems are necessary. In order to traverse the complexities of this disease, medical professionals, support groups, and social services are crucial in offering direction, treatment, and emotional support. The conventional and recently approved medicines for the management of Huntington's disease are covered in detail in this chapter (Sun, 2023; Frank, 2014).

The Pathophysiology of Huntington's Disease

A very disabling neurodegenerative condition with a complex and intricate pathogenesis is Huntington's disease (HD). It results from a genetic mutation in the chromosome 4 HTT gene. The CAG repeat sequence within the gene has grown due to this mutation. Unaffected people typically have 10-35 CAG repeats, but HD patients typically have 36 or more repeats. The severity and age of start of HD symptoms are correlated with the length of this expansion. A mutant huntingtin protein (mHTT) with an extended polyglutamine (polyQ) tract results from this genetic mutation. According to Ghosh and Tabrizi (2018), the pathophysiological cascade in HD is intricate and involves a number of crucial processes.

Initially harmful protein aggregates can form inside of neurons as a result of mHTT's propensity for misfolding and aggregation. Cellular dysfunction and neuro-inflammation are caused by these aggregates, which interfere with normal cellular processes (Wanker et al., 2019). The main targets are neurons, notably those in the striatum of the brain. The typical motor symptoms of HD, such as chorea (jerky, uncontrollable movements) and dystonia (abnormal muscle contractions), are exacerbated by the loss of neurons that occurs as the disease advances see in Figure 1 (Gil and Ana, 2008).

Additionally, mHTT impairs axonal transport, causes mitochondrial dysfunction, modifies neurotransmitter release, and messes up synaptic transmission among other aspects of cellular function in neurons. Collectively, these biological abnormalities cause neuronal damage and eventual death. Neuroinflammation is a vital component of HD's pathogenesis. The brain's immune cells, microglia and astrocytes, get activated as neurons are harmed and mHTT aggregates build up, resulting in persistent neuroinflammation.

According to (Ghosh and Tabrizi, 2018), this inflammatory response exacerbates neuronal damage and contributes to the disease's progressive character.

HD has a broad range of clinical manifestations, including not just motor dysfunction but also cognitive decline, mental symptoms (such as anxiety and sadness), and behavioral problems. Although there are cases of early-onset HD where symptoms first present in childhood or adolescence, these symptoms commonly appear in mid-adulthood (Morales et al., 2023).

Symptoms of Huntington's Disease

A neurodegenerative condition known as Huntington's disease (HD) is characterized by a variety of symptoms that worsen over time. The three main types of these symptoms are motor, cognitive, and psychiatric. It's crucial to remember that different HD sufferers may experience different levels of symptom intensity and development. As shown in Figure 2.

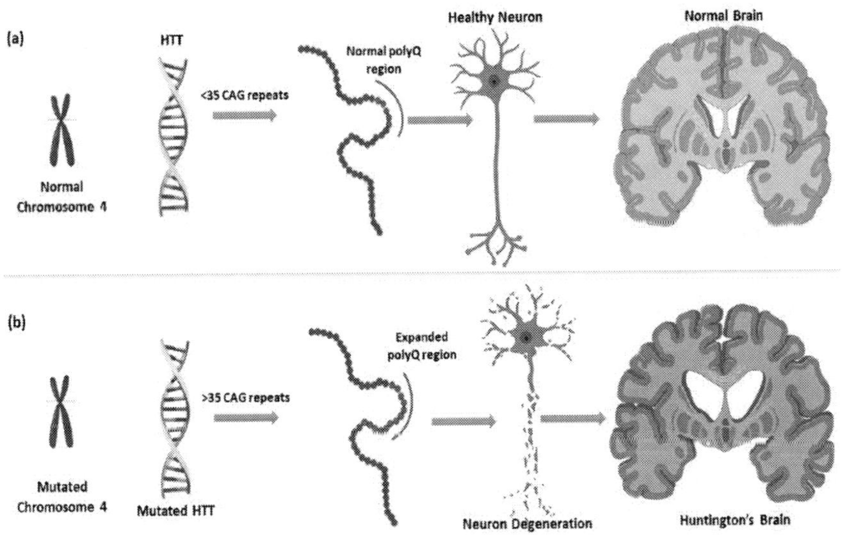

Figure 1. Pathophysiology of Huntington Disease: Illustration of a) normal brain, b) huntington's brain.

Motor Symptoms

Chorea

Chorea describes uncontrollable, jerky, and frequently unpredictable movements, one of the defining motor symptoms of HD. The arms, legs, face, and trunk are just a few of the body areas that might be impacted by these movements. As the condition worsens, chorea frequently does as well.

Dystonia

Dystonia is characterized by persistent muscle spasms that cause aberrant postures or habitual twisting motions.

Impaired Coordination

The coordination, balance, and fine motor skills issues that people with HD frequently encounter make simple things like walking and writing increasingly difficult.

Bradykinesia

Bradykinesia, or slowness of movement, can make doing routine tasks more challenging and time-consuming (Palaiogeorgou et al., 2023).

Cognitive Symptoms

Cognitive Decline

As HD worsens, people may experience cognitive decline, including memory issues, focus issues, and decreased judgment.

Executive Dysfunction

Task organization, planning, and completion may be challenging. The ability to make decisions and solve problems may also be impacted.

Reduced Digesting Speed

Those who have HD may think more slowly and have trouble digesting information rapidly (Bonner-jackson et al., 2013; Tyebji and Hannan, 2017).

Psychiatric Symptoms

Depression

Depression is a frequent symptom of HD and presents as protracted melancholy, a loss of interest in activities, and a sense of hopelessness.

Anxiety

People with HD frequently exhibit anxiety symptoms such excessive concern, agitation, and fear.

Irritability and Agitation

A large portion of HD patients experience irritability, mood fluctuations, and agitation, which can make it challenging to maintain relationships and function in daily life.

Psychosis

People with HD occasionally hallucinate, delusions, or paranoia (Epping et al., 2013).

Behavioral Symptoms

Apathy

The absence of desire or interest in pursuits, even those once enjoyed, is a sign of apathy.

Social Withdrawal

HD patients may experience increased social isolation as their condition worsens.

Impulsivity

Some HD sufferers may act impulsively or have poor impulse control.

Obsessive-Compulsive Features

Sometimes, there may be obsessive thoughts and compulsive activities (Loi et al., 2018).

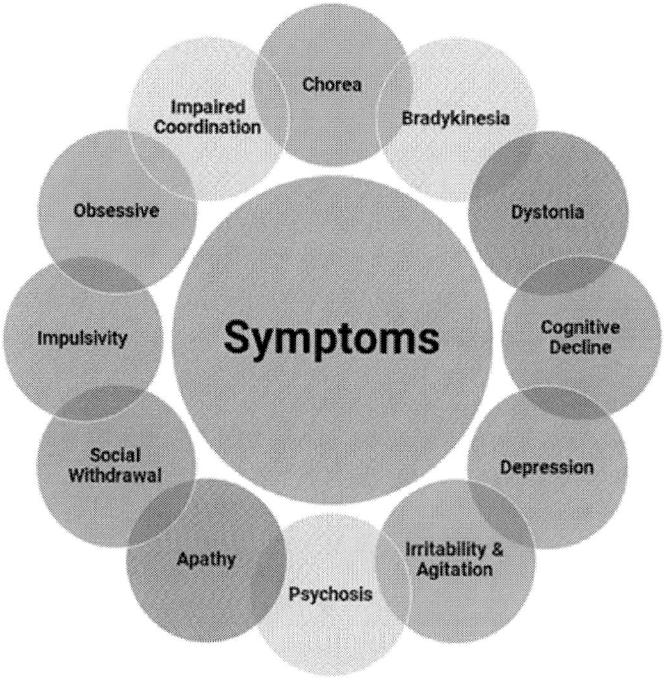

Figure 2. Symptoms of Huntington disease.

Causes of Huntington's Disease

A hereditary mutation in a particular gene called the HTT gene is the main genetic cause of Huntington's disease (HD). The main contributing elements and causes of Huntington's disease are listed below:

Genetic Mutation

The HTT gene, also called the huntingtin gene, is the primary genetic source of Huntington's disease. On chromosome 4 is where this gene is found. The gene's CAG (cytosine-adenine-guanine) repeat sequence has expanded due to the mutation (Dos and Do, 2020).

CAG Repeat Expansion

The HTT gene normally has between 10 and 35 CAG repeats in HD-unaffected people. However, there is an aberrant amplification of the CAG repeats in HD patients, typically with 36 or more repetitions. The genetic signature of HD is this enlarged CAG repeat sequence (McGarry et al., 2015).

Autosomal Dominant Inheritance

Huntington's disease is inherited in an autosomal dominant manner, which means that only one copy of the defective gene (from either parent) is required for the development of the condition. A person is at risk of developing HD if they inherit a single mutant allele of the HTT gene, and they typically have a 50% chance of transferring the mutation to their progeny (Germain and Jurcasimina, 2018).

Anticipation

Genetic anticipation, in which the quantity of CAG repeats tends to increase more in succeeding generations, is a noteworthy characteristic of HD. As a result, affected people from succeeding generations frequently experience earlier symptom start and worsening illness severity (Migliore et al., 2019).

Polyglutamine Expansion

A mutant huntingtin protein (mHTT) with an extended polyglutamine (polyQ) tract is produced as a result of the HTT gene's expanded CAG repeat. According to Wanker et al., (2019), this mutant protein is prone to misfolding and aggregation inside of neurons.

Protein Aggregation

Misfolded mHTT proteins cluster together within neurons to generate hazardous protein clumps. According to Gandhi et al., (2019), these aggregates impair typical cellular processes, resulting in cellular malfunction and neurodegeneration.

Neuronal Dysfunction and Neuroinflammation

The presence of mHTT impairs a number of cellular functions in neurons, including synaptic signaling, axonal transport, and mitochondrial function. Neuronal malfunction and death are the results of this disturbance. Neuroinflammatory processes are triggered in reaction to this protein aggregation and destruction, which aids in the course of the illness (Kumar *et al.*, 2021).

Neurological Mechanisms in the Progression of Huntington's Disease

Dopaminergic Impairment

Huntington's disease (HD), a fatal neurodegenerative condition, is characterized by dopaminergic dysfunction. Dopamine transmission in the brain is delicately balanced, but HD causes a gradual loss of dopaminergic neurons, mostly in the striatum. The irregular dopamine release and altered receptor function that characterize HD motor symptoms like chorea and dystonia are a result of this disruption. There is presently no cure for HD, which highlights the need for continued study into the intricate brain mechanisms underlying the disease. Treatments for HD try to reduce symptoms, especially those related to dopamine (Shiino et al., 2023).

Excitotoxicity

It has an impact on the pathogenesis of the complicated neurodegenerative condition Huntington's disease (HD). This phenomenon includes the neurotransmitter glutamate overstimulating and subsequently harming nerve cells (neurons). Excitotoxicity is believed to develop in HD as a result of the existence of mutant huntingtin protein, a defining feature of the condition. By interacting with glutamate receptors and transporters and causing an excessive glutamate release, mutant huntingtin protein can impair normal neurotransmission. This overabundance of glutamate overwhelms the neighboring neurons, causing an influx of calcium ions into these cells. This, in turn, starts intracellular processes that harm the neurons and ultimately cause their death. A variety of HD symptoms, such as motor dysfunction, cognitive deterioration, and mental symptoms are influenced by excitotoxicity (Smith-Dijak et al., 2019).

Autophagy Instability

Autophagy, the cellular process responsible for degrading and recycling damaged or dysfunctional components, plays a critical role in maintaining cellular homeostasis and preventing the accumulation of toxic proteins. In the context of Huntington's disease (HD), a devastating neurodegenerative disorder characterized by the progressive loss of motor and cognitive functions, autophagy instability emerges as a significant factor in disease pathology.

In healthy cells, autophagy helps clear misfolded proteins and aggregates, such as mutant huntingtin protein, which is the hallmark of HD. However, in

HD, there is mounting evidence of autophagy dysfunction. The mutant huntingtin protein itself appears to interfere with the normal autophagic process. It disrupts autophagosome formation, inhibits the fusion of autophagosomes with lysosomes (where degradation occurs), and impairs the turnover of cellular waste. As a result, toxic protein aggregates accumulate within neurons, contributing to their dysfunction and eventual death (Rangel et al., 2022).

Mitochondrial Dysfunction and Oxidative Stress

These two are interconnected factors that play a significant role in the pathogenesis of Huntington's disease (HD). The vital cellular organelles known as mitochondria are in charge of generating adenosine triphosphate (ATP), which is used as an energy source. There is growing evidence that mitochondrial function is impaired in HD. The hallmark of HD, mutant huntingtin protein, disturbs mitochondrial dynamics and reduces their capacity to make ATP effectively. Because of this malfunction, neurons have lower energy levels, which makes them more susceptible to harm and degeneration. Furthermore, mitochondrial dysfunction is closely linked to oxidative stress in HD. Oxidative stress occurs when there is an imbalance between the production of reactive oxygen species (ROS) and the cell's ability to neutralize them with antioxidants. As a result of their poor energy generation, dysfunctional mitochondria overproduce ROS in HD. These ROS can subsequently cause harm to DNA, proteins, and lipids in cells, which accelerates the degeneration of neurons (Golpich et al., 2017).

In HD, oxidative stress and mitochondrial dysfunction work in opposition to one another. The creation of ROS by damaged mitochondria exacerbates the damage to those organelles, further impairing cellular energy production and raising the level of oxidative stress. According to Elfawy and Das (2019), this vicious loop eventually results in neuronal malfunction and death.

Trophic support is the term used to describe the vital nutrients and growth substances that neurons need to stay healthy and perform properly. Several mechanisms underlie this decrease in trophic support in HD. One key aspect is the disruption of signaling pathways that promote neuronal survival and growth. Mutant huntingtin protein, which is the hallmark of HD, interferes with these pathways, particularly those mediated by *brain-derived neurotrophic factor* (BDNF) and other neurotrophic factors. BDNF is essential for the survival and maintenance of neurons, and its reduced levels and impaired signaling in HD contribute to neuronal dysfunction and death (Mo et al., 2015). Additionally, the diminished trophic support in HD is linked to disrupted transport of crucial molecules within neurons.

Disruptions in Huntington's Disease

Motor Disturbance

It typically begins by affecting the MSNs (Medium Spiny Neurons) in the indirect pathway before impacting those in the direct pathway. This two-phase pattern is a hallmark of the condition (Plotkin and Surmeier, 2015). Unlike chorea, which tends to ease off, this phase's movement issues are more closely connected to how long someone has had the illness and the length of their CAG repeat expansion (McColgan and Tabrizi, 2018).

To assess dystonia, chorea, walking, eye movements, speech, alternating hand movements, and other motor problems in Huntington's disease, healthcare professionals rely on two tools: the Universal Huntington Disease Rating Scale (UHDRS) and the Total Motor Score (TMS). It's important to note that the UHDRS TMS can be influenced by differences in how different evaluators rate it, but it remains responsive to detecting changes in a patient's condition over time (Hogarth et al., 2005).

Cognitive Disturbance

Several years before symptoms become evident, it is possible to identify a specific cognitive impairment pattern in the brain that affects emotion recognition, processing speed, visuospatial abilities, and executive functions. To monitor changes during the early stages of the disease over a period of 12 to 24 months, various tests can be employed. These include the symbol digit modalities test, which evaluates psychomotor speed, the indirect circle tracing test, the Stroop word reading test, and the emotion recognition test. The Stroop word reading test has been shown to be the most sensitive indication of cognitive abnormalities, in the premanifest stage of Huntington's disease (Andrews et al., 2021).

Neuropsychiatric Disturbance

Neuropsychiatric symptoms, including apathy, anxiety, rage, melancholy, compulsive behavior, and psychosis, are present in Huntington's disease (HD). According to Anderson et al., (2011), people with the disorder's apparent form frequently experience these symptoms. Many years before the manifestation of observable symptoms, mental instability is typically seen in the premanifest stage. According to the most recent Registry cohort research, which includes both premanifest and manifest cases, apathy affects 28% of people. Furthermore, 13% of individuals say they have melancholy, irritability, or obsessive-compulsive traits. Only 1% of people experience psychosis, which is a far less frequent occurrence (Van, 2014). Only apathy has consistently shown a worsening trend as the illness progresses among the various neuropsychiatric symptoms. This phenomenon could be attributed to the limited availability of effective treatments for apathy, unlike the options available for managing conditions like depression, anxiety, and anger, where antidepressants and antipsychotic medications are more commonly employed (Tabrizi et al., 2013).

Clinical Approaches for the Management of Huntington's Disease

Conventional Method

Huntington's disease (HD) is a progressive neurodegenerative disorder that currently has no cure. However, there are conventional methods of treatment and management aimed at alleviating symptoms and improving the quality of life for individuals with HD. See in Table 1.

Medications

Typical Antipsychotic Drugs

Typical antipsychotic drugs are not the primary treatment for Huntington's disease (HD), a neurodegenerative disorder affecting motor and cognitive function. Instead, HD management involves a multidisciplinary approach.

Atypical Antipsychotic Drugs

These atypical antipsychotic medications are often preferred over typical antipsychotics like haloperidol because they may have a lower risk of movement-related side effects (extrapyramidal symptoms), which can be particularly problematic for individuals with HD who already experience movement difficulties.

Table 1. Antipsychotic drugs used in management of Huntington disease (Unti et al., 2017)

Typical Antipsychotic Drugs		
	Class	Drug
1	*Phenothiazines*	Thiopropazate, fluphenazine, perfenazine
2	*Butyrophenones*	Haloperidol, trifluperidol
3	*Thioxanthines*	Flupentixol
4	*Diphenylpiperidine*	Pimozide, loxapine
5	*Benzamide*	Tiapride, amisulpiride
Atypical Antipsychotic Drugs		
	Atypical Antipsychotics	Olanzapine, risperidone, clozapine, quetiapine, ziprasidone

Novel Therapeutic Approaches

Dopaminergic Modulation

Tetrabenazine (TBZ)

TBZ is a VMAT2 inhibitor employed to manage chorea in individuals with Huntington's disease, and it works by diminishing dopamine stores. Ongoing research (NCT02509783) is investigating TBZ's effects on behavioral symptoms like depression in HD patients. Furthermore, this study is exploring if TBZ's impact on serotonin levels might also help address impulsivity, offering a more holistic approach to managing the diverse symptoms of Huntington's disease and enhancing patients' well-being (Wyant et al., 2017).

Deutetrabenazine

Deutetrabenazine is like a tweaked version of TBZ, where they've replaced some hydrogen with deuterium to make it last longer in the body and require fewer daily doses. Right now, there are two clinical studies underway involving Deutetrabenazine. One, identified as NCT04713982, is looking into how it affects speech and walking abilities. The other, NCT04301726, is focused on its effectiveness in relieving difficulties with swallowing in Huntington's disease. These investigations could potentially offer new ways to improve the lives of individuals with HD.

Valbenazine

The most specialized version of VMAT2 inhibition is valbenazine, derived from TBZ's alpha isomer. Valbenazine has already received FDA approval for addressing tardive dyskinesia. Given its chemical similarity to TBZ and TBZ's success in managing HD-related chorea, there's an ongoing clinical trial (NCT04102579) checking if valbenazine can also effectively help ease chorea in individuals with Huntington's disease. This research could potentially provide another promising option for HD patients (Rodrigues and Wild, 2020).

Glutamatergic Modulation

Dextromethorphan

Dextromethorphan, an NMDA antagonist, undergoes rapid metabolism into dextrorphan by the enzyme cytochrome P450 2D6 (CYP2D6). To increase its presence in the bloodstream, dextromethorphan is administered alongside the CYP2D6 inhibitor quinidine. The clinical trial with identifier NCT03854019 is currently investigating the potential therapeutic benefits of this drug combination for managing Huntington's disease-related chorea. This research is based on dextromethorphan's ability to block NMDA receptors and its potential to reduce excitotoxicity in the brains of individuals with Huntington's disease (Bhatnagar et al., 2023; Taylor et al., 2016).

Mitochondrial Function and Biogenesis

Fenofibrate

Fenofibrate, which is a PPAR agonist, can activate PGC-1 (*Proliferator Activated Receptor Gamma Co-Activator 1-Alpha*) and promote the creation of new mitochondria. The purpose of the clinical trial with the identifier NCT03515213 is to investigate whether boosting PGC-1 through pharmacological means could be a valuable approach for treating Huntington's disease. This research stems from the belief that the impaired production of mitochondria in HD may be linked to improper expression of PGC-1 (Valero et al., 2014).

Triheptanoin

Triheptanion is a type of C7 fatty acid that, when processed by the liver, produces acetyl-CoA and propionyl-CoA. Individuals with Huntington's disease (HD) often exhibit reduced levels of branched-chain amino acids, possibly due to changes in mitochondrial oxidation necessary for generating acetyl-CoA and succinyl-CoA, essential for the Krebs cycle. Triheptanoin is thought to provide substrates for the Krebs cycle, potentially increasing ATP availability and improving the overall energy profile of the HD brain, (Rodrigues and Wild, 2018). To assess its impact on motor and cognitive functions, as well as the overall quality of life for patients, an ongoing clinical study with identifier NCT02453061 is currently investigating Triheptanoin. This study will utilize brain energy metabolism and volumetric magnetic resonance imaging to measure caudate volume.

Metformin

Metformin a medication that activates AMP-activated protein kinase (AMPK) and is commonly used to manage type 2 diabetes, has demonstrated potential benefits in Huntington's disease (HD) research. In laboratory studies using *in vitro* HD models and C. elegans expressing polyQ, metformin showed preventive effects (Vazquez et al., 2016). Treatment with metformin extended the lifespan of male R6/2 HD transgenic mice and alleviated motor and neuropsychiatric symptoms in zQ175 mice (Sanchis et al., 2019). Moreover, an analysis of the Enroll-HD database revealed a link between metformin use and better cognitive performance in HD patients (Garcia et al., 2022). Based on these results, an ongoing clinical research (NCT04826692) is examining the security and effectiveness of metformin therapy in halting cognitive deterioration in HD patients.

Antibody Therapy

A monoclonal antibody called ANX005 has been studied in relation to Huntington's disease (HD). The complement system protein C1q, which has been linked to neuroinflammation and synapse loss in HD, is the goal of ANX005's formulation, which aims to decrease its levels. According to certain studies (Lansita et al., 2017; Carpanini et al., 2019), ANX005 inhibits complement system activation and may lessen the inflammatory response in the brain, which can be harmful in HD. The safety and tolerability of ANX005 in those with Huntington's disease or those at risk of developing the disorder are now being studied (NCT04514367).

Gene Manipulations

Gene silencing methods like RNA interference (RNAi) and antisense oligonucleotides (ASOs) are used in gene manipulation. These methods aim to reduce the production of mHTT by targeting and selectively inhibiting the HTT gene's expression. Promising research and clinical trials have shown the potential of such therapies in lowering mHTT levels and mitigating HD symptoms (Mestre, 2019; Germain et al., 2023).

Another avenue of genetic manipulation is gene editing using technologies like CRISPR-Cas9. Researchers are exploring ways to precisely edit the HTT gene to correct the mutation responsible for mHTT production. While this approach holds great promise, it also presents technical and safety challenges that need to be carefully addressed in clinical development (Alkanli et al., 2023).

AMT-130

AMT-130 is designed to deliver a small piece of genetic material called microRNA to the brain, which aims to reduce the production of the toxic mutant huntingtin (mHTT) protein associated with HD. The therapy works by using an adeno-associated virus (AAV) vector to transport the microRNA into brain cells, where it silences the expression of the mutant HTT gene. By lowering the levels of mHTT, AMT-130 seeks to slow down or potentially halt the progression of HD and alleviate its associated symptoms. Adults who are in the early stages of Huntington's disease are currently being recruited for participation in an ongoing proof-of-concept (POC) study. This study, identified as NCT04120493, aims to assess the safety of administering AMT-130 directly into the striatum of the brain (Spronck et al., 2021; Caron et al., 2020).

Combined Pharmacological Therapies

The potential benefits of combining several medications (deutetrabenazine, risperidone, Zoloft, and idebenone) to manage symptoms at different stages of Huntington's disease (HD) progression in an ongoing clinical trial (NCT04071639). Idebenone, which is a synthetic derivative of coenzyme Q10 known for its antioxidant properties, differs from deutetrabenazine and risperidone, as it primarily acts as an antioxidant rather than a dopaminergic modulator. Importantly, prior research has already assessed how idebenone affects HD patients in a year-long, double-blind clinical study with parallel groups. The study explored the potential synergistic effects of this medication combination in a more holistic approach to treating HD symptoms. When it comes to the important measures of the Quantified Neurologic Examination (QNE) and the Activities of Daily Living Scale (ADL), which assess functional status in Huntington's disease, there weren't any noticeable differences between the groups. Nevertheless, there's a good chance that idebenone might show improved results when used alongside risperidone, deutetrabenazine, or both medications (Islam et al., 2023; Kim et al., 2021).

Stem Cell Therapies

Studies have demonstrated the potential effectiveness of using neural progenitor cell therapies, derived from induced pluripotent stem cells (iPSCs), in the treatment of neurodegenerative conditions like HD (Wenceslau et al., 2017). It revealed that human neural progenitor cells generated from iPSCs have the capacity to successfully integrate into animal brains and mature into typical neurons. This transformation has shown promise in enhancing both behavioral and motor functions (Mu et al., 2014). These discoveries offer hope for improved treatments for neurodegenerative diseases like HD. Three ongoing clinical trials, identified as NCT03252535, NCT02728115, and NCT04219241, are currently investigating the safety, effectiveness, and appropriate dosages of intravenous stem cell therapy for individuals affected by Huntington's disease (HD).

Multiple research studies have shown that transplanting induced pluripotent stem cells (iPSCs) generated from somatic cells can lead to enhancements in both behavior and motor skills in rodent models of Huntington's disease (HD). For instance, in one study, striata of 10-month-old YAC128 mice were transplanted with mouse iPSCs derived from a healthy mouse, which led to appreciable improvements. Additionally, this intervention significantly increased the levels of BDNF protein and its receptors in the striatum (Conner et al., 2023; Saha et al., 2022).

Deep Brain Stimulation

In order to modify neural activity, DBS entails the surgical insertion of electrodes into particular brain regions, generally the globus pallidus internus (GPi) or the sub thalamic nucleus (STN). In HD, DBS is being investigated for its potential to treat psychiatric disorders like depression and impulsivity as well as motor symptoms like chorea and dystonia. According to Kaczyska et al., (2022), the precise mechanism of action is still not entirely understood. The three ongoing clinical trials (NCT02535884, NCT04244513, and NCT04429230) have as their main objectives to ascertain the effectiveness of this specific strategy (Cif et al., 2023).

Nanotechnology and Nanoparticles

For the diagnosis and treatment of neurological illnesses like Huntington's disease (HD), nanotechnology provides intriguing possibilities. Nanoparticles, which are very small particles with diameters between 1 and 100 nanometers, are essential to these developments. As carriers for therapeutic agents including siRNAs, stem cells, antioxidants, and medications, a variety of natural and synthetic nanomaterials are being researched, including polymers, metals, proteins, lipids, and polysaccharides (Singh et al., 2022).

These nanoparticles are special because of their small size, large surface area, hydrophobicity, high capacity for adsorption, and capacity for surface modification. Nanoparticles with a size between 20 and 100 nm are particularly suitable for addressing neurodegenerative conditions as they can cross the blood-brain barrier (BBB). One significant application is in small interfering RNA (siRNA)-based gene therapies for silencing the expression of genes like HTT in HD. Nanoparticles enhance siRNA's circulation time, cellular absorption, and accumulation, ensuring effective gene silencing. Nanoparticles can be tailored with specific ligands to target cells or organelles, improving drug permeability through the BBB. This targeted delivery minimizes interactions with other cellular components, reducing adverse effects. Nanoparticles also demonstrate potential in combating oxidative stress in neurodegenerative disorders. See in Figure 3 Their ability to scavenge reactive oxygen species (ROS) and restore antioxidant properties protects neural cells during neurodegeneration (Mustafa et al., 2023).

Furthermore, nanoparticles interfere with protein aggregation, which is a hallmark of HD progression. They bind to protein monomers and fibrils, preventing their aggregation and stabilizing their structures. Various types of nanoparticles, including polymeric nanoparticles, lipid-based nanoparticles, liposomes, dendrimers, nanogels, solid lipid nanoparticles, micelles, metal nanoparticles, quantum dots, magnetic nanoparticles, nanocrystals, and fullerenes, serve as drug delivery systems in HD treatments. Polymeric nanoparticles, for instance, have low toxicity, adjustable degradation rates, high loading capacities, and surface modification abilities. They are employed to deliver medications and siRNAs for HD treatment and stimulate stem cell expansion and differentiation. Dendrimers, with their highly branched structures and numerous functional groups, are attractive for gene and drug delivery, as they can penetrate the BBB and offer targeted drug delivery (Valadão et al., 2022).

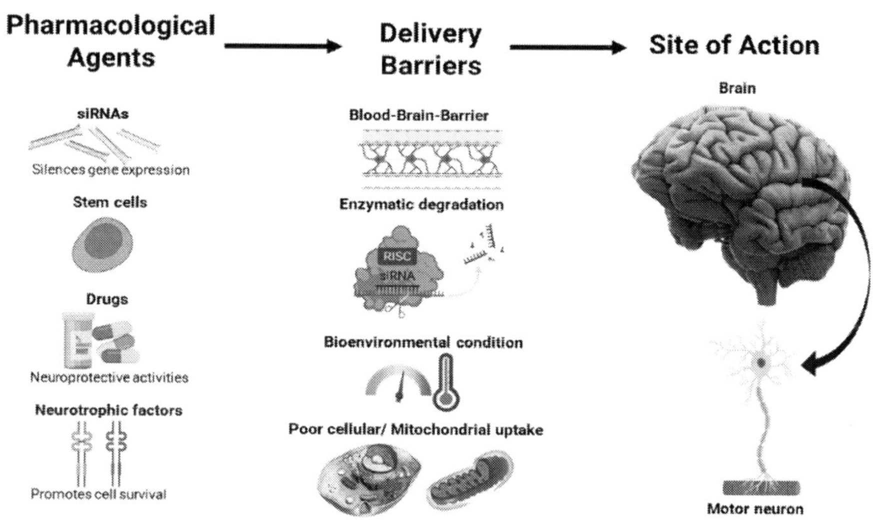

Figure 3. Nanoparticles as delivery systems for different therapeutic agents: Illustration of 1) the most promising therapeutic agents for the treatment of Huntington's disease (HD): siRNAs, stem cells, drugs, and neurotrophic factors, 2) the main barriers (BBB, enzymatic degradation, bioenvironmental conditions, and poor cellular/mitochondrial uptake), and 3) the target site of the therapeutic molecules to exert their ameliorative activity.

Other nanoparticle options like micelles, nanogels, liposomes, and solid lipid nanoparticles provide controlled drug release, enhanced stability, and improved drug delivery to specific brain regions. Carbon-based nanomaterials, such as fullerenes, carbon nanotubes, and graphene, are explored for their antioxidant properties and potential to inhibit protein aggregation. However, their reactivity and potential neurotoxicity require careful consideration. Metallic nanoparticles like gold, cerium, iron, and molybdenum offer unique physicochemical properties, enabling site-specific drug delivery and reducing ROS and protein aggregation (Mustafa et al., 2023).

Conclusion

Huntington's disease (HD) is a rare genetic disorder caused by an HTT gene mutation, leading to toxic huntingtin protein production. It follows autosomal dominant inheritance, causing progressive mid-adulthood symptoms like chorea and cognitive decline. HD's pathophysiology involves mutant protein aggregation, leading to neuronal dysfunction. HD's progression involves complex mechanisms, including dopaminergic impairment, excitotoxicity, autophagy instability, mitochondrial dysfunction, oxidative stress, and decreased trophic support. Neuropharmacology manages symptoms and genetic testing is crucial for at-risk individuals. Support systems are essential for affected individuals and families. Clinical approaches aim to alleviate symptoms, including dopaminergic and glutamatergic modulations, gene manipulation, stem cell therapy, and nanotechnology. Ongoing research offers hope for improved treatments and care for the persons affected with Huntington's disease.

References

Alkanli, S. S., Alkanli, N., Ay, A., and Albeniz, I. 2023. CRISPR/Cas9 Mediated Therapeutic Approach in Huntington's Disease. *Molecular Neurobiology,* 60(3): 1486-1498.

Anderson, K., Craufurd, D., Edmondson, M. C., Goodman, N., Groves, M., van Duijn, E. and Goodman, L. 2011. An international survey-based algorithm for the pharmacologic treatment of obsessive-compulsive behaviors in Huntington's disease. *PLoS currents,* 3.

Andrews, S. C., Langbehn, D. R., Craufurd, D., Durr, A., Leavitt, B. R., Roos, R. A. and TRACK-HD Investigators. 2021. Apathy predicts rate of cognitive decline over 24 months in premanifest Huntington's disease. *Psychological medicine*, 51(8): 1338-1344.

Bhatnagar, A., Parmar, V., Barbieri, N., Bearoff, F., Elefant, F. and Kortagere, S. 2023. Novel EAAT2 activators improve motor and cognitive impairment in a transgenic model of Huntington's disease. *Frontiers in behavioral neuroscience,* 17: 1176777.

Bonner-Jackson, A., Long, J. D., Westervelt, H., Tremont, G., Aylward, E., Paulsen, J. S. and Coordinators of the Huntington Study Group. 2013. Cognitive reserve and brain reserve in prodromal Huntington's disease. *Journal of the International Neuropsychological Society*, 19(7): 739-750.

Caron, N. S., Southwell, A. L., Brouwers, C. C., Cengio, L. D., Xie, Y., Black, H. F. and Hayden, M. R. 2020. Potent and sustained huntingtin lowering via AAV5 encoding miRNA preserves striatal volume and cognitive function in a humanized mouse model of Huntington disease. *Nucleic acids research,* 48(1): 36-54.

Carpanini, S. M., Torvell, M. and Morgan, B. P. 2019. Therapeutic inhibition of the complement system in diseases of the central nervous system. *Frontiers in immunology,* 10: 362.

Cif, L., Demailly, D., Gehin, C., Seng, E. C., Dornadic, M., Huby, S. and Coubes, P. 2023. Deep brain stimulation effect in genetic dyskinetic cerebral palsy: The case of ADCY5-related disease. *Molecular Genetics and Metabolism,* 138(1): 106970

Conner, L. T., Srinageshwar, B., Bakke, J. L., Dunbar, G. L. and Rossignol, J. 2023. Advances in stem cell and other therapies for Huntington's disease: An update. *Brain Research Bulletin*, 110673.

Dos Santos, N. T. H. and Do Bomfim, F. R. C. 2020. Gene editing by CRISPR/CAS9 for treatment of Huntington disease. *International Journal of Development Research,* 10: 38631-38635.

Eje, O. E., Ogbonna, C. V., Onoyima, C. S. and Nduka, F. O. 2023. Huntington Disease: Mechanism of Pathogenesis and Recent Developments in Its Therapeutic Strategies: A Review. *J. Chem. Rev,* 5(2): 129-142.

Elfawy, H. A. and Das, B. 2019. Crosstalk between mitochondrial dysfunction, oxidative stress, and agerelated neurodegenerative disease: Etiologies and therapeutic strategies. *Life sciences,* 218: 165-184.

Epping, E. A., Mills, J. A., Beglinger, L. J., Fiedorowicz, J. G., Craufurd, D., Smith, M. M. and Coordinators of the Huntington Study Group. 2013. Characterization of depression in prodromal Huntington disease in the neurobiological predictors of HD (PREDICT-HD) study. *Journal of psychiatric research,* 47(10): 1423-1431.

Frank, S. 2014. Treatment of Huntington's disease. *Neurotherapeutics,* 11: 153-160.

Gandhi, J., Antonelli, A. C., Afridi, A., Vatsia, S., Joshi, G., Romanov, V. and Khan, S. A. 2019. Protein misfolding and aggregation in neurodegenerative diseases: a review of pathogeneses, novel detection strategies, and potential therapeutics. *Reviews in the Neurosciences,* 30(4): 339-358.

García-Puga, M., Saenz-Antoñanzas, A., Matheu, A. and López de Munain, A. 2022. Targeting myotonic dystrophy type 1 with metformin. *International Journal of Molecular Sciences,* 23(5): 2901.

Germain, D. P. and Jurca-Simina, I. E. 2018. Principles of human genetics and Mendelian inheritance. *Neurometabolic hereditary diseases of adults*: 1-28.

Germain, N. D., Chung, W. K. and Sarmiere, P. D. 2023. RNA interference (RNAi)-based therapeutics for treatment of rare neurologic diseases. *Molecular Aspects of Medicine*, 91, 101148.

Ghosh, R. and Tabrizi, S. J. 2018. Huntington disease. *Handbook of clinical neurology*, 147: 255-278.

Gil, J. M., and Ana C. R. 2008. Mechanisms of neurodegeneration in Huntington's disease." *European Journal of Neuroscience* 27, no. 11: 2803-2820.

Golpich, M., Amini, E., Mohamed, Z., Azman Ali, R., Mohamed Ibrahim, N. and Ahmadiani, A. 2017. Mitochondrial dysfunction and biogenesis in neurodegenerative diseases: pathogenesis and treatment. *CNS neuroscience & therapeutics,* 23(1): 5-22.

Hogarth, P., Kayson, E., Kieburtz, K., Marder, K., Oakes, D., Rosas, D. and Huntington Study Group. 2005. Interrater agreement in the assessment of motor manifestations of Huntington's disease. *Movement disorders*, 20(3): 293-297.

Islam, M. R., Jony, M. H., Thufa, G. K., Akash, S., Dhar, P. S., Rahman, M. M. and Venkidasamy, B. 2023. A clinical study and future prospects for bioactive compounds and semi-synthetic molecules in the therapies for Huntington's disease. *Molecular Neurobiology,* 1-34.

Jimenez-Sanchez, M., Licitra, F., Underwood, B. R. and Rubinsztein, D. C. 2017. Huntington's disease: mechanisms of pathogenesis and therapeutic strategies. *Cold Spring Harbor perspectives in medicine,* 7: 7.

Kaczyńska, J., Sitek, E. J., Witkowski, G., Rudzińska-Bar, M., Janik, P., Sławek, J. and Zielonka, D. 2022. Is deep brain stimulation effective in Huntington's Disease? - a systematic literature review. *Neurologia i Neurochirurgia Polska.*

Kim, A., Lalonde, K., Truesdell, A., Gomes Welter, P., Brocardo, P. S., Rosenstock, T. R. and Gil-Mohapel, J. 2021. New avenues for the treatment of Huntington's disease. *International Journal of Molecular Sciences,* 22(16): 8363.

Kumar, V., Singh, C. and Singh, A. 2021. Zebrafish an experimental model of Huntington's disease: Molecular aspects, therapeutic targets and current challenges. *Molecular biology reports,* 1-14.

Lansita, J. A., Mease, K. M., Qiu, H., Yednock, T., Sankaranarayanan, S. and Kramer, S. 2017. Nonclinical development of ANX005: a humanized anti-C1q antibody for treatment of autoimmune and neurodegenerative diseases. *International Journal of Toxicology,* 36(6): 449-462.

Loi, S. M., Walterfang, M., Velakoulis, D. and Looi, J. C. 2018. Huntington's disease: Managing neuropsychiatric symptoms in Huntington's disease. *Australasian Psychiatry,* 26(4): 376-380.

McColgan, P. and Tabrizi, S. J. 2018. Huntington's disease: a clinical review. *European journal of neurology,* 25(1): 24-34.

McGarry, A. J., Biglan, K. and Marshall, F. 2015. Huntington disease. In *Rosenberg's Molecular and Genetic Basis of Neurological and Psychiatric Disease*, 861-868.

Mestre, T. A. 2019. Recent advances in the therapeutic development for Huntington disease. *Parkinsonism & Related Disorders*, 59: 125-130.

Migliore, S., Jankovic, J. and Squitieri, F. 2019. Genetic counseling in Huntington's disease: potential new challenges on horizon?. *Frontiers in neurology*, 10: 453.

Mo, C., Hannan, A. J. and Renoir, T. 2015. Environmental factors as modulators of neurodegeneration: Insights from gene–environment interactions in Huntington's disease. *Neuroscience and Biobehavioral Reviews*, 52: 178-192.

Morales, E., Herrera, C., Montaño, L., Martínez, K., Meza, M., Del Villar, N. and Rodríguez, A. 2023. Current knowledge and future directions in Huntington's disease. *Archivos de Neurociencias,* 27(4): 31-43.

Mu, S., Wang, J., Zhou, G., Peng, W., He, Z., Zhao, Z. and Zhang, J. 2014. Transplantation of induced pluripotent stem cells improves functional recovery in Huntington's disease rat model. *PLoS One,* 9: 7, e101185.

Mustafa, G., Hassan, D., Zeeshan, M., Ruiz-Pulido, G., Ebrahimi, N., Mobashar, A. and Díez-Pascual, A. M. 2023. Advances in nanotechnology versus stem cell therapy for the theranostics of Huntington's disease. *Journal of Drug Delivery Science and Technology*, 87, 104774.

Palaiogeorgou, A. M., Papakonstantinou, E., Golfinopoulou, R., Sigala, M., Mitsis, T., Papageorgiou, L. and Vlachakis, D. 2023. Recent approaches on Huntington's disease. *Biomedical Reports,* 18(1): 1-7.

Plotkin, J. L. and Surmeier, D. J. 2015. Corticostriatal synaptic adaptations in Huntington's disease. *Current opinion in neurobiology*, 33: 53-62.

Rangel, M., Kong, J., Bhatt, V., Khayati, K. and Guo, J. Y. 2022. Autophagy and tumorigenesis. *The FEBS Journal*, 289(22): 7177-7198.

Rodrigues, F. B. and Wild, E. J. 2018. Huntington's disease clinical trials corner: February 2018. *Journal of Huntington's disease*, 7(1): 89-98.

Rodrigues, F. B. and Wild, E. J. 2020. Huntington's disease clinical trials corner. *Journal of Huntington's disease*, 9(2): 185-197.

Ross, C. A. and Tabrizi, S. J. 2011. Huntington's disease: from molecular pathogenesis to clinical treatment. *The Lancet Neurology*, 10(1): 83-98.

Saha, S., Manami, J. D., Salman, K. P. and Yusha A 2022. Pathogenesis and potential therapeutic application of stem cells transplantation in Huntington's disease. *Regenerative Therapy*, 21: 406-412.

Sanchis, A., García-Gimeno, M. A., Cañada-Martínez, A. J., Sequedo, M. D., Millán, J. M., Sanz, P. and Vazquez-Manrique, R. P. 2019. Metformin treatment reduces motor and neuropsychiatric phenotypes in the zQ175 mouse model of Huntington disease. *Experimental and molecular medicine,* 51(6): 1-16.

Shiino, S., van Wouwe, N. C., Wylie, S. A., Claassen, D. O. and McDonell, K. E. 2023. Huntington disease exacerbates action impulses. *Frontiers in Psychology*, 14: 1186465.

Singh, S., Hema., Sharma, N., Sachdeva, M., Behl, T., Zahoor, I. and Fuloria, N. k 2022. "Focusing the pivotal role of nanotechnology in Huntington's disease: an insight into the recent advancements." *Environmental Science and Pollution Research* 29, no. 49 : 73809-73827.

Smith-Dijak, A. I., Sepers, M. D. and Raymond, L. A. 2019. Alterations in synaptic function and plasticity in Huntington disease. *Journal of neurochemistry*, 150(4): 346-365.

Spronck, E. A., Vallès, A., Lampen, M. H., Montenegro-Miranda, P. S., Keskin, S., Heijink, L. and Haan, M. D. 2021. Intrastriatal administration of AAV5-miHTT in non-human primates and rats is well tolerated and results in miHTT transgene expression in key areas of Huntington disease pathology. *Brain Sciences*, 11(2): 129.

Sun, X. 2023. Diagnosis and treatment for Huntington's disease. *In International Conference on Modern Medicine and Global Health (ICMMGH 2023)* (Vol. 12789, pp. 154-157). SPIE.

Tabrizi, S. J., Scahill, R. I., Owen, G., Durr, A., Leavitt, B. R., Roos, R. A. and Langbehn, D. R. 2013. Predictors of phenotypic progression and disease onset in premanifest and early-stage Huntington's disease in the TRACK-HD study: analysis of 36-month observational data. *The Lancet Neurology*, 12(7): 637-649.

Taylor, C. P., Traynelis, S. F., Siffert, J., Pope, L. E. and Matsumoto, R. R. 2016. Pharmacology of dextromethorphan: Relevance to dextromethorphan/quinidine (Nuedexta®) clinical use. *Pharmacology and therapeutics*, 164: 170-182.

Tyebji, S. and Hannan, A. J. 2017. Synaptopathic mechanisms of neurodegeneration and dementia: insights from Huntington's disease. *Progress in Neurobiology*, 153: 18-45.

Unti, E., Mazzucchi, S., Palermo, G., Bonuccelli, U. and Ceravolo, R. 2017. Antipsychotic drugs in Huntington's disease. *Expert review of neurotherapeutics,* 17(3): 227-237.

Valadão, K. M. G., Luizeti, B. O., Yamaguchi, M. U., Issy, A. C. and Bernuci, M. P. 2022. Nanotechnology in Improving the Treatment of Huntington's Disease: a Systematic Review. *Neurotoxicity Research,* 40(2): 636-645.

Valero, T. 2014. Editorial (thematic issue: Mitochondrial biogenesis: Pharmacological approaches). *Current pharmaceutical design*, 20(35): 5507-5509..

Van Duijn, E., Craufurd, D., Hubers, A. A., Giltay, E. J., Bonelli, R., Rickards, H., Landwehrmeyer, G. B. and European Huntington's Disease Network Behavioural Phenotype Working Group. 2014. Neuropsychiatric symptoms in a European Huntington's disease cohort (REGISTRY). *J Neurol Neurosurg Psychiatry*, 85: 1411-1418.

Vázquez-Manrique, R. P., Farina, F., Cambon, K., Dolores Sequedo, M., Parker, A. J., Millán, J. M. and Neri, C. 2016. AMPK activation protects from neuronal dysfunction and vulnerability across nematode, cellular and mouse models of Huntington's disease. *Human molecular genetics,* 25(6): 1043-1058.

Wanker, E. E., Ast, A., Schindler, F., Trepte, P. and Schnoegl, S. 2019. The pathobiology of perturbed mutant huntingtin protein–protein interactions in Huntington's disease. *Journal of Neurochemistry,* 151(4): 507-519.

Wenceslau, C. V., Kerkis, I., Pompeia, C. and Haddad, M. S. 2017. Pluripotent stem cells to model and treat huntington's disease. *Huntington's Disease - Molecular Pathogenesis and Current Models.*

Wyant, K. J., Ridder, A. J. and Dayalu, P. 2017. Huntington's disease - update on treatments. *Current neurology and neuroscience reports,* 17: 1-11.

Chapter 6

Emerging Therapeutic Approaches for Amyotrophic Lateral Sclerosis (ALS)

Vipin Kesharwani[1,*],
Shikhar Verma[1],
Prakash Deep[1],
Anupama Singh[1],
Shrishti Verma[1],
Shashank Patel[1],
Mohit Agrawal[2]
and Shivendra Kumar[3]
[1]School of Pharmaceutical Sciences, Maharishi University of Information Technology, Lucknow, Uttar Pradesh, India
[2]School of Medical & Allied Sciences, K. R. Mangalam University, Gurugram, Haryana, India
[3]Department of Pharmacology, Rajiv Academy for Pharmacy, Mathura, UP, India

Abstract

The neurodegenerative disease amyotrophic lateral sclerosis (ALS) is deadly and is characterized by degeneration of both upper and lower motor neurons, gradual loss of muscle function and death, in 2 to 5 years following the onset of symptoms. The quality of life is nevertheless significantly improved by symptomatic treatments such reducing salivation, easing muscle cramps and relieving pain and spasticity. The

* Corresponding Author's Email: vipinkesharwani1610@gmail.com.

In: Neurogenerative Disorders
Editors: Mohit Agrawal, Manmohan Singhal, Amit Kumar Nayak et al.
ISBN: 979-8-89530-143-2

discovery of disease-modifying medicines has proven hard for a number of reasons, as it has with all other neurodegenerative illnesses. But among the few neurodegenerative illnesses for which disease-modifying treatments have been licensed, ALS is one of them. To target particular pathogenic processes found in ALS, new developing therapeutics such as antisense oligonucleotides, autologous mensenchymal stem cells and kinase inhibitors are being developed. Currently, the FDA has reported four therapies for ALS that can either decrease the course of the disease or increase survival. The first three drugs (Riluzole, Edaravone, and PB-TURSO) had only a minor impact on survival and illness progression, necessitating the development of additional disease-modifying medicines. Toferson, the fourth drug, was just recently approved for treating SOD1-mediated ALS. Recent developments in our knowledge of the genetics, pathology and molecular mechanisms underlying ALS have allowed us to identify fresh targets and approaches that are now being applied in novel therapeutic therapies for the disease. We believe that this method for treating ALS will have a significant effect on the wider field of medication discovery for neurodegenerative diseases.

Keywords: amyotrophic lateral sclerosis, stem cell, neurodegenerative illness, pathology

Introduction

Upper and lower motor neurons (MNs) both are affected by the progressive neurodegenerative disease known as amyotrophic lateral sclerosis (ALS), popularly referred to as "Lou Gehrig's disease," which can cause paralysis and finally lead to death from respiratory failure (Oskarsson et al., 2018; Hobson et al., 2016; and Paez-Colasante et al., 2015). There is a significant geographic variation in the incidence of ALS, which has been estimated to vary from 0.8 to 3.6 per million individuals every year (Longinetti et al., 2019). ALS usually has two subtypes: familial ALS (fALS), that impacts to family members and sporadic ALS (ALS), which impacts individuals without a documented family history of the illness. In 85-90% of patients, ALS is present. The remaining 10-15% of the instances of ALS are the familial variety (Tiwari et al., 2005: Siddique T and Dellafave L, 2006). The most common ALS-causing mutation identified to date, accounting for roughly 40% of fALS cases and 6-8% of ALS occurrences in Caucasian groups, is a G4 C2 hexanucleotide repeated mutation in the C9 or f72 gene. There are at least 50 genes associated with ALS that may be disease-causing or disease-modifying. Some additional genes which are usually mutated in ALS include SOD1, TARDPB, or FUS; although changes among other disease linked proteins that cause ALS, are rather rare (Mathis et al., 2019: Chia R and Chio A, 2018). Despite evidence from research suggesting that many genetic and environmental factors may facilitate the beginning of ALS, neither one ecological nor genomic risk factor has been proven to be associated with the progression of sporadic ALS. The primary pathogenic characteristics of the disease involve regression of upper and lower axons and cytons, destruction of cortico-bulbar and cortico-spinal circuits. Majorly the ALS patients (97%) have TDP-43, a proteinopathy that links to TAR DNA. As motor neurons are injured, a protein (TDP-43) is removed via nucleus and as a result, the cytoplasm aggregates into complexes with dense or skein-like shapes as shown in Figure 1 (Ling et al., 2013; Tanet al., 2017). Despite the existence of cytoplasmic protein aggregates with different compositions, ALS brought on by alterations affecting the SOD1 (Cu-Zn Superoxide Dismutase) and FUS (Fused in Sarcoma) genes is certainly not a TDP- 43 proteino-pathy (Kato, 2001). However, research into genetic forms of ALS has connected numerous dysfunctional biochemical processes to ALS development; the actual mechanism of the condition is still unknown. A consensus criterion for the diagnosis of ALS, known as the El Escorial criteria, was first developed in 1994 and updated by Brooks in 2000 (Brooks, 1914; Brooks et al., 2000). This criterion combines information from the clinical examination, nerve conduction, electromyography and laboratory tests to rule out other potential diagnosis. In general, respiratory insufficiency causes the death of most individuals in between 2-5 years of the occurrence of clinical signs; however, some people live for more than 10 years after diagnosis. Understanding the complexity of the disease, which includes mental retardation and cognitive abnormalities, is crucial for the prognosis since it will influence caregiving assistance and decision making. Additionally, recently created models, levels and evaluation can give people with amyotrophic lateral sclerosis and their doctors a greater picture of the trajectory of their disease. The glutamate inhibitor Riluzole, the antioxidant Edaravone and the recently suggested Sodium phenylbutyrate/Taurursodiol are 3 medications with an effect on illness progression that are not approved and vary by nation to nation (Paganoni et al., 2020; Abeet al., 2014). Oxidative strain, excito-toxicity, malfunctioning of mitochondria, ribonucleic acid biotransformation, impaired synapse integrity defect in axon transportation and neural inflammation are additional pathways that are hypothesised to be important in the development of ALS condition (Mejzini et al., 2019; Mead et al., 2023). However, the only two mechanisms that are current FDA-approved medications address oxidative stress and excitotoxicity. While much current research aims to find new medications, others concentrate on enhancing medication delivery and efficacy (Johnson et al., 2022). Clinical trials in ALS 20 have assessed more than 50 substances with various modes of action. In addition to them, other medicines that directly target disease-causing genes or suspected disease pathways have been studied in ALS patients or animal models, showing significant promise for future clinical application. We provide an overview of ALS treatment at the moment. We go into great detail on medical therapy since, in our opinion, it is integral to the management of the ALS disease and cannot be separated from current disease therapy. Addressing the emerging therapeutic strategies and in progress scientific investigations, along with concerning small-molecule therapies, in addition to clinical investigations examining gene-targeted treatment (antisense oligonucleotides along with virus vectors causing RNA dysfunction and CRISPR/Cas9), Monoclonal antibodies (MA) and stem-cell therapy.

Genetic Factors Contributing to ALS

The majority of ALS cases are sporadic (without a definite family history) and just 5 to 10% are familial, meaning they are passed down owing to particular genetic abnormalities. Numerous genes are connected to the disease in families.

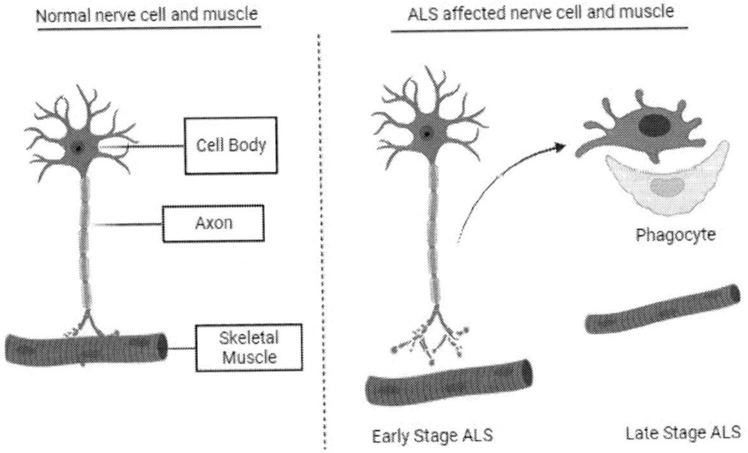

Figure 1. Normal and Affected nerve cells and muscles with ALS.

Mutations in Superoxide Dismutase (SOD1)

The most frequent SOD1 gene mutations are D90A, A4V and G93A. The least frequent but extensively studied of these three mutations is a Glycine-93 conversion into Alanine (G93A). The first mutation discovered to induce motor neuron disease in a transgenic mice model was G93A. On the other hand, an alanine-valine shift at the 4th codon is a prevalent alteration discovered among the North American ALS individuals (Valentine J. S. and Hart P. J, 2003). Reactive oxygen species (ROS) build up and mitochondrial dysfunction are caused by the mitochondrial build-up of aberrant SOD1 masses, which leads to neuronal death and mitochondrial damage (Muyderman H and Chen T, 2014; Harraz M. M et al., 2008; Sasaki et al., 2007).

TARD-BP Mutation

Alterations affecting the TAR DNA-binding protein (TARD-BP) are being identified in small subset of individuals for four percent of fALS cases and one percent of sALS cases (Zou Z. Y et al., 2017). The typical microsatellite sequence (GU/GT) present within DNA and RNA interacts with TDP- 43 that is one of transcription modulator with a high degree of selectivity (Buratti E. and Baralle F. E., 2008). The depletion of operational TDP-43 had been seen in ALS patients. The development of protein complexes in the cytosol which causes neurotoxicity has been connected to this loss, which has negative consequences on RNA metabolism (Cascella R. et al., 2016).

C9 or f72 Mutation

The C9 or f72 alteration, that occurs in around 5% of sALS patients along with 30% of all fALS instances, is the most significant mutation connected to the aetiology of ALS. Over 50% of ALS individuals with C9 or f72 and TDP43 alterations have been found to exhibit cognitive problems and dementia (Cooper-Knock J. et al., 2012; Seltman R. E. and Matthews B. R., 2012). An earlier age at commencement and shorter duration of survival help identify patients with hexa-nucleotide repeated expansions (Majouni E et al., 2012).

TBK1 Mutation

Optineurin (OPTN) and p62 represent two instances of the multi-functional kinases that the TBK1 protein is known for binding and phosphorylation, and both have been associated with the onset of ALS (Li F. et al., 2018: Pottier C et al., 2015). These are included in innate immunity and auto-phagy. A functional mutation in TBK1 may result in decreased protein expression or lack of interaction with its adaptors, respectively.

Environmental Factors Contributing to ALS

Although the precise origin of ALS is still unknown, a number of environmental factors have been investigated for their potential roles in the onset or progression of the condition.

Hazardous Metals

Subjection to heavier metals including that to lead, arsenic, selenium and mercury, were examined extensively. Lead exposure measures in ALS patients suggest that lead exposure may be one of the key environmental variables contributing to the development of the disease, according to earlier studies. The records of ALS patients who had previously been exposed to lead sparked worries about a link between lead exposure and the disease. According to Trojsi and colleagues, numerous studies have been conducted on the potential contribution of a number of heavy metals to the molecular processes causing motor neuron degeneration.

BMI and Nutritional State

ALS Individuals with BMI from 30 to 35, possess a good prognosis of surviving than people with BMI of 35 or lower, according to research by Paganoni and colleagues (Riech-Slotky R. et al., 2013). Greater pre-morbid BMI has been found to be associated with a lower incidence of ALS, as determined by O'Reilly and colleagues, as well as better performance on the ALSFRS-R (ALS Functional Rating Scale) (O'Rielly E. J. et al., 2013). It is commonly known as that ALS is substantially impacted by having decreased body mass (Lindauer E. et al., 2013).

Pesticides

Pesticides cause oxidative damage, malfunctioning of mitochondria, storage of synuclein, and death of neurons; at larger levels, they are probably a factor in the onset of ALS. The development of other neurodegenerative diseases has also been linked to pesticides (Bozzoni V. et al., 2016), making it more difficult to isolate their role in ALS. It should be mentioned that the development of the disease is, also influenced by a combination of genetic susceptibility and long-term impacts of pesticide exposure.

Molecular Mechanisms Underlying Disease Progression

Excitotoxicity

Excessive postsynaptic glutamate receptor activation is thought to be a primary pathogenic factor in ALS (King A. E. et al., 2016), which results in excitotoxicity. Long-term synaptic glutamate elevation leads to excessive neuronal activity, which raises intracellular calcium levels and has subsequent neurotoxic effects as shown in Figure 2 (Van Damme P. et al., 2005). Long-lasting pathogenic alterations brought on by excitotoxicity include ER damage and mitochondrial calcium overload (Kazama M, 2020). By blocking the glutamate-cysteine antiporter, lowering cytoplasmic glutathione concentrations and raising indicators of intracellular oxidative stress, high glutamate exposure also reduces cysteine import (Lewerenz, J. 2013).

Mitochondrial Dysfunction

It has been shown that many abnormal ALS disease-associated proteins that communicate with mitochondrial functionality and disrupts it as showing in Figure 3. Through a number of processes, alterations in certain ALS markers were linked to compromised activity of mitochondria. For instance, aberrant SOD1 agglomerates, present around the inter-membrane region of mitochondria and declines functioning of the electron-transfer chains (ETC) subunits. The pathophysiology of ALS has been postulated to be largely determined by mitochondrial malfunction. Alterations to energy production, excessive ROS production interference with axon transportation, changes to mitochondrial framework and interactions, interference with Ca^{2+} interruptions, and activation of apoptosis; are all factors that were discussed in ALS research models and individual bio-samples (Jhanji R., 2021). Impairment within specialised regions of endoplasmic reticulum-mitochondria linked phospholipid bilayers, which impact neural calcium equilibrium, mitochondrial interactions, endoplasmic reticulum functioning and autophagy, have been linked to axonal degeneration.

Dysfunctional Protein Homeostasis

An intricate structure that includes the production, bending, deterioration of protein molecules that act to stressful indications, such as the unfolded protein's reactions within mitochondria along with ER and the cytoplasmic heat-shock reaction, controls and appropriate equilibrium within protein synthesis & depletion. Age related neurological disorders may be exacerbated by the decline of proteomic accuracy, formation of protein agglomerates and oxidised protein entities in senescent cells as showing Figure 4. Numerous studies have suggested that aberrant proteostasis has an involvement in the onset of the disease (Montibeller, L. 2020).

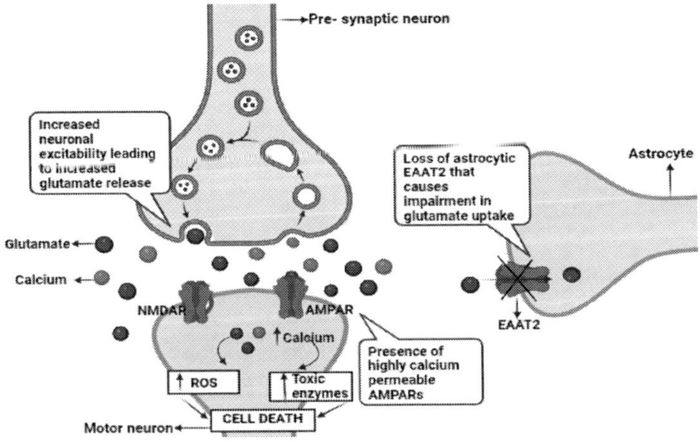

Figure 2. Excitotoxicity occurs in ALS neuron.

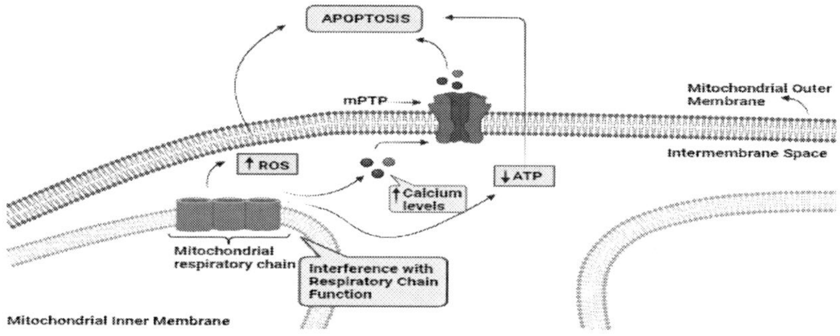

Figure 3. Mitochondrial Dysfunction occur in ALS neuron.

Disturbed RNA Metabolism and RBPs

Build-up of protein and other pathological interactions in ALS are closely tied to changes in RNA processing. Improper operation of RNA-binding proteins (RBPs) is the cause of the abnormal processing of RNA. Proteins known as RNA-binding proteins join with double- or single-stranded RNA, in cells to create ribonucleoprotein complexes. The RBP regulates the suppression of multiple genes' transcription in ALS patients, including TARDP. Interference with mRNA synthesis and suppression, result in flawed splicing, along with negative impact on local translation and RNA transport as showing Figure 5. Additionally, oxidative substances, which were found elevated in cerebro-spinal fluid and serum of patients (Mitsumoto, H. 2009), may cause this RNA dysfunction.

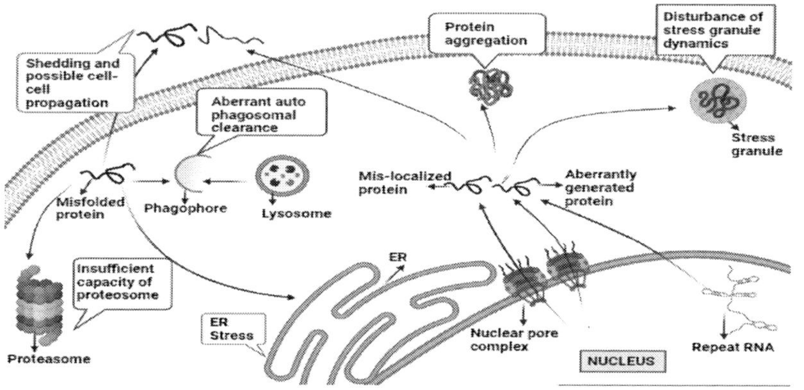

Figure 4. Impaired protein homeostasis occurs in ALS neuron.

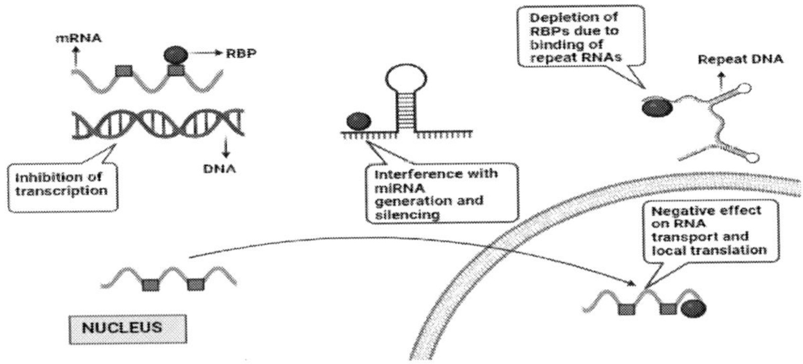

Figure 5. Disturbed RNA metabolism and RBPs occur in ALS neuron.

Neuroinflammation and Astrogliosis

A typical pathogenic occurrence of neurodegenerative illnesses is neuroinflammation. Microglia, astrocytes and the complement system are all activated as a result of MTNs destruction in ALS, which furthers the neurodegeneration as shown in Figure 6. It is widely acknowledged that nearby glial cells regulate the course of ALS-related motor neuron deterioration by regulating the disease's course. Additionally, inflammation-causing agents such prostaglandin E2, leukotriene B4 and NO are secreted by astrocytes under both basal (not activated) and activated settings.

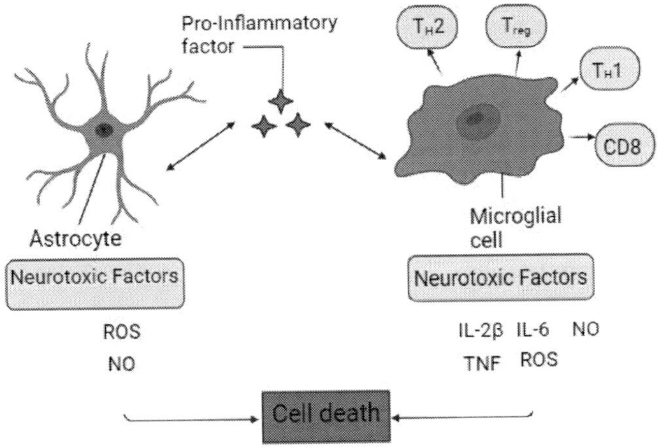

Figure 6. Neuroinflammation process occur in ALS neuron

Impaired Axonal Transport and Integrity

One of the important findings revealing axon transmission deficiencies related to neuro-degeneration is the build-up of organelles along with additional proteins in axons and cell bodies seen in human neuro-degenerative illness, specifically deposition of neurofilament and flawed proteins as showing Figure 7. Axon transport deficiencies, however, might develop separately from MN deterioration. Axons can endure despite persistent transport deficiencies, (Mancuso, R. and Navarro, X. 2015). The Dynein/dynactin complex perturbation is another compelling idea. This complex helps, maintain axons by transporting misfolded and aggregated proteins, damaged organelles and vesicles from axon to the cell structures. In both fALS and sALS, the gene that codes for dynactin has undergone several point mutations. The largest dynactin component (DCTN1), which enables the dynactin-dynein communication, is an essential component if it is complete dynactin/dynein complex. Alterations that occur in the genes, that encode this component, results in a fast MN deterioration that resembles ALS in both people and animals.

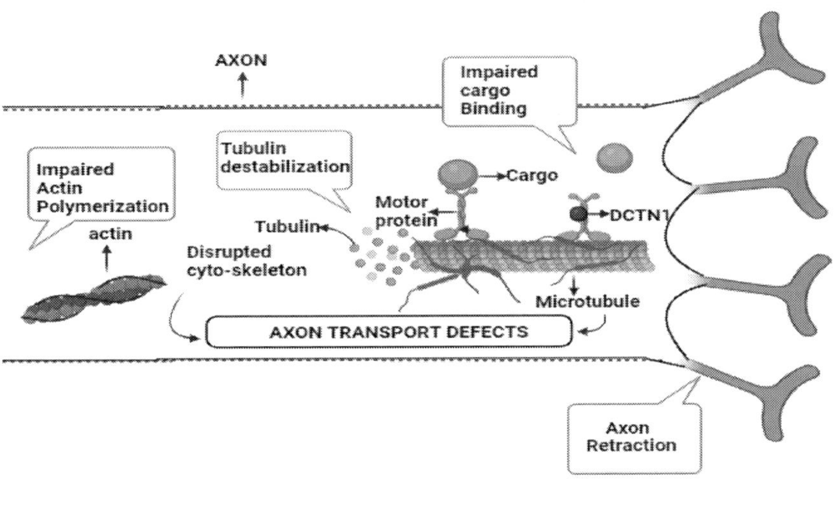

Figure 7. Impaired axonal transport and integrity occur in ALS neuron.

Current Therapeutic Approaches

The available ALS treatments are in scarce. Only four FDA-approved medications have been available recently (riluzole, edaravone, Taurursodiol, and Tofersen), aimed at managing symptoms, improving quality of life, and potentially slowing the progression of the disease.

Riluzole

The FDA and EMA both approved riluzole in 1995 and 1996, respectively. For a very long time, the only treatment for ALS sufferers, was riluzole (6-(trifluoromethoxy)-2-aminobenzothiazole). The main goal of the targeted pathway was to lessen excitotoxicity, particularly glutamate's excitotoxicity. It reduces glutamate release into the synaptic cleft by acting as a sodium channel blocker on presynaptic neurons, which is the first effect. Additionally, the activation of excitatory amino acid transporter 2 (EAAT2) channels in astrocytic cells increases glutamate absorption. There is a non-competitive inhibition of the glutamate receptors for aminomethylphosphonic acid (AMPA) and N-methyl-D-aspartate (NMDA) on postsynaptic neurons. Finally, it appears that GABA receptors are potentiated and gamma-aminobutyric acid (GABA) reuptake is decreased (Albo, F. et al., 2004: Kretschmer, B. D. et al., 1998: Fumagali, E. et al., 2008 et al.). In the initial investigation, 155 people took part in an unborn, double-blind, placebo-controlled experiment to examine the use of Riluzole in the treatment of ALS. The recommended dosage of Riluzole for the intervention group was 100 mg per day, which is still the case today. A considerable delay in the course of the disease was observed after a year of treatment (Bensimon, G. et al., 1994). A second multicenter, double-blind, placebo-controlled study with 959 individuals in 1996 (Lacomblez, L. et al., 1996) supported these findings. The greatest chance of survival may come from taking riluzole at earlier, steady levels (Masrori, P. and Van Damme, P. 2020). Riluzole has also recently been created in an oral-film formulation, offering yet another way to make administration easier and guarantee the continuity of medical care (Qureshi, I. et al., 2020; Wymer, J. et al., 2023).

Edaravone

Edaravone (3-methyl-1-phenyl-2-pyrazoline-5-one) was approved for use in Japan and South Korea. after the FDA's endorsement in 2017. By scavenging free radicals, it was intended to lessen oxidative stress and the neuroinflammatory response (Ikeda, K. et al., 2015; Watanabe, 1994: Yamamoto, T. et al., 1997). Based on a phase III trial with 137 individuals that was randomized, double-blind and placebo controlled, it is used to treat ALS. In two clinical trials, edaravone was unable to demonstrate any benefit. Edaravone may be beneficial for a subgroup of patients with early disease, based on a post hoc review of the 2nd study and an additional stage 3 trial, which found a 33% reduction in disease development at 6 months (Paganoni, S. et al., 2020). Edavarone is now administered intravenously at a dose of 60 milligrams per day. The subsequent monthly cycles all last for ten days, as opposed to the initial administration, which lasts for fourteen days. But compared to taking a medicine orally, this therapy procedure is less convenient. In 2022, the FDA granted approval for a 105 mg/day oral solution.

Sodium Phenylbutyrate and Taurusodiol

Newly, Taurursodiol (also known as PB-TUDCA [tauroursodeoxycholic acid] or PB-TURSO) have been made available as a fixed dosage combination of sodium 4-pheylbutanoate and 2- [(3-, 7-dihydroxy-24-oxo-5-cholan-24-yl) amino] ethane sulfonicacid, dihydrate]. Both of the ingredients in this medication have previously received medical use approval from the FDA. While hyperammonemia brought on by urea cycle abnormalities can be treated with sodium phenylbutyrate (Peña-Quintana, L. et al., 2017). The FDA then approved the product based on the results of CENTAUR, 137 people took part in a stage II multicenter, randomized, double-blinded trial that evaluated the safety and effectiveness of a fixed-dose combination (Paganoni, S. et al., 2020; Paganoni, Set al., 2021; Paganoni, S. et al., 2022). After a phase 2 trial showed a slowdown of the Amyotrophic Lateral Sclerosis Functional Rating Scale-revised (ALSFRS-R) progression and an increase in survival, it was approved in 2022. It targets endoplasmic reticular stress and mitochondria (Abe et al., 2014; Cedarbaum, J. M. et al., 1999). In February 2023, 664 participants in a phase III trial of the fixed-dose combination were fully enrolled (NCT05021536). The oral suspension of sodium phenylbutyrate/taurussol was prepared using a powder and water that was at room temperature. Following three weeks of once-day dosing, Taurursodiol, 1 g, and 3 g of sodium phenylbutyrate, given twice day is the recommended dosage.

Tofersen

For the treatment of ALS patients with a known SOD1 mutation, Ionis Pharmaceuticals developed Tofersen, and Biogen co-developed it under license. Tofersen is believed to inhibit the creation of the SOD1 protein by binding to the SOD1 mRNA, as a result, mutant SOD1's detrimental increase of function is decreased. Tofersen is injected intrathecally once in every month. The tofersen trial involved a total of 72 participants; 36 received a placebo. With Tofersen as opposed to a placebo, SOD1 levels in the CSF and neurofilament light chains in the plasma both dropped. The ALSFRS-R score changed by -6.98 with tofersen and -8.14 with placebo up to week 28 in the subgroup with speedier advancement. Secondary clinical outcomes between the two groups did not differ significantly. The open label extension had 95 participants in all. For the remaining end points, early-start tofersen was favored by differences that were not multiplicity-adjusted. For the early-start group and the delayed-start cohort, the ALSFRS-R score had altered by 6.0 and 9.5, respectively, at 52 weeks. Adverse events associated to lumber punctures were frequent. 7% of people who received tofersen experienced neurologic severe adverse effects. The FDA had added three months to the NDA for tofersen's review period, according to a statement released by Biogen in October 2022. Tofersen was given the FDA's blessing on April 25, 2023, for the treatment of ALS as showing Table 1.

Emerging Directions in ALS Treatment

Numerous treatments have undergone, or are currently through, various preclinical and clinical evaluation stages. They can be categorized based on the disease's pathophysiology models.

Table 1. Therapeutic methods for Amyotrophic Lateral Sclerosis that have received FDA approval (Doreen Ho et al., 2023)

Drugs	Mode of Action	Dosage Form	Efficacy	Side Effects	Brand Name	Reference
Riluzole	Glutamate-induced excitotoxicity	50 mg two times in a day	extends life by 60 to 90 days	digestive, lightheadedness, and elevated liver enzymes	Tiglutik	Doreen Ho et al., 2023
Edaravon	Free-radical scavenger	60 mg IV for 14 days	33% of ALSFRS-R's slowdown at 6 months.	Injection site contusion, Git disturbance, Headache, Allergic reaction	Radicava	Doreen Ho et al., 2023
PB-TURSO	Histone deacetylase inhibitor and mitochondrial integrity	3–1 g three times in a day x 3 weeks and then two times in a day	25% slowing on ALSFRS-R per month	nausea, a URT infection, diarrhea, and abdominal pain Heart failure and renal disease require caution	Relyvrio	Doreen Ho etal., 2023
Tofersen	SOD1-ALS	After that, 100 mg/15 mL IT will be given every 14 days for the next 28 days.	Plasma NfL and CSF SOD1 levels are decreased	Inflammation of the papillae, aseptic meningitis, aseptic fatigue, arthralgia, myelitis, and radiculitis	Qalsody	Doreen Ho et al., 2023

RNA-Based Therapies (Antisense Oligonucleotides)

Single-stranded DNA antisense oligonucleotides (ASOs) have enhanced technology for high affinity and stable binding to target RNA. A kind of motor neuron disease called spinal muscular atrophy has shown that ASOs can effectively reduce the disease's course. ASOs in development for ALS function by cleaving the target RNA in a manner dependent on RNase H. Currently, ataxin-2, stathmin-2, SOD1, C9 or f72 and FUS are among the genes that ASOs in ALS target, with several other targets being researched.

Stem Cell Therapy

Stem cells, which may develop into any particular cell type when directed in the appropriate direction by growth hormones, may be used as a treatment for ALS. Numerous preclinical studies have looked at how it can favor neuronal survival and target numerous pathways. One dose of autologous mesenchymal stem cells from bone marrow has been used in clinical trials. After mesenchymal stem cell transplantation, CSF indicators of inflammation reduced, and improvements in ALSFRS-R slope up to six months later were linked with increased monocyte chemoattractant protein-1 (MCP-1) levels. The most prevalent types of them are hematopoietic or mononuclear cells, mesenchymal stem cells, neural stem cells and induced pluripotent stem cells. Additional research is being done on this safe and well-tolerated therapy.

Neuroinflammation Modulators

Neuroinflammation is another hallmark of the ALS pathogenesis, the muscular denervation and loss of motor neurons (Lewerenz, J. 2013; Williams, T. L. et al., 1997). Many anti-inflammatory drugs have not demonstrated therapeutic efficacy, numerous trials are still underway and various immune system functions are being targeted (Lewerenz, J. 2013, Lamanauskas, N. et al., 2008). A large number of the medications now undergoing clinical trials to modulate abnormal microglial activity. The immune cells that live inside the CNS permanently are known as microglia and they can be either in their resting or active stages. The term "disease associated microglia" is increasingly widely used to describe microglia, since they are thought to have a "toxic" character when they release proinflammatory cytokines (Battaglia, G. and Bruno, V. 2018). When microglia release anti-inflammatory cytokines and phagocytose cell waste, they simultaneously exhibit neuroprotective properties (Battaglia, G. and Bruno, V. 2018). Anti-inflammatory medications are therefore being investigated as potential therapeutics that decrease microglia activation or generate a protective microglia phenotype (Lewerenz, J. 2013; Dyer, A. M. and Smith, A. 2017).

Conclusion

The improvement of present treatments and potential new treatment options seem to be of utmost importance, as the number of ALS patients globally is predicted to increase to over 380,000 by 2040, partly as a result of aging populations (Hobson, E. V. and McDermott, C. J. 2016: Qureshi, I. et al.,

2020). Environmental and genetic risk factors are involved in the complex disease known as ALS. The potential pathogenic pathways involve several genes. In recent years, an increasing number of additional genes have been found that are probably involved in the etiology of ALS. Given the complexity and heterogeneity of ALS, creating effective treatments has proven to be difficult. New therapies are being created to focus on specific pathogenic ALS mechanisms, contain kinase inhibitors, mesenchymal stem cells, integrated stress response inhibitors, antisense oligonucleotidesand endoplasmic reticulum stress inhibitors, among others. More research is required in this area to clarify the important impacts. Given the extensive array of compounds currently being examined and the rising number of clinical studies in recent years, future therapies to treat or perhaps even cure, ALS are highly anticipated.

Disclaimer

None.

References

Abe, K., Itoyama, Y., Sobue, G., Tsuji, S., Aoki, M., Doyu, M., ... & Edaravone ALS Study Group. (2014). Confirmatory double-blind, parallel-group, placebo-controlled study of efficacy and safety of edaravone (MCI-186) in amyotrophic lateral sclerosis patients. *Amyotrophic Lateral Sclerosis and Frontotemporal Degeneration*, 15(7-8), 610-617.

Albo, F., Pieri, M., & Zona, C. (2004). Modulation of AMPA receptors in spinal motor neurons by the neuroprotective agent riluzole. *Journal of neuroscience research*, 78(2), 200-207.

Battaglia, G., & Bruno, V. (2018). Metabotropic glutamate receptor involvement in the pathophysiology of amyotrophic lateral sclerosis: new potential drug targets for therapeutic applications. *Current opinion in pharmacology*, 38, 65-71.

Bensimon, G., Lacomblez, L., Meininger, V. A. L. S., & ALS/Riluzole Study Group. (1994). A controlled trial of riluzole in amyotrophic lateral sclerosis. *New England Journal of Medicine*, 330(9), 585-591.

Bozzoni, V., Pansarasa, O., Diamanti, L., Nosari, G., Cereda, C., & Ceroni, M. (2016). Amyotrophic lateral sclerosis and environmental factors. *Functional neurology*, 31(1), 7.

Brooks, B. R. (1994). El Escorial World Federation of Neurology criteria for the diagnosis of amyotrophic lateral sclerosis. Subcommittee on Motor Neuron Diseases/Amyotrophic Lateral Sclerosis of the World Federation of Neurology Research Group on Neuromuscular Diseases and the El Escorial" Clinical limits of amyotrophic lateral sclerosis" workshop contributors. *Journal of the neurological sciences*, 124, 96-107.

Brooks, B. R., Miller, R. G., Swash, M., & Munsat, T. L. (2000). El Escorial revisited: revised criteria for the diagnosis of amyotrophic lateral sclerosis. *Amyotrophic lateral sclerosis and other motor neuron disorders*, 1(5), 293-299.

Buratti, E., & Baralle, F. E. (2008). Multiple roles of TDP-43 in gene expression, splicing regulation, and human disease. *Front Biosci*, 13(8), 10-2741.

Cascella, R., Capitini, C., Fani, G., Dobson, C. M., Cecchi, C., & Chiti, F. (2016). Quantification of the Relative Contributions of Loss-of-function and Gain-of-function Mechanisms in TAR DNA-binding Protein 43 (TDP-43) Proteinopathies. *Journal of Biological Chemistry*, 291(37), 19437-19448.

Cedarbaum, J M., Stambler, N., Malta, E., Fuller, C., Hilt, D., Thurmond, B. and Nakanishi, A. 1999. The ALSFRS-R: A revised ALS functional rating scale that incorporates assessments of respiratory function. BDNF ALS Study Group (Phase III). *J. Neurol. Sci.* 169, 13–21. [CrossRef].

Chia, R., Chiò, A., & Traynor, B. J. (2018). Novel genes associated with amyotrophic lateral sclerosis: diagnostic and clinical implications. *The Lancet Neurology*, 17(1), 94-102.

Cooper-Knock, J., Hewitt, C., Highley, J. R., Brockington, A., Milano, A., Man, S., ... & Shaw, P. J. (2012). Clinico-pathological features in amyotrophic lateral sclerosis with expansions in C9ORF72. *Brain*, 135(3), 751-764.

Doreen, Ho., Vincent Picher-Martel., Sarah, Luppino., N. P., Katherine., M. Burke., (2023). *New therapies - including antisense oligonucleotides, mesenchymal stem cells, and kinase inhibitors are in development to target specific pathogenic mechanisms identified in ALS.*59-63.

Dyer, A. M., & Smith, A. (2016). Riluzole 5 mg/mL oral suspension: for optimized drug delivery in amyotrophic lateral sclerosis. *Drug design, development and therapy*, 59-64.

Fumagalli, E., Funicello, M., Rauen, T., Gobbi, M., & Mennini, T. (2008). Riluzole enhances the activity of glutamate transporters GLAST, GLT1 and EAAC1. *European journal of pharmacology*, 578(2-3), 171-176.

Harraz, M. M., Marden, J. J., Zhou, W., Zhang, Y., Williams, A., Sharov, V. S., ... & Engelhardt, J. F. (2008). SOD1 mutations disrupt redox-sensitive Rac regulation of NADPH oxidase in a familial ALS model. *The Journal of clinical investigation*, 118(2), 659-670.

He, Y., Benz, A., Fu, T., Wang, M., Covey, D. F., Zorumski, C. F., & Mennerick, S. (2002). Neuroprotective agent riluzole potentiates postsynaptic GABAA receptor function. *Neuropharmacology*, 42(2), 199-209.

Hobson, E. V., & McDermott, C. J. (2016). Supportive and symptomatic management of amyotrophic lateral sclerosis. *Nature Reviews Neurology*, 12(9), 526-538.

Ikeda, K., Iwasaki, Y., & Kaji, R. (2015). Neuroprotective effect of ultra-high dose methylcobalamin in wobbler mouse model of amyotrophic lateral sclerosis. *Journal of the Neurological Sciences,* 354(1-2), 70-74.

Jhanji, R., Behl, T., Sehgal, A. and Bungau, S. 2021. Mitochondrial dysfunction and trafic jams in amyotrophic lateral sclerosis. *Mitochondrion* 58, 102–110.

Johnson, S. A., Fang, T., De Marchi, F., Neel, D., Van Weehaeghe, D., Berry, J. D. and Paganoni, S. 2022. Pharmacotherapy for Amyotrophic Lateral Sclerosis: A Review of Approved and Upcoming Agents. *Drugs* 82, 1367–1388. [CrossRef].

Kato, S., Sumi-Akamaru, H., Fujimura, H., Sakoda, S., Kato, M., Hirano, A., ... & Ohama, E. (2001). Copper chaperone for superoxide dismutase co-aggregates with superoxide dismutase 1 (SOD1) in neuronal Lewy body-like hyaline inclusions: an immunohistochemical study on familial amyotrophic lateral sclerosis with SOD1 gene mutation. *Acta neuropathologica,* 102, 233-238.

Kazama, M., Kato, Y., Kakita, A., Noguchi, N., Urano, Y., Masui, K., ... & Shibata, N. (2020). Astrocytes release glutamate via cystine/glutamate antiporter upregulated in response to increased oxidative stress related to sporadic amyotrophic lateral sclerosis. *Neuropathology,* 40(6), 587-598.

King, A. E., Woodhouse, A., Kirkcaldie, M. T., & Vickers, J. C. (2016). Excitotoxicity in ALS: overstimulation, or overreaction?. *Experimental neurology,* 275, 162-171.

Kretschmer, B. D., Kratzer, U., & Schmidt, W. J. (1998). Riluzole, a glutamate release inhibitor, and motor behavior. *Naunyn-Schmiedeberg's archives of pharmacology,* 358, 181-190.

Lacomblez, L., Bensimon, G., Leigh, P. N., Guillet, P., Powe, L., Durrleman, S., ... & Meininger, V. (1996). A confirmatory dose-ranging study of riluzole in ALS. *Neurology,* 47(6_suppl_4), 242S-250S.

Lamanauskas, N., & Nistri, A. (2008). Riluzole blocks persistent Na+ and Ca2+ currents and modulates release of glutamate via presynaptic NMDA receptors on neonatal rat hypoglossal motoneurons *in vitro*. *European Journal of Neuroscience*, 27(10), 2501-2514.

Lewerenz, J., Hewett, S. J., Huang, Y., Lambros, M., Gout, P. W., Kalivas, P. W., ... & Maher, P. (2013). The cystine/glutamate antiporter system xc− in health and disease: from molecular mechanisms to novel therapeutic opportunities. *Antioxidants & redox signaling,* 18(5), 522-555.

Lewerenz, J., Hewett, S. J., Huang, Y., Lambros, M., Gout, P. W., Kalivas, P. W., ... & Maher, P. (2013). The cystine/glutamate antiporter system xc− in health and disease: from molecular mechanisms to novel therapeutic opportunities. *Antioxidants & redox signaling*, 18(5), 522-555.

Li, F., Xu, D., Wang, Y., Zhou, Z., Liu, J., Hu, S., ... & Pan, L. (2018). Structural insights into the ubiquitin recognition by OPTN (optineurin) and its regulation by TBK1-mediated phosphorylation. *Autophagy,* 14(1), 66-79.

Lindauer, E., Dupuis, L., Müller, H. P., Neumann, H., Ludolph, A. C., & Kassubek, J. (2013). Adipose tissue distribution predicts survival in amyotrophic lateral sclerosis. *PloS one,* 8(6), e67783.

Ling, S. C., Polymenidou, M., & Cleveland, D. W. (2013). Converging mechanisms in ALS and FTD: disrupted RNA and protein homeostasis. *Neuron,* 79(3), 416-438.

Longinetti, E., & Fang, F. (2019). Epidemiology of amyotrophic lateral sclerosis: an update of recent literature. *Current opinion in neurology,* 32(5), 771-776.

Majounie, E., Renton, A. E., Mok, K., Dopper, E. G., Waite, A., Rollinson, S., ... & Traynor, B. J. (2012). Frequency of the C9orf72 hexanucleotide repeat expansion in patients with amyotrophic lateral sclerosis and frontotemporal dementia: a cross-sectional study. *The Lancet Neurology,* 11(4), 323-330.

Mancuso, R., & Navarro, X. (2015). Amyotrophic lateral sclerosis: Current perspectives from basic research to the clinic. *Progress in Neurobiology*, 133, 1-26.

Masrori, P., & Van Damme, P. (2020). Amyotrophic lateral sclerosis: a clinical review. *European journal of neurology,* 27(10), 1918-1929.

Mathis, S., Goizet, C., Soulages, A., Vallat, J. M., & Le Masson, G. (2019). Genetics of amyotrophic lateral sclerosis: A review. *Journal of the Neurological Sciences,* 399, 217-226.

Mead, R. J., Shan, N., Reiser, H. J., Marshall, F., & Shaw, P. J. (2023). Amyotrophic lateral sclerosis: a neurodegenerative disorder poised for successful therapeutic translation. *Nature Reviews Drug Discovery*, 22(3), 185-212.

Mead, R. J., Shan, N., Reiser, H. J., Marshall, F., & Shaw, P. J. (2023). Amyotrophic lateral sclerosis: a neurodegenerative disorder poised for successful therapeutic translation. *Nature Reviews Drug Discovery*, 22(3), 185-212.

Mejzini, R., Flynn, L. L., Pitout, I. L., Fletcher, S., Wilton, S. D., & Akkari, P. A. (2019). ALS genetics, mechanisms, and therapeutics: where are we now?. *Frontiers in neuroscience,* 13, 1310.

Mitsumoto, H. (2009). The clinical features and prognosis of amyotrophic lateral sclerosis. *Amyotrophic lateral sclerosis: A guide for patients and families*, 21-44.

Montibeller, L., Tan, L. Y., Kim, J. K., Paul, P., & de Belleroche, J. (2020). Tissue-selective regulation of protein homeostasis and unfolded protein response signalling in sporadic ALS. *Journal of Cellular and Molecular Medicine,* 24(11), 6055-6069.

Muyderman, H., & Chen, T. (2014). Mitochondrial dysfunction in amyotrophic lateral sclerosis–a valid pharmacological target?. *British journal of pharmacology*, 171(8), 2191-2205.

Nowicka, N., Juranek, J., Juranek, J. K., & Wojtkiewicz, J. (2019). Risk factors and emerging therapies in amyotrophic lateral sclerosis. *International journal of molecular sciences,* 20(11), 2616.

O'Reilly, É. J., Wang, H., Weisskopf, M. G., Fitzgerald, K. C., Falcone, G., McCullough, M. L., ... & Ascherio, A. (2013). Premorbid body mass index and risk of amyotrophic lateral sclerosis. *Amyotrophic Lateral Sclerosis and Frontotemporal Degeneration,* 14(3), 205-211.

Oskarsson, B., Gendron, T. F., & Staff, N. P. (2018, November). Amyotrophic lateral sclerosis: an update for 2018. In *Mayo clinic proceedings* (Vol. 93, No. 11, pp. 1617-1628). Elsevier.

Paez-Colasante, X., Figueroa-Romero, C., Sakowski, S. A., Goutman, S. A., & Feldman, E. L. (2015). Amyotrophic lateral sclerosis: mechanisms and therapeutics in the epigenomic era. *Nature Reviews Neurology,* 11(5), 266-279.

Paganoni, S., Hendrix, S., Dickson, S. P., Knowlton, N., Berry, J. D., Elliott, M. A., ... & Cudkowicz, M. (2022). Effect of sodium phenylbutyrate/taurursodiol on tracheostomy/ventilation-free survival and hospitalisation in amyotrophic lateral sclerosis: long-term results from the CENTAUR trial. *Journal of Neurology, Neurosurgery & Psychiatry,* 93(8), 871-875.
Paganoni, S., Hendrix, S., Dickson, S. P., Knowlton, N., Berry, J. D., Elliott, M. A., ... & Cudkowicz, M. (2022). Effect of sodium phenylbutyrate/taurursodiol on tracheostomy/ventilation-free survival and hospitalisation in amyotrophic lateral sclerosis: long-term results from the CENTAUR trial. *Journal of Neurology, Neurosurgery & Psychiatry,* 93(8), 871-875.
Paganoni, S., Macklin, E. A., Hendrix, S., Berry, J. D., Elliott, M. A., Maiser, S., ... & Cudkowicz, M. E. (2020). Trial of sodium phenylbutyrate–taurursodiol for amyotrophic lateral sclerosis. *New England Journal of Medicine*, 383(10), 919-930.

Peña-Quintana, L., Llarena, M., Reyes-Suarez, D., & Aldamiz-Echevarria, L. (2017). Profile of sodium phenylbutyrate granules for the treatment of urea-cycle disorders: patient perspectives. *Patient preference and adherence,* 1489-1496.

Pottier, C., Bieniek, K. F., Finch, N., van de Vorst, M., Baker, M., Perkersen, R., ... & Rademakers, R. (2015). Whole-genome sequencing reveals important role for TBK1 and OPTN mutations in frontotemporal lobar degeneration without motor neuron disease. *Acta neuropathologica,* 130, 77-92.

Qureshi, I., Lovegren, M., Wirtz, V., Larouche, R., Tanguay, M., Anderson, M. S., ... & Berman, R. M. (2020). A pharmacokinetic bioequivalence study comparing sublingual riluzole (BHV-0223) and oral tablet formulation of riluzole in healthy volunteers. *Clinical pharmacology in drug development,* 9(4), 476-485.

Reich-Slotky, R., Andrews, J., Buchsbaum, R., Levy, D., Kaufmann, P., & Thompson, J. (2013). *Body mass index (BMI) as predictor of ALSFRS-r score decline in ALS patients* (P07. 085).

Sasaki, S., Horie, Y., & Iwata, M. (2007). Mitochondrial alterations in dorsal root ganglion cells in sporadic amyotrophic lateral sclerosis. *Acta neuropathologica,* 114, 633-639.

Seltman, R. E., & Matthews, B. R. (2012). Frontotemporal lobar degeneration: epidemiology, pathology, diagnosis and management. *CNS drugs*, 26, 841-870.

Tan, R. H., Ke, Y. D., Ittner, L. M., & Halliday, G. M. (2017). ALS/FTLD: experimental models and reality. *Acta neuropathologica,* 133(2), 177-196.

Theile, J. W., & Cummins, T. R. (2011). Inhibition of Navβ4 peptide-mediated resurgent sodium currents in Nav1. 7 channels by carbamazepine, riluzole, and anandamide. *Molecular pharmacology,* 80(4), 724-734.

Tiwari, A., Xu, Z., & Hayward, L. J. (2005). Aberrantly Increased Hydrophobicity Shared by Mutants of Cu, Zn-Superoxide Dismutase in Familial Amyotrophic Lateral Sclerosis. *Journal of Biological Chemistry,* 280(33), 29771-29779.

Valentine, J. S., & Hart, P. J. (2003). Misfolded CuZnSOD and amyotrophic lateral sclerosis. *Proceedings of the National Academy of Sciences*, 100(7), 3617-3622.

Van Cutsem, P., Dewil, M., Robberecht, W., & Van Den Bosch, L. (2006). Excitotoxicity and amyotrophic lateral sclerosis. *Neurodegenerative diseases,* 2(3-4), 147-159.

Watanabe, T., Yuki, S., Egawa, M., & Nishi, H. (1994). Protective effects of MCI-186 on cerebral ischemia: possible involvement of free radical scavenging and antioxidant actions. *Journal of Pharmacology and Experimental Therapeutics*, 268(3), 1597-1604.

Williams, T. L., Day, N. C., Ince, P. G., Kamboj, R. K., & Shaw, P. J. (1997). Calcium-permeable α-amino-3-hydroxy-5-methyl-4-isoxazole propionic acid receptors: A molecular determinant of selective vulnerability in amyotrophic lateral sclerosis. *Annals of Neurology: Official Journal of the American Neurological Association and the Child Neurology Society,* 42(2), 200-207.

Wymer, J., Apple, S., Harrison, A., & Hill, B. A. (2023). Pharmacokinetics, bioavailability, and swallowing safety with riluzole oral film. *Clinical Pharmacology in Drug Development*, 12(1), 57-64.

Yamamoto, T., Yuki, S., Watanabe, T., Mitsuka, M., Saito, K. I., & Kogure, K. (1997). Delayed neuronal death prevented by inhibition of increased hydroxyl radical formation in a transient cerebral ischemia. *Brain research*, 762(1-2), 240-242.

Zou, Z. Y., Zhou, Z. R., Che, C. H., Liu, C. Y., He, R. L., & Huang, H. P. (2017). Genetic epidemiology of amyotrophic lateral sclerosis: a systematic review and meta-analysis. *Journal of Neurology, Neurosurgery & Psychiatry*, 88(7), 540-549.

Chapter 7

Multiple Sclerosis: Pathophysiology and Clinical Approaches

Bhavana Singh[1],
Anurag Verma[2],
Vaibhav Rastogi[2],
Deepika Joshi[3],
Nidhi Semwal[4],
Urvashi Saxena[2]
and Gauree Kukreti[5]

[1]School of Pharmacy, Sharda University, Plot no 32, 34, Knowledge Park III, Greater Noida, Uttar Pradesh, India
[2]Teerthanker Mahaveer College of Pharmacy, Teerthanker Mahaveer University, Moradabad (UP), India
[3]Siddhartha Institute of Pharmacy, Sahastradhara Road, Dehradun, Uttarakhand, India
[4]School of Pharmaceutical Science, Shri Guru Ram Rai University, Dehradun, India
[5]School of Pharmaceutical Sciences and Technology, Sardar Bhagwan Singh University, Balawala, Dehradun, UK, India

Abstract

Multiple Sclerosis (MS) is a chronic neuroinflammatory disorder characterized by demyelination and axonal damage in the central nervous system (CNS), resulting in progressive neurological disability. Although its etiology remains elusive, the prevailing hypothesis posits a multifactorial origin, involving a complex interplay of genetic predisposition and environmental factors, leading to a dysregulated immune response against CNS antigens. The pathophysiology of MS

In: Neurogenerative Disorders
Editors: Mohit Agrawal, Manmohan Singhal, Amit Kumar Nayak et al.
ISBN: 979-8-89530-143-2

involves focal inflammatory infiltration, glial activation, oxidative stress, and mitochondrial dysfunction, culminating in neuronal and axonal damage.
Clinical approaches to managing MS have undergone significant advancements, primarily focusing on controlling the inflammatory process, managing symptoms, and improving quality of life. Recent developments in disease-modifying therapies (DMTs) show promise in slowing disease progression and reducing relapses, although they do not offer a cure for MS. The debate between escalation and early aggressive treatment strategies continues. In this review, we present an overview of current understanding of MS pathophysiology and discuss the latest advances in clinical treatment approaches, along with potential challenges and future directions.
The exploration of novel therapeutics targets, like neuroprotective and remyelination agents, alongside personalized medicine approaches, underscores the necessity for further research. Future advancements in understanding the pathophysiology of MS and improvements in clinical approaches can pave the way for effective treatments and the potential to alter the course of this complex and debilitating disease.

Keywords: multiple sclerosis, central nervous system, disease-modifying therapies, pathophysiology, neuroprotective

Introduction

Multiple Sclerosis (MS) is a chronic, autoimmune disease primarily affecting the central nervous system (CNS), which encompasses the intricate network involving the brain and spinal cord. Despite extensive medical research, the precise origins and causal mechanisms remain enigmatic.

At the core of MS lies the body's immune system, typically acting as the body's defense against foreign pathogens. In MS, however, this system turns against its host, mistakenly attacking the protective myelin sheath that wraps around nerve fibers. This assault on the myelin leads to the formation of scar tissue or sclerosis, hence the term "Multiple Sclerosis" reflecting the presence of multiple areas of scarring. The damaged myelin impedes the smooth flow of electrical impulses along nerve fibers resulting in a myriad of symptoms, ranging from mild to severe, depending on the affected part of the CNS (Albert M et al., 2007).

While the exact cause of MS remains elusive, prevailing theories suggest a combination of genetic and environmental factors may render certain individuals more susceptible. Some researchers propose the potential of a viral trigger, theorizing that a virus, possibly common in the environment, could initiate the immune response in genetically predisposed individuals. However, to date, no single virus has been conclusively identified as the causative agent (Aloso A. and Hernan M. A., 2008).

It's crucial to acknowledge that MS isn't a one-size-fits-all condition. Instead, it is classified into four primary types, each with distinct characteristics:

Relapsing-Remitting MS (RRMS): This represents the most common form of MS. Patients with RRMS encounters episodes of new or escalating symptoms, followed by periods of partial or complete recovery. Secondary-Progressive MS (SPMS): Individual with SPMS typically starts with RRMS. Over time, symptoms progressively worsenwith or without periods of flare-ups or remission. Primary-Progressive MS (PPMS): PPMS entails a steady deterioration of symptoms from the onset, without relapses. Progressive-Relapsing MS (PRMS): This rare variant of MS combines the continuous progression of PPMS with the relapses of RRMS. Symptoms of MS are diverse and can be unpredictable, ranging from physical symptoms like fatigue, difficulty walking, numbness, and muscle spasms, to cognitive and emotional symptoms such as memory issues, mood swings, and depression.

Diagnosing MS is not straight forward as there isn't a single definitive test. Neurologists rely on a combination of methods, including clinical evaluation of symptoms, magnetic resonance imaging (MRI) scans to detect areas of demyelination, spinal fluid analysis for markers of inflammation, and evoked potentials to measure electrical activity in the CNS. While a cure for MS remains elusive, several treatments are available to manage symptoms and slow disease progression. Disease-modifying therapies (DMTs) are drugs that can reduce the frequency and severity of relapses. Additionally, symptomatic treatments, physical therapy, and lifestyle interventions play a crucial role in enhancing the quality of life for individual with MS (Astier AL et al., 2006). Interestingly, MS exhibits geographical and gender biases, being more prevalent in colder regions and more common among women. The disease also shows a gender bias, being more common among women. Typically, MS first manifests in individuals between the ages of 20 and 40 (Baecher-Allan C et al., 2018).

Pathophysiology of Multiple Sclerosis

Genetic and Environmental Factors

Multiple Sclerosis (MS) is a multifactorial disease, arising from a combination of genetic and environmental factors (Figure 1) (Omar Deeb et al., 2022). Understanding the intricate interactions between these factors can help elucidate the pathophysiology of MS. Here's a breakdown of both:

Genetic Factors

Genetic Predisposition
Individuals with a family history of Multiple Scleorosis (MS) face a higher risk of developing the disease, indicating the involvement of genetic factors in susceptibility.

HLA-DRB1
The most prominent genetic risk factor for MS is the HLA-DRB1*1501 allele, located within the major histocompatibility complex (MHC) class II region on chromosome 6. This region plays a critical role in the immune system's capacity to distinguish between self and non-self.

Other Genes
Numerous other genes outside the MHC region have also been identified as minor risk factors for MS. Many of these genes are involved in immune system function (Baranzini S. E. and Oksenberg J. R., 2017).

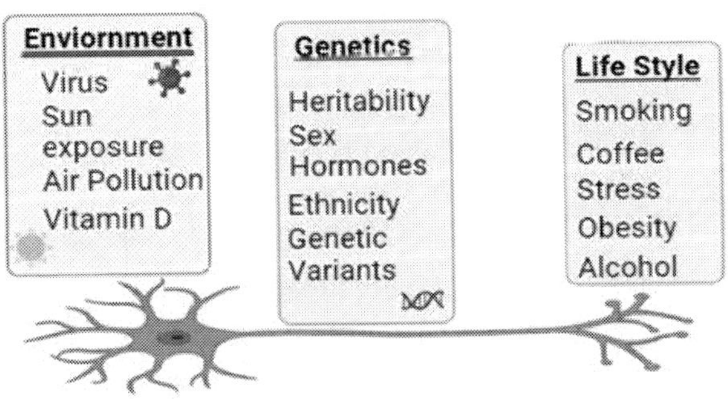

Figure 1. Effect of Environment, Genetic and Lifestyle factors on Multiple Sclerosis.

Environmental and Genetic Interplay in MS

Multiple sclerosis (MS) is influenced by environmental factors and genetic predisposition. Sunlight exposure, often associated with vitamin D, correlates inversely with MS prevalence. Additionally, infections, particularly the Epstein-Barr virus (EBV), may trigger MS in genetically susceptible individuals. Risk factors such as smoking and childhood obesity also elevate the risk of MS. Precise pathophysiology involves inflammation, demyelination, axonal damage, and gliosis. Understanding this interplay between genes and the environment is crucial for developing targeted therapies for MS.

Dysregulated Immune Response

Our immune system, when malfunctioning, can manifest as either hyperactive, leading to allergies or autoimmune diseases like MS, or hypoactivity resulting in increased susceptibility to infections due to primary or acquired deficiencies. Mechanisms underlying these dysfunctions include loss of tolerance, chronic inflammation, faulty signaling, and barrier disruption. Immune dysregulation can lead to tissue damage, heightened susceptibility to infections, or even the development of cancers (Compston A. and Coles A., 2002). Treatments range from immune suppressants to immunostimulatory therapies, highlighting the significance of comprehending these mechanisms.

Inflammatory Infiltration

Inflammation's hallmark is "inflammatory infiltration," where immune cells migrate to sites of injury. Cells such as neutrophils, macrophages, and lymphocytes play significant rolesin this processThey are guided by chemokines, adhere to blood vessels, and migrate to the affected tissue. This process ideally leads to threat neutralization and healing, but in certain conditions, such as MS, immune infiltration can result in chronic inflammation and damage, where immune cells attack the central nervous system (CNS).

Glial Activation in the CNS

Glial cells play a vital role in supporting and protecting neurons. In response to stimuli, particularly microglia and astrocytes become activated. Microglial activation releases pro-inflammatory substances, which may contribute to neurodegenerative diseases (Chen A. Y. et al., 2017). Astrocyte activation, known as reactive astrogliosis, has complex roles in CNS diseases, sometimes providing protection and other times exacerbating damage.

Oxidative Stress and Mitochondrial Dysfunction

Oxidative stress occurs when there is an imbalance between the production of reactive oxygen species (ROS) and their detoxification. Mitochondria, often referred to as cell "powerhouses," malfunction, leading to an increased generation of ROS. This creates a feedback loop: more ROS further impairs mitochondrial function. Both oxidative stress and mitochondrial dysfunction are central to diseases such as Alzheimer's, cardiovascular issues, and metabolic syndromes. Understanding their interconnected roles offers promising therapeutic targets for these conditions.

Neuronal and Axonal Damage in Neurological Conditions

Neurons play a crucial role in transmitting signals throughout our body, and damage to them is observed in numerous neurological disorders. This damage can arise from various factors, including excitotoxicity, oxidative stress, mitochondrial dysfunction, inflammation, physical trauma, demyelination, neurotrophic factor deprivation, and protein misfolding. Understanding these mechanisms is vital for effectively managing and treating these conditions (Figure 2).

Consequences of Neuronal and Axonal Damage

Loss of Function: Damage to neurons can lead to loss of specific functions, depending on the affected neuronal population. For example, damage to motor neurons can result in muscle weakness or paralysis. Retrograde and

Anterograde Degeneration: Following axonal damage, degeneration can occur in two directions retrograde, which involves degeneration backwards towards the cell body, and anterograde, which involves degeneration beyond the point of injury.

Compensatory Mechanisms: Some neurons may undergo synaptic plasticity, forming new connections to compensate for lost function, although this adaptive process is often limited. Clinical Mamifestation: Depending on the brain region or neuronal population affected, symptoms can vary widely, ranging from cognitive decline, sensory deficits, movement disorders, to mood disturbances.

In summary, neuronal and axonal damage plays central roles in the the pathology of many neurological conditions. Understanding the underlying mechanisms and consequences is essential for accurate diagnosis, prognosis, and the development of therapeutic strategies (Dutta R. and Trapp B. D., 2014).

Clinical Manifestations and Diagnosis

Symptomatology

Multiple Sclerosis (MS) is a complex characterized by a broad spectrum of symptoms that can vary greatly from one individual to another. These symptoms arise from inflammation, demyelination, and axonal damage within the central nervous system (CNS). Here are the primary symptoms of MS: *Motor Symptoms:*

- Muscle Weakness: Frequently one of the initial indicators of MS, it can impact any part of the body.
- Spasticity: Refers to sensations of rigidity and a variety of involuntary muscle contractions.
- Tremor: Individual with MS may develop tremorswhich can affect the hands, arms, and legs.
- Gait Difficulties: Many factors of MS can contribute to this, including muscle weakness, spasticity, loss of balance, and fatigue.

Sensory Symptoms

- Numbness and Tingling: Often among the first signs of MS or a relapse.
- Neuropathic Pain: May present as burning, itching, stabbing, or tearing pains.
- Lhermitte's Sign: Characterized by a brief, stabbing, electric-shock-like sensation that runs down the back and/or limbs upon flexing the neck.
- Decreased Sensation of Pain or Temperature: Particularly noticeable in the extremities.

Visual Symptoms

- Optic Neuritis: Inflammation of the optic nerve resulting in pain and temporary vision loss.
- Diplopia: Perception of double vision.
- Nystagmus: Uncontrolled eye movements.

Coordination and Balance

- Ataxia: Lack of coordination affecting walking, speech, or limb movements.
- Vertigo and Dizziness: A false sensation that one's surroundings are spinning.

Autonomic and Sexual Symptoms

- Bladder Dysfunction: Including urgency, hesitancy, incomplete emptying, or incontinence.
- Bowel Dysfunction: Constipation and, less frequently, incontinence.
- Sexual Dysfunction: Including altered sensation, reduced libido, and difficulties in achieving orgasm.

Cognitive and Emotional Symptoms

- Cognitive Dysfunction: Affecting memory, attention, processing speed, and executive functions.
- Depression: Common in people with MS.
- Mood Swings: Including irritability and symptoms of anxiety.

Other Symptoms

- Fatigue: A prevalent and difficult symptom often experienced by MS patients.
- Hearing Loss: Though rare, some people with MS may experience this.
- Dysphagia: Difficulty in swallowing.
- Dysarthria: Slurred speech due to impaired motor control of speech muscles.

Diagnosis

The diagnosis of MS is typically based on a combination of clinical evaluation, imaging studies, and other tests:

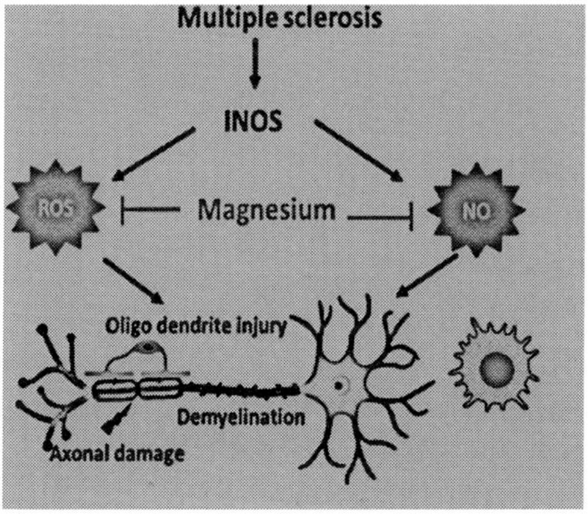

Figure 2. Neuronal damage in Multiple Sclerosis (Dutta R and Trapp BD, 2014).

MRI (Magnetic Resonance Imaging)

Displays regions of demyelination (lesions) within the brain and spinal cord.

Lumbar Puncture

Examination of cerebrospinal fluid (CSF) may reveal increased concentrations of immunoglobulin G (IgG) and the occurrence of oligoclonal bands, markers of immune responses in the CNS.

Evoked Potentials

These tests gauge the brain's electrical responses to various stimuli (such as visual or electrical prompts) and can detect irregularities or delays in nerve transmission.

Clinical Criteria

The McDonald criteria are commonly used, which consider the number of neurological episodes a patient has had, the appearance of lesions in the CNS, and progression of symptoms (Frohman E. M. et al., 2006).

It's important to note that MS can mimic many other conditions, so a thorough differential diagnosis is crucial. Furthermore, given the heterogeneity of MS, two patients can experience very different symptom profiles. Regular follow-ups and monitoring are essential, as the disease can evolve over time.

Diagnostic Criteria and Tools

The process of diagnosing Multiple Sclerosis (MS) involves a combination of clinical evaluation, imaging, and other tests to ascertain the presence of disseminated lesions in time and space (meaning lesions appear in different locations and at different times). Since no single test can definitively diagnose MS, a variety of diagnostic criteria and tools are used.

Diagnostic Criteria

McDonald Criteria

This is the most widely accepted set of criteria for the diagnosis of MS. It has been revised multiple times, with the most recent revision (as of my last training cut-off in September 2021) being in 2017. The McDonald criteria consider.

Clinical Attacks
Episodes of neurological symptoms.

MRI Findings
The presence and distribution of lesions in the CNS.

Evidence of Dissemination in Time (DIT)
Indicating that lesions have formed at different times.

Evidence of Dissemination in Space (DIS)
Indicating that lesions are present in more than one location in the CNS.

The criteria aim to streamline the diagnosis, potentially allowing for an earlier and more accurate diagnosis of MS (Filippi M. et al., 2018).

Diagnostic Tools

MRI (Magnetic Resonance Imaging)

This is the most valuable tool for diagnosing MS. It visualizes areas of demyelination (lesions or plaques) in the brain and spinal cord.

Gadolinium-Enhanced MRI

A contrast agent that can help highlight active inflammation and differentiate between old and new lesions.

Lumbar Puncture (Spinal Tap)

This method entails obtaining a cerebrospinal fluid (CSF) sample from the spinal canal. The fluid is analyzed for oligoclonal bands, specific immunoglobulin patterns seen in approximately 85-95% of individuals with MS.

Evoked Potentials

These assessments capture the brain's electrical reactions to stimuli. They can identify discrepancies in nerve routes that might seem typical during a clinical evaluation.

Visual Evoked Potentials (VEP)

The most commonly used evoked potential test in MS diagnosis, it measures the transmission of visual stimuli.

Blood Tests

Although there isn't a conclusive blood test for MS, blood analyses can assist in excluding conditions with symptoms similar to MS, facilitating the differentiation process.

Neurological Examination

A detailed examination by a neurologist can detect changes in eye movements, coordination, reflexes, and other motor and sensory functions.

Optical Coherence Tomography (OCT)

An imaging test that looks at the retina and can identify thinning of the retinal nerve fiber layer, which is often present in MS (Giorgio A et al., 2011).

Diagnosing MS is a process of piecing together multiple pieces of evidence while also excluding other potential causes for the symptoms. Given that MS has such a wide range of symptoms and can mimic other diseases, this comprehensive approach is essential to ensure an accurate diagnosis. Regular monitoring and reassessment are also vital, as the disease can evolve over time.

Therapeutic Approaches to Multiple Sclerosis

Disease-Modifying Therapies (DMTs) play a pivotal role in managing Multiple Sclerosis (MS), targeting the disease's core processes to reduce relapse frequency, decelerate disability progression, and optimize long-term outcomes. These medications largely function by modulating or suppressing the immune system (Gilmore CP et al., 2009). Among the first DMTs approved were injectable Interferon Betas, such as Avonex and Rebif (Interferon beta-1a) and Betaseron and Extavia (Interferon beta-1b), which are believed to decrease inflammation by modifying the immune system. Another injectable option, Glatiramer Acetate (like Copaxone and Glatopa), acts as an immune decoy, potentially diverting the system from attacking myelin. The therapeutic landscape has expanded with oral DMTs like Fingolimod (Gilenya) that prevents specific immune cells from reaching the CNS, Dimethyl Fumarate (Tecfidera) that counteracts inflammation, Teriflunomide (Aubagio) which inhibits certain immune cell multiplication, and Cladribine (Mavenclad), an immunosuppressant. Infused DMTs have emerged, with monoclonal antibodies like Natalizumab (Tysabri), which blocks immune cells from entering the CNS, and Ocrelizumab (Ocrevus) and Alemtuzumab (Lemtrada), both targeting specific proteins on immune cells, leading to their depletion. Table 1 The field also witnesses experimental therapies, including stem cell treatments and novel immunomodulators. While the efficacy of DMTs is notable, potential side effects mandate regular patient monitoring, involving blood tests and MRIs. In decision-making, the balance between treatment benefits and potential risks is central, emphasizing the importance of patient-healthcare provider discussions (Gustavsson A et al., 2011).

Table 1. Overview of Therapeutic Approaches to Multiple Sclerosis (Sidara S et al., 2019)

S.No.	Therapeutic Approach	Primary Focus	Description	Example
1.	Disease-Modifying Therapies (DMTs)	Disease progression	Drugs designed to reduce relapses and slow the progression of MS.	Interferon beta-1a, Glatiramer acetate
2.	Symptomatic Treatments	Symptom relief	Medications targeting specific MS symptoms.	Baclofen (for spasticity), Modafinil (for fatigue)
3.	Physical Therapy	Mobility & Function	Exercises and routines to improve mobility, strength, and balance.	Stretching routines, walking exercises
4.	Rehabilitation	Function & Independence	Strategies to improve cognitive and physical functions impaired by MS.	Cognitive rehabilitation, Occupational therapy
5.	Lifestyle Interventions	Overall well-being	Approaches that focus on diet, stress management, and overall health.	Vitamin D supplements, Exercise routines

Emerging Trends and Future Directions

Novel Therapeutic Targets

Research in Multiple Sclerosis (MS) continues to expand, yielding insights into the disease's underlying mechanisms and identifying novel therapeutic targets. Here are some emerging targets and their mechanisms.

B Cells

While earlier treatments focused primarily on T cells, B cells have been recognized as significant contributors to the pathogenesis of MS.

Ocrelizumab and Ofatumumab: These are anti-CD20 monoclonal antibodies that deplete B cells. Ocrelizumab, in particular, is the first drug approved for both relapsing and primary progressive forms of MS. They target the CD20 marker on B cells, leading to B cell depletion (Li R et al., 2018).

Sphingosine-1-Phosphate (S1P) Receptors

S1P receptors play a role in lymphocyte (a type of white blood cell) migration and function.

Fingolimod (Gilenya): The first S1P receptor modulator approved for MS. It prevents lymphocytes from exiting lymph nodes, reducing their number in the bloodstream and CNS.

Siponimod (Mayzent) and Ponesimod: Are newer S1P receptor modulators. Siponimod is approved for secondary progressive MS (Krieger SC et al., 2016).

Bruton's Tyrosine Kinase (BTK) Inhibitors

BTK is essential for B cell receptor signaling.

Evobrutinib and Tolebrutinib: These are BTK inhibitors currently being investigated for MS. By inhibiting BTK, these drugs can reduce B cell activity and possibly other immune cell types involved in MS.

Remyelination Targets

Strategies that promote remyelination are of great interest, as they address the repair of damaged nerves, not just inflammation.

Anti-LINGO-1 (Opicinumab): LINGO-1 is a protein that inhibits remyelination. By targeting LINGO-1, this drug aims to promote remyelination and potentially improve nerve function.

Neuroprotection

Strategies aim to protect neurons from damage, which can help in slowing disease progression.

Alpha-lipoic acid: An antioxidant that has shown potential neuroprotective properties and is being researched for its role in slowing brain atrophy in MS (Luchetti S. et al., 2018).

Modulation of the Gut Microbiome

There's increasing evidence linking the gut microbiome to autoimmune diseases, including MS.

Probiotics and dietary interventions: Research is ongoing to determine if manipulating the gut microbiome can influence the course of MS.

Targeting Metabolism

Certain metabolic pathways might be altered in MS, and targeting these can be a potential therapeutic strategy.

Dimethyl Fumarate (Tecfidera): While its exact mechanism isn't fully understood, it might exert its effects through the modulation of the NRF2 pathway, which plays a role in cellular response to oxidative stress (Lublin FD et al., 2014).

Stem Cell Therapies

Hematopoietic stem cell transplantation (HSCT) is being studied as a treatment for MS. It involves high-dose immunosuppression followed by transplantation of the patient's own stem cells to "reset" the immune system.

While some of these novel targets have led to approved treatments, others are still in experimental stages. The continuous exploration of these targets and the development of new drugs reflect the evolving understanding of MS and the commitment of the scientific community to finding effective therapies. As always, the benefits and risks of each therapy need to be carefully considered, and decisions should be tailored to the individual's specific circumstances (Mahad D. H. et al., 2015).

Neuroprotective Agents

Neuroprotection refers to strategies and mechanisms that protect the central nervous system (CNS) neurons from degeneration or injury. In the context of Multiple Sclerosis (MS), neuroprotective agents are of immense interest because they aim to prevent the progression of disability by directly protecting neurons and axons from the damaging effects of inflammation, demyelination, and other pathological processes.

Here are some neuroprotective agents or strategies that have been investigated for potential use in Multiple Sclerosis.

Laquinimod

Mechanism

Though its exact mechanism is not entirely understood, laquinimod is believed to have both immunomodulatory and direct neuroprotective effects. In animal models, it has demonstrated a capacity to reduce neurodegeneration and promote CNS repair.

Clinical Status

Clinical trials have shown potential benefits in reducing brain atrophy, but its effectiveness in comparison to other available MS treatments remains a topic of discussion.

Clemastine Fumarate

Mechanism

Originally an antihistamine, clemastine fumarate has shown potential remyelinating capabilities, which indirectly provide neuroprotection.

Clinical Status

Early-phase clinical trials have suggested potential benefits in promoting remyelination and thus neuroprotection in MS patients (Rosati G., 2001).

Ongoing Research in Neuroprotective Mechanisms

Mitochondrial Protectors

Mitochondrial dysfunction is believed to be involved in axonal damage in MS. Agents that protect mitochondrial function could offer neuroprotection.

Ion Channel Modulators

Dysfunction of ion channels in demyelinated axons is another mechanism leading to axonal damage. Modulating these channels can potentially offer neuroprotection.

Growth Factors

Molecules like BDNF (brain-derived neurotrophic factor) support neuron survival and health. Enhancing their activity or levels could provide neuroprotective benefits (Peterson J. W. et al., 2001).

Lifestyle and Complementary Approaches

Diet and Nutrition

Diets rich in antioxidants, such as the Mediterranean diet, could offer neuroprotective benefits by reducing oxidative stress.

Exercise

Regular physical activity has been shown to have neuroprotective effects, possibly by promoting neuroplasticity and releasing neurotrophic factors.

Neuroprotective strategies represent a crucial area of MS research, given their potential to halt or even reverse disability progression. As research evolves, it's hoped that more effective neuroprotective agents will be identified and integrated into the comprehensive management of MS (Scalfari A. et al., 2013).

Personalized Medicine Approaches

Personalized medicine, often termed precision medicine, involves tailoring medical care and therapeutic strategies to the individual characteristics of each patient. The approach leverages genetic, clinical, environmental, and lifestyle information to make informed treatment and prevention strategies for individual patients. In the context of Multiple Sclerosis (MS), personalized medicine approaches can be particularly beneficial due to the highly variable disease course and patient responses to therapies.

Here are some of the personalized medicine approaches being explored or adopted in the management of Multiple Sclerosis.

Genetic Profiling

By understanding specific genetic markers or mutations, physicians may predict disease course or response to certain treatments. While no specific gene has been identified as the singular cause of MS, several genetic variations have been linked to disease susceptibility and may influence disease progression or treatment response (Sundgvist E. et al., 2012).

Biomarker Identification

Neurofilament Light Chain (NFL)

Elevated levels of NFL in the blood or cerebrospinal fluid (CSF) can indicate neural damage and may be used to monitor disease activity or predict disease progression.

MRI-Based Markers

Advanced imaging techniques can help identify patterns of lesion development or brain atrophy, guiding treatment decisions based on disease activity.

Pharmacogenomics

By analyzing how genes affect a person's response to drugs, it may be possible to predict which medications a patient will respond best to, ensuring more effective treatments and reducing potential side effects.

Monitoring Disease Activity

Frequent monitoring using MRI, optical coherence tomography (OCT) for retinal nerve fiber layer thickness, or other tests can help adjust treatments based on disease activity and progression.

Lifestyle and Environmental Factors

Evaluating an individual's lifestyle habits, such as diet, exercise, and exposure to potential environmental triggers, can help tailor recommendations and interventions to reduce the risk of disease flares.

Comprehensive Symptom Assessment

Given the wide range of symptoms in MS, personalized symptom management is crucial. Regularly assessing symptoms ensures that treatments address each patient's unique challenges.

Integrative Medicine Approaches

Tailoring complementary therapies, such as diet, physical therapy, stress-reduction techniques, and supplements, based on the individual needs and preferences of the patient.

Advanced Imaging

Using cutting-edge imaging techniques, such as functional MRI or PET scans, to gain insights into disease activity and neural connectivity, aiding in more precise treatment strategies.

Patient Engagement and Feedback

Encouraging patients to actively participate in their care, providing feedback on treatment efficacy and side effects, ensures a tailored approach based on real-time patient experience (Rocca M. A. et al., 2015).

The advancement of personalized medicine in MS requires collaboration between researchers, clinicians, and patients. As technology and our understanding of MS evolve, the hope is to refine these personalized approaches further, optimizing treatment outcomes, minimizing side effects, and enhancing the quality of life for individuals with MS (Yeshokumar A. K. et al., 2017).

Conclusion

In conclusion, the landscape of Multiple Sclerosis (MS) research and treatment has been evolving rapidly over the past decades, reflecting both the complexity of the disease and the relentless commitment of the scientific community to improving patient outcomes. The shift towards personalized medicine is emblematic of a broader move in healthcare: recognizing the uniqueness of each patient and tailoring interventions accordingly. From understanding the intricate genetic, environmental, and immunological underpinnings of MS to the development of novel therapeutic agents targeting remyelination and neuroprotection, the advances are promising. While challenges persist, especially in understanding the root causes of MS and developing treatments for its progressive forms, the progress made instills hope. Incorporating personalized approaches, like genetic profiling, biomarker identification, and patient-centric feedback mechanisms, underscores the importance of individualized care. As science continues to merge with technology and patient advocacy, the MS community can remain optimistic about a future where the disease is more manageable, if not curable. Ultimately, as with many areas in medicine, collaboration – between researchers, clinicians, patients, and advocates – will be the keystone to further breakthroughs and improved quality of life for those living with MS.

Disclaimer

None.

References

Albert, M., Antel, J., Bruck, W., & Stadelmann, C. (2007). Extensive cortical remyelination in patients with chronic multiple sclerosis. *Brain Pathology,* 17, 129-138.

Alonso, A., & Hernan, M. A. (2008). Temporal trends in the incidence of multiple sclerosis: a systematic review. *Neurology,* 71, 129-135.

Astier, A. L., Meiffren, G., Freeman, S., & Hafler, D. A. (2006). Alterations in CD46-mediated Tr1 regulatory T cells in patients with multiple sclerosis. *Journal of clinical investigation,* 116, 3252-3257.

Baecher-Allan, C., Kaskow, B. J., & Weiner, H. L. (2018). Multiple sclerosis: mechanisms and immunotherapy. *Neuron,* 97, 742-768.

Baranzini, S. E., & Oksenberg, J. R. (2017). The genetics of multiple sclerosis: from 0 to 200 in 50 years. *Trends in Genetics,* 33, 960-970.

Chen, A. Y., Chonghasawat, A. O., & Leadholm, K. L. (2017). Multiple sclerosis: frequency, cost, and economic burden in the United States. *Journal of clinical neuroscience,* 45, 180-186.

Compston, A., & Coles, A. (2002). Multiple sclerosis. *Lancet,* 359, 1221-1231.

Dutta, R., & Trapp, B. D. (2014). Relapsing and progressive forms of multiple sclerosis: insights from pathology. *Current opinion in neurology,* 27, 271-278.

Filippi, M. (2018). Prediction of a multiple sclerosis diagnosis in patients with clinically isolated syndrome using the 2016 MAGNIMS and 2010 McDonald criteria: a retrospective study. *Lancet Neurology,* 17, 133-142.

Frohman, E. M., Racke, M. K., & Raine, C. S. (2006). Multiple sclerosis — the plaque and its pathogenesis. *The New England journal of medicine*, 354, 942-955.

Gilmore, C. P. (2009). Regional variations in the extent and pattern of grey matter demyelination in multiple sclerosis: a comparison between the cerebral cortex, cerebellar cortex, deep grey matter nuclei and the spinal cord. *Journal of Neurology, Neurosurgery, and Psychiatry,* 80, 182-187.

Giorgio, A. (2011). Cortical lesions in radiologically isolated syndrome. *Neurology,* 77, 1896-1899.

Gustavsson, A. (2011). Cost of disorders of the brain in Europe 2010. *European Neuropsychopharmacology,* 21, 718-779.

Krieger, S. C., Cook, K., De Nino, S., & Fletcher, M. (2016). The topographical model of multiple sclerosis: a dynamic visualization of disease course. *Neurol. Neuroimmunology & Neuroinflamation,* 3, e279.

Li, R., Patterson., & K, Bar-Or A. (2018). Reassessing the contributions of B cells in multiple sclerosis. *Nature Reviews Immunology,* 19, 696-707.

Lublin, F. D. (2014). Defining the clinical course of multiple sclerosis: the 2013 revisions. *Neurology,* 83, 278-286.

Luchetti, S. (2018). Progressive multiple sclerosis patients show substantial lesion activity that correlates with clinical disease severity and sex: a retrospective autopsy cohort analysis. *Acta Neuropathology,* 135, 511-528.

Mahad, D. H., Trapp, B. D., & Lassmann, H. (2015). Pathological mechanisms in progressive multiple sclerosis. *Lancet Neurology,* 14, 183-193.

Omar, D. (2022). Exploring the effect of Genetic, Enviornmental and Lifestyle Factors on multiple sclerosis susceptibility. Multiple Sclerosis-Genetics, Disease Mechanism and Clinical Developments. *Intech Open,* 1-20.

Peterson, J. W., Bo, L., Mork, S., Chang, A., & Trapp, B. D. (2001). Transected neurites, apoptotic neurons, and reduced inflammation in cortical multiple sclerosis lesions. *Annals of Neurology*, 50, 389-400.

Rocca, M. A. (2015). Clinical and imaging assessment of cognitive dysfunction in multiple sclerosis. *Lancet Neurology,* 14, 302-317.

Rosati, G. (2001). The prevalence of multiple sclerosis in the world: an update. *Neurological sciences,* 22, 117-139.

Scalfari, A. (2013). Mortality in patients with multiple sclerosis. Neurology, 81, 184-192.

Sidara, S. (2019). An Overview of Therapeutic Options in Relapsing-remitting Multiple Sclerosis. *Cureus,* 11, 1-11.

Sundqvist, E. (2012). Epstein-Barr virus and multiple sclerosis: interaction with HLA. *Genes Immunology,* 13, 14-20.

Yeshokumar, A. K., Narula, S., & Banwell, B. (2017). Pediatric multiple sclerosis. *Current opinion in neurology,* 30, 216-221.

Chapter 8

Therapeutic Interventions for Spinal Muscular Atrophy

Saurav Sarkar[1],
Soumik Laha[2]
and Soma Das[2,*]
[1]Division of Pharmaceutics, Department of Pharmaceutical Technology, University of North Bengal, Raja Rammohunpur, Dist-Darjeeling, India
[2]Department of Pharmaceutical Technology, School of Health and Medical Sciences, Adamas University:Barasat - West Bengal, India

Abstract

Spinal muscular atrophy (SMA) is a hereditary condition characterised by the degeneration of the neurological system, resulting in a gradual decline in muscle strength and deterioration. Spinal Muscular Atrophy (SMA) still lacks a definitive treatment; nevertheless, various therapeutic strategies exist that aim to enhance the overall quality of life for individuals affected by this disorder. Conventional therapy methods for spinal muscular atrophy (SMA) primarily emphasise the alleviation of symptoms and the provision of supportive care. The potential interventions encompass physical therapy, occupational therapy, and speech therapy, as well as the utilization of orthotics and other adaptable equipment.

The field of gene therapy has witnessed significant progress in the treatment of spinal muscular atrophy (SMA), hence presenting a promising outlook for individuals affected by this condition.

* Corresponding Author's Email: somapharma@gmail.com.

In: Neurogenerative Disorders
Editors: Mohit Agrawal, Manmohan Singhal, Amit Kumar Nayak et al.
ISBN: 979-8-89530-143-2

The field of therapeutic interventions for spinal muscular atrophy (SMA) is characterized by ongoing advancements, with the continuous development of novel treatment modalities.
This chapter presents an engaging examination of therapeutic advancements, highlighting the progress made in combating SMA. The extensive examination and persuasive data provided in this document serve as a source of optimism, encouraging researchers, doctors, and the wider medical community to intensify their endeavours in pushing forward the boundaries of spinal muscular atrophy (SMA) treatment.

Keywords: *SMN1, SMN2,* spinal muscular atrophy, survival motor neuron gene, motor neurons

Introduction

Spinal Muscular Atrophy: An Overview

Spinal Muscular Atrophy (SMA) is a hereditary condition characterized by muscle weakening, resulting in difficulties with body movement. Alpha motor neuron loss is the underlying cause of this neurogenetic disease. This condition is uncommon and impacts approximately one child out of every 6,000 to 10,000.,

The primary cause of spinal muscular atrophy (SMA) is the expression of the survival motor neuron 1 (SMN1) gene, which encodes the SMN protein essential for motor neuron activity and locomotion. Motor neuron degeneration results in muscle weakness, muscle atrophy, and reduced muscle tone in the shoulders, hips, and back. SMA is classified into various subtypes ranging from SMA 0 to SMA 4 (Prior et al., 2020).

The Importance of Therapeutic Interventions

Before 2016, there were no specific therapeutic interventions available for SMA.

Following that, Antisense Oligonucleotides (ASOs) and virus-mediated gene therapy were granted permission for therapeutic application. Furthermore, the FDA has approved Nusinersen, Onasemnogene, and Risidiplam as therapies specifically for SMA. These medications are delivered through several routes of administration.

The primary goals of these therapies are to enhance the synthesis of SMN protein, hence enhancing motor function. Due to the unpredictable nature of SMA, finding a solution for this condition is exceedingly challenging (Nicolau et al., 2021, D'Amico et al., 2011).

Understanding the Pathophysiology of Spinal Muscular Atrophy

Spinal muscular atrophy is a neurological condition characterized by the degeneration of alpha motor neurons, resulting in muscle weakness and atrophy. The majority of cases of spinal muscular atrophy (SMA) occur as a result of a mutation in the SMN1 gene. The SMN1 gene encodes the SMN protein, which is essential for the normal functioning and maintenance of motor neurons. Patients affected by SMA experience issues in the SMN1 gene due to either a missing section of the gene or gene alterations. The insufficient production of SMN proteins due to eliminating or mutations of the SMN1 gene leads to the shrinking and death of motor neurons. An individual can have a maximum of eight copies of the SMN2 gene. The presence of several copies of the SMN2 gene can mitigate symptoms of SMA by compensating for the absence of the SMN1 protein (Baranello et al., 2021; Nicolau et al., 2021).

Genetic Basics of SMA

The SMA 1 gene is predominantly linked to the gene located on chromosome 5.

The proximal spinal muscular atrophy (SMA) is caused by a mutation in the MN gene, resulting in the highest possible level of the condition. Infantile SMA variations refer to types of spinal muscular atrophy that are not associated with the SMN1 gene. SMA with respiratory disease (SMARD1) is a form of juvenile SMA that is caused by a mutation in the IGHMBP2 gene.

Beside that UBE1, SCO2, EXOSC3, TSEN54, RARS2, VRK1, DYNC1H1, BICD2, PLEKHG5, VAPB, LMNA, MAPT, AR, HSPB1, HSPB8, GARS, DYNC1H1, HSPB3, FBXO38, 11Q13, GARS, REFP1, BSCL2, IGHMBP2, SLC5A7, DCTN1, GARS, REFP1, BSCL2, IGHMBP2, SLC5A7, DCTN1, DNAJB2, SETX, ATP7A, LASIL, TRPV4 genes or locus are associated fully or partially with Spinal muscular atrophy (Wirth, 2021).

Motor Neuron Degeneration and Muscle Atrophy

People with spinal muscular atrophy (SMA) suffer from a lack of the survival motor neuron (SMN) protein, which causes their muscles to deteriorate and weaken.

This muscle weakness predominantly presents in the muscles of the chest, arm, and upper leg, leading to a severe disease. Muscle atrophy is a result of genetic abnormalities in the same gene due to its hereditary nature.

For rare cases SMA occurred due to inheritance in an autosomal recessive method where afflicted individual has two defective gene and commonly inheriting one form each parent (Farrar et al., 2017).

Disease Progression and Clinical Variability

The diagnosis of MA is conducted through the evaluation of patient history and genetic testing. Since there are five forms of SMA that can arise in patients, it is crucial to identify the specific gene responsible for SMA. Previously, muscle biopsy and electromyography (EMG) were commonly employed for detecting spinal muscular atrophy (SMA). However, molecular testing is now frequently utilized for this purpose.

Diagnosis and Classification of Spinal Muscular Atrophy

The diagnosis of MA is conducted through the evaluation of patients by analyzing their medical history and performing genetic testing. Since there are five different kinds of SMA that can develop in patients, it is crucial to identify the specific gene responsible for SMA. Previously, muscle biopsy and electromyography (EMG) were commonly used for detecting spinal muscular atrophy (SMA). However, molecular testing is now widely employed for this purpose (Angilletta I. et al., 2023).

Clinical Evaluation and Symptomatology

As homozygous loss of function of the SMN1 gene is caused by SMA patients, genetic testing will reveal proof of confirmation of SMA.

Some general outcomes include proximal predominance weakness, reduction of absent refluxes, tongue fasciculations, limb tremor is typical with SMA. In SMA weakens the muscles including hips, shoulders, thighs with progressions in SMA it might impact breathing and swallowing which is life threatening for patient (Burglen L. et al., 1996).

As this sickness is associated to genetic disorder. For evaluation of presence of SMA. Molecular diagnostics is done to detect SMN1 gene deletion. If homozygous deletion is identified by SMN1 gene deletion testing, then it is proven the presence of SMA. If it is not passed, then SMN dosage testing and sequencing of SMN gene is done to detect mutation of gene (Mendell et al., 2017).

Genetic Testing and Diagnostic Tools

The SMN1 gene is primarily responsible for causing spinal muscular atrophy (SMA). Patients must undergo genetic testing to diagnose the deletion of the SMN1 gene. Genetic testing can be used to identify and prevent mortality or disability in newborns affected with SMA. If parents possess this gene, genetic testing is conducted based on the family history record to identify the defective gene (Darras B. T. et al., 2017, Jedrzejowska M. et al., 2008).

Classification of SMA Types (Type 0, Type 1, Type 2. Type 3. Type 4)

As per phenotype variation SMA can classified into several types (Type 0 to type 5).

Type 0

This is also called Congenital SMA. Age of onset of this type of SMA is before birth. This is a rare phenotype where respiratory problem occurs at first and rather it leads to death within some weeks (Dubowitz V., 1999).

Type 1

This is also classified into Ia, Ib (Onset <3 months), Ic (Onset 3-6 months) as per onset of age. This type of SMA presents in the first six months of life. Severe hypotonia occurs and which ultimately made action to unable to sit or roll. The weakness of intercostals muscle leads to breathing pattern dysfunction and bell-shaped chest. It can also lead to death within 2 years.

Type 2

It is known as dubowitz disease which occurs generally at 6 months to 8 months old. In this type, patient can sit but proximal weakness affects legs over arms which can cause problem in walking. Around 70% patients survive until age of 25 years.

Type 3

It is known as Kugelberg-Welander Disease which occurs after 18 months. Like type 2, proximal weakness occurs which affects legs over arms. Patients may loses ability to walk. Type 3 subdivided into IIIa (<3 years onset), IIIb (>3 years onset), IIIc (>1 years onset).

Type 4

It is the mild phenotype of SMA occurs in patients >30 years or 0-30 years old. Mild motor impairment occurs in this stage (Groen et al., 2018).

Supportive Care and Symptomatic Management

SMA sufferers require supportive care from healthcare experts and other individuals in order to manage their condition and live with SMA. Patients with spinal muscular atrophy who rely on wheelchairs may encounter numerous obstacles when traveling to the clinic or engaging in other activities. Professionals should undergo thorough training and possess significant expertise in order to effectively handle individuals with Spinal Muscular Atrophy (SMA) (Darras B. T. et al., 2019).

Respiratory Care and Pulmonary Support

As SMA is related with muscle weakening and atrophy, respiratory muscles are also connected with this type of symptom, which further advances to cough difficulty due to poor clearance of airway secretions.

Breathing problems occur. Regular respiratory tests need to be done for SMA patients by pulmonologists. One or a combination of therapies is needed to keep airways clear.

Nutritional Support and Gastrointestinal Management

Nutritional support is very much essential to maintain proper nutritional intake. Sufficient levels of calcium and vitamin D must be taken to maintain body mass index. Several gastrointestinal consequences are connected with SMA patients, include constipation, delayed stomach emptying, dysphagia, and GER. These symptoms can induce an increased risk of aspiration, which leads to mortality. SMA patients who are non-sitters are assessed by VFSS (videofluoroscopic swallowing study) if dysphagia arises. Food that increases GER should be avoided to get rid of malnutrition and other issues (Ross & Kwon, 2019).

Orthopedic Considerations and Physical Therapies

Muscle weakness and muscle atrophy are the major problem related with SMA. Muscle strength can be enhanced via physical treatments. Aquatherapy and hippotherpy are done as physical therapy which helps to increase the body mobility (Fujak A. et al., 2010).

Psychological Support for Patients and Families

SMA is juvenile disease and patient can suffer from the beginning phase of his existence, family support is very much important for this situation. As the patient is unable to movement, physically he needs a substantial support from the family for move within dwelling. Beside that family members need to make assist patients to enhance his vitality for live. This will help sufferers to live (Sari, D. M. et al., 2022).

Disease Modifying Therapies

Therapy of SMA is extremely complex since different forms of functional motor impairment develops during therapy procedure. The Food and Drug Administration (FDA) has approved three therapies: Nusinersen, Onasemnogene abeparvovec, Risidiplam. Nusinersin is intrathecally administrated, Onasemnogene abeparvovec is administrated intravenously whilst ridiplasm is administrated orally to treat SMA patients (Tisdale S., 2015).

Nusinersen (Spinarza): Mechanism of Action and Clinical Efficacy

Nusinersen is first approved USFDA medicine to treat children and adults with SMA. This is sold as Spinarza which is intrathecally administrated used to treat SMA. Nusinersen is a survival motor neuron 2 (SMN2) antisense oigonucleotie (ASO). As SMA occurs due to shortage of SMN protein, nusinersen has an influence on SMN2 mRNA by boosting exon inclusion and help to produce full length of SMN protein. It help to replenish the SMN protein. Nusinersen aid to replace the SMN protein shortage for SMA patients by acting as a splice altering oligonucleotide. It directly works as targeting sequence on SMN2 pre mRNA by displacing heterogenous ribonucleoproteins at intronic splice silencing site 1 (ISS1). It demonstrates biphasic pharmacokinetics in plasma. Beside that its processed by hydrolysis and removed by urine excretion and it has no known interaction with CYP450 enzymes. (Messina & Sframeli, 2020, Chiriboga C. A. et al., 2019, De Vivo D. C., et al., 2019).

Risdiplam (Evrysdi): A Novel Treatment Approach

Ridiplasm is the first oral FDA-approved medication to treat SMA. It is licensed for the treatment of children as well as adults. Risdiplam enhances the SMN protein concentration by enhancing the effectiveness of SMN2 gene transcription.

The key advantage of Risdiplam rather than Nusinersen, that is administrated by oral route where Nusinersen need to administer through intrathecal route. It has been proven that, in clinical trails that risdiplam enhanced motor function greatly in newborns with SMA1 and for the adult patients with SMA type 2 or 3. Risdiplam operates by binding in two places in SMN2 pre mRNA in the exonic splicing enhancer 2 in exon 7 and 5' splice site in intron 7. It act by extending full length of SMN2 mRNA and enhancing functional SMA protein and also stimulates the inclusion of exon 7' (Parente & Corti, 2018).

Onasemnogene Abeparvovec (Zolgensma): Gene Replacement Therapy

Onasemnogene Abeparvovec is USFDA authorized medicine which is administrated intravenously for treatment of SMA. This medicine is developed by Novartis under trade name of Zolgensma. Onasemnogene Abeparvovec is a adenoassociated virus vector based gene therapy that can copy human SMN gene into specific motor neuron cells. This one-time intravenous injection can enhance muscle mobility and function for SMA sufferers. It can be provided for the youngsters more than 2 years age. It exhibited a significant improvement in motor functioning. But it has harmful effects like vomiting and liver impairment. For that reason, liver dysfunction should be checked for at least after 3 months of administration (Parente & Corti, 2018, Strauss K. A., et al., 2022).

Emerging Therapies and Future Directions

Beside this medicines now-a-days new effective therapies are introduced for challenging in SMA. Olesoxime a newly created steroid similar chemical has demonstrated its great usefulness in mice model and later in human model to enhance neurological factor on SMA patients. Docosahexaenoic acid (DHA) also help in neural growth. Dietary dietary treatments also assisted to improve in neuroprotection (Ramdas S., 2020, DiDonato C. J. et al., 1997).

Adjunctive Therapies and Complementary Approaches

Spinal Muscular Atrophy (SMA) is a hereditary condition distinguished by muscular weakness and atrophy as a result of the progressive deterioration of motor neurons. The comprehensive care of spinal muscular atrophy (SMA) necessitates the implementation of a multidisciplinary strategy, wherein physical therapy and occupational therapy assume crucial roles in augmenting the overall quality of life, promoting functional independence, and mitigating the occurrence of problems (Mercuri et al., 2020, Rao V. K., 2018).

Physical and Occupational Therapy

Physical treatment has the potential to enhance muscle strength, range of motion, and endurance among those diagnosed with spinal muscular atrophy (SMA). Additionally, it has the potential to aid in the prevention or correction of scoliosis, a spinal curvature that frequently occurs in individuals diagnosed with SMA (Scoto et al., 2017).

Occupational therapy has been shown to be beneficial in facilitating the acquisition of essential skills related to activities of daily living for those diagnosed with spinal muscular atrophy (SMA). These skills encompass various self-care tasks, including but not limited to dressing, bathing, and eating. Additionally, it can assist individuals in modifying their residential surroundings to enhance accessibility (Arnold & Fischbeck, 2018).

Assistive Devices and Mobility Aids

Assistive equipment and mobility aids play a crucial role in augmenting the autonomy and overall well-being of individuals diagnosed with spinal muscular atrophy (SMA). Mobility difficulties frequently manifest as a result of muscle weakness. Wheelchairs, braces, and orthotics serve as assistive devices that offer assistance in facilitating movement and maintaining proper posture. Powered mobility devices facilitate increased independence and self-sufficiency. Customized adaptations, such as the installation of ramps and the provision of accessible vehicles, serve to enhance accessibility. The involvement of occupational therapists in the process of device selection and training is essential to provide optimal outcomes. These assistive devices enable individuals with Spinal Muscular Atrophy (SMA) to surmount physical constraints, actively partake in everyday tasks, and achieve complete involvement in their respective communities (Mercuri et al., 2022).

Speech and Swallowing Therapy

The implementation of speech and swallowing therapy is of utmost importance for patients diagnosed with spinal muscular atrophy (SMA). The presence of muscle weakness in the throat and mouth region can give rise to challenges in both the act of speaking and the process of swallowing, so impacting an individual's ability to effectively communicate and maintain enough nutrition. Speech therapists evaluate these difficulties and create customized exercises to enhance vocal regulation, articulation, and coordination of swallowing. The techniques employed encompass modifications in posture, exercises aimed at strengthening the relevant muscles, and the implementation of adaptive measures to ensure safe swallowing. The implementation of speech and swallowing treatment has been shown to improve the overall quality of life for individuals by facilitating efficient communication and reducing the risk of issues associated with aspiration and malnutrition (Iftikhar et al., 2021).

Nutritional Supplements and Dietary Interventions

The utilization of nutritional supplements and dietary modifications plays a crucial role in the management of spinal muscular atrophy (SMA). Nutritional status might be adversely affected by the presence of muscle weakness and difficulty with swallowing. High-calorie, high-protein supplements have been found to be beneficial in meeting energy requirements and supporting muscle preservation. Customized dietary plans take into account the presence of dysphagia, providing appropriate food consistencies to mitigate the risk of aspiration. Dietitians engage in collaborative efforts with healthcare teams to develop individualized dietary regimens, while also overseeing the progress of growth and nutritional well-being. These interventions aim to maximize health outcomes, facilitate growth, and mitigate potential consequences. When incorporated into the care provided by SMA, these interventions have a substantial impact on the overall well-being and quality of life of persons (Govoni et al., 2018).

Gene Therapies and Gene Editing Strategies

Spinal muscular atrophy (SMA) exhibits potential for therapeutic intervention through the utilization of gene therapies and gene editing methods. Gene treatments, such as onasemnogene abeparvovec (Zolgensma), are designed with the objective of introducing a functional SMN gene into the body to rectify the hereditary defect responsible for spinal muscular atrophy (SMA). Gene editing technologies, such as CRISPR-Cas9, have the capability to accurately manipulate the defective SMN gene present in the cells of individuals. Nevertheless, there are still other issues that need to be addressed, including the optimization of delivery methods, the examination of long-term consequences, and the careful evaluation of ethical implications. Ongoing research endeavours aim to further enhance these methodologies, presenting novel opportunities for the therapy of spinal muscular atrophy (SMA) by targeting the fundamental genetic factors contributing to the development of the disorder (Rao et al., 2018, Lefebvre S. et al., 1995).

CRISPR-Cas9 and Other Gene Editing Techniques

The potential therapeutic applications of CRISPR-Cas9 and other gene editing methodologies in the treatment of spinal muscular atrophy (SMA) are considerable. The utilization of CRISPR-Cas9 facilitates the accurate alteration of the defective SMN gene, which is accountable for spinal muscular atrophy (SMA), with the potential to rectify the genetic mutation and reinstate the manufacture of normal SMN protein. Additional gene editing techniques, such as base editing and prime editing, provide more precise alterations to DNA without the requirement of introducing exogenous genetic material (Li et al., 2020).

Nevertheless, there are several problems that need to be addressed in order to achieve success in this endeavor. These challenges encompass the need to ensure precise targeting, minimize any unintended effects on non-targeted areas, and build a long-term safety and efficacy profile. The ethical implications surrounding germline editing and its potential unintended consequences necessitate thorough evaluation (Zhou et al., 2018).

The establishment of strong partnerships among researchers, physicians, and regulatory entities is vital in order to progress these methodologies and facilitate their transformation into secure and efficacious therapies for individuals and families impacted by spinal muscular atrophy (SMA) (McMillan et al., 2022).

Challenges and Ethical Considerations

The application of gene treatments and gene editing techniques in the context of spinal muscular atrophy (SMA) poses significant obstacles and raises ethical concerns. The rigorous nature of ensuring therapeutic safety, efficacy, and long-term consequences arises from the quick rate of developments. The issue of affordability and healthcare inequities arises in relation to ensuring equitable access to medicines such as Zolgensma. There are ethical considerations that arise in relation to prenatal testing, germline editing, and the possibility for unforeseen repercussions. The conundrum of reconciling intrusive therapies with the preservation of quality of life poses ethical challenges for both patients and caregivers. The involvement and cooperation of researchers, doctors, policymakers, ethicists, and patient advocates are essential in order to effectively tackle these difficulties. The advancement of SMA treatments will be guided by values of transparency, open discourse, and ethical adherence, with a primary focus on promoting the well-being of persons and families impacted by the condition (Burgart et al., 2018, Schmalbruch H., 2001).

Stem Cell-Based Therapies

The utilization of stem cell-based therapies presents a potentially advantageous approach in the treatment of spinal muscular atrophy (SMA). Researchers have the ability to create motor neurons and muscle cells using pluripotent stem cells, namely induced pluripotent stem cells (iPSCs), with the aim of potentially replacing or providing support to impaired cells. The objective of these transplanted cells is to enhance motor function and mobility through the restoration of neurons that are lacking. Despite the existence of hurdles such as the need for effective integration, regulation of immune responses, and assuring long-term safety, these techniques demonstrate promise in tackling the fundamental underlying factors of spinal muscular atrophy (SMA). These endeavours hold promise for groundbreaking treatments that have the potential to significantly enhance the quality of life for those afflicted with Spinal Muscular Atrophy (SMA) (Han et al., 2020).

Stem Cell Transplantation: Current Research and Applications

The science of stem cell transplantation is experiencing fast advancements and holds significant promise for the treatment of spinal muscular atrophy (SMA). Contemporary scholarly investigations are mostly centered around the utilization of induced pluripotent stem cells (iPSCs) for the purpose of generating motor neurons and muscle cells, with the aim of replacing those that have been compromised or impaired. The objective of these transplanted cells is to reinstate motor function and enhance muscular strength. Furthermore, there is ongoing research into the utilization of exosome-based therapies originating from stem cells with the aim of promoting the release of therapeutic factors that can enhance the survival of motor neurons. Clinical trials play a crucial role in substantiating the safety and effectiveness of stem cell transplantation, thereby providing a promising avenue for groundbreaking therapeutic interventions that have the potential to transform the management of spinal muscular atrophy (SMA) by directly addressing the fundamental cellular deficiencies associated with the disease (Adami & Bottai, 2019; Scoto et al., 2017).

Induced Pluripotent Stem Cells (iPSCs) and Their Potential in SMA

The utilization of induced pluripotent stem cells (iPSCs) exhibits significant potential in the domain of spinal muscular atrophy (SMA) investigation and therapy. The aforementioned cells, which have undergone reprogramming from mature cells, have the capacity to undergo differentiation into motor neurons that closely resemble the cells damaged by spinal muscular atrophy (SMA). Induced pluripotent stem cells (iPSCs) offer a highly valuable platform for investigating the underlying mechanisms of diseases, conducting drug screening experiments, and gaining insights on individual variations (Zhou et al., 2018).

Researchers have the ability to utilize these tools in order to advance and refine treatment methodologies, such as gene editing and drug testing, that are specifically customized to suit the distinct genetic composition of individual patients (Adami & Bottai, 2019; Ando et al., 2017).

Furthermore, induced pluripotent stem cells (iPSCs) have the capacity to create motor neurons that can be utilized for transplantation purposes, thereby refilling the diminished pool of neurons in individuals affected with spinal muscular atrophy (SMA). With the progression of research, induced pluripotent stem cells (iPSCs) have emerged as a promising route for exploring Spinal Muscular Atrophy (SMA), providing valuable insights into the disease and presenting novel opportunities for developing personalized therapeutic interventions that address the fundamental cellular deficits associated with SMA (Lin et al., 2017).

Clinical Trials and Research Initiatives

The importance of clinical trials and research endeavours in the field of spinal muscular atrophy (SMA) cannot be overstated, as they play a pivotal role in the advancement of our comprehension and therapeutic approaches to this hereditary condition. These endeavours involve a range of methods, comprising gene therapies such as onasemnogene abeparvovec (Zolgensma) and small molecule medications like risdiplam and nusinersen (Spinraza). The research also places emphasis on the optimization of supportive care measures, including respiratory assistance and physical treatments, with the aim of improving the overall quality of life.). The establishment of collaborative partnerships between research institutions, pharmaceutical firms, and advocacy groups plays a crucial role in ensuring the effective execution of clinical trials. These attempts possess the potential to enhance therapeutic interventions and offer a more optimistic outlook for individuals impacted by Spinal Muscular Atrophy (SMA) (Pechmann et al., 2019).

Overview of Current Clinical Trials

The present clinical studies in the field of spinal muscular atrophy (SMA) involve a wide range of therapies. Gene treatments, such as onasemnogene abeparvovec (commonly known as Zolgensma), have the objective of substituting the defective SMN1 gene. The research also places emphasis on the use of supportive care measures, such as interventions targeting respiratory function and physical therapies. The trials are evaluating the efficacy of assistive devices, rehabilitation programs, and medications targeted towards certain subtypes of spinal muscular atrophy (SMA). The establishment of effective partnerships between research institutions, pharmaceutical corporations, and patient advocacy groups is crucial for the successful implementation of clinical trials. These clinical trials provide optimism for the development of efficacious therapies and contribute to the advancement of our comprehension of spinal muscular atrophy (SMA) and its intricacies (Shorrock et al., 2018, Issa S. S. et al., 2023).

Promising Research Areas and Innovations

The field of spinal muscular atrophy (SMA) is now witnessing significant advancements in research fields and inventions, which have the potential to greatly transform treatment options. Gene therapies, encompassing gene replacement and editing methodologies, possess the capacity to rectify the fundamental genetic anomaly. The primary objective of stem cell therapies is to reinstate motor function, and the advancement in comprehending various subtypes of spinal muscular atrophy (SMA) is facilitating the development of individualized therapeutic approaches. The aforementioned improvements collectively instill a sense of optimism regarding the potential for enhanced therapies, results, and overall well-being among persons and families impacted by SMA (Ramdas & Servais, 2020; Scoto et al., 2017).

Comprehensive Care and a Multidisciplinary Approach

The provision of comprehensive care for spinal muscular atrophy (SMA) necessitates the adoption of a multidisciplinary strategy, wherein a collective of medical professionals, therapists, and caretakers work together to effectively address the intricate requirements of patients. A collaborative effort is undertaken by medical practitioners, including neurologists, pulmonologists, therapists, and social workers, with the aim of enhancing the overall well-being of individuals, addressing symptoms, and offering comprehensive assistance throughout the course of the illness. The implementation of a comprehensive, collaborative strategy guarantees a holistic and individualized care plan that encompasses the physiological, psychological, and sociological aspects of SMA (Ropars et al., 2020).

Establishing SMA Care Centers

The establishment of care facilities dedicated to spinal muscular atrophy (SMA) is of utmost importance in order to enhance the quality of care provided to those affected by this condition. These specialized centers facilitate the collaboration of diverse medical specialists, therapists, and support workers to deliver comprehensive care that is specifically designed to address the intricate requirements of individuals with SMA. Additionally, these centers foster a collaborative atmosphere, facilitating the development of tailored treatment programs that encompass disease-modifying medications, symptom alleviation, and rehabilitation services. In addition, these centers play a crucial role in promoting research, providing educational opportunities, and offering essential support services for both patients and caregivers. Through the consolidation of knowledge and allocation of resources, care centers for spinal muscular atrophy (SMA) strive to achieve optimal standards of care and enhance outcomes for persons affected by SMA (Mercuri et al., 2018; Pechmann et al., 2019).

Collaboration Between Healthcare Providers and Support Organizations

The establishment of effective collaboration between healthcare providers and support groups is of utmost importance in the context of spinal muscular atrophy (SMA). Healthcare providers deliver comprehensive medical knowledge, develop individualized treatment strategies, and administer therapeutic measures. The establishment of this collaboration facilitates the development of an all-encompassing support network that amplifies the availability of specialized healthcare services, educational resources, and community involvement opportunities. The provision of holistic care for individuals with Spinal Muscular Atrophy (SMA) is facilitated, hence promoting a sense of community and shared understanding among patients, caregivers, and healthcare providers. Collectively, they collaborate in pursuit of enhanced results and an enhanced standard of living for individuals impacted by SMA (Murrell et al., 2018; Ropars et al., 2020).

Addressing the Lifelong Challenges of SMA

A comprehensive strategy is necessary to effectively address the enduring problems associated with spinal muscular atrophy (SMA). The use of early intervention strategies including disease-modifying medications, such as gene therapy or small molecules, has the potential to affect the trajectory of disease progression. The optimization of quality of life and independence can be achieved through the collaborative efforts of medical specialists, therapists, and caretakers. Furthermore, the continuous investigation and advocacy initiatives by researchers and patient advocates contribute to the development of therapies and the promotion of knowledge, guaranteeing that individuals affected by spinal muscular atrophy (SMA) obtain the essential healthcare and support required to effectively manage the distinct obstacles they face throughout their lifespan (Wan et al., 2019, Ottesen E. W. et al., 2023).

Enhancing Quality of Life for SMA Patients and Families

Improving the overall well-being of individuals with Spinal Muscular Atrophy (SMA) and their families necessitates the implementation of a holistic strategy. The enhancement of physical well-being is facilitated by disease-modifying therapies, the collaboration of multidisciplinary care teams, and the utilization of assistive technologies. Psychological needs are effectively addressed through the provision of emotional support, counseling services, and the establishment of peer networks. t. Through the integration of medical interventions, comprehensive support systems, and continuous research efforts, individuals diagnosed with Spinal Muscular Atrophy (SMA) and their families are able to effectively negotiate the challenges associated with the condition, thereby experiencing enhanced autonomy, greater emotional welfare, and a heightened sense of interconnectedness and self-empowerment (Aksaralikitsunti & Sanmaneechai, 2022).

The Importance of Palliative Care

Palliative care assumes a critical function in the management of spinal muscular atrophy (SMA) by offering comprehensive assistance to individuals and their families as they confront the difficulties associated with a degenerative and intricate ailment. The primary objective of this approach is to improve the overall well-being of individuals by addressing symptoms, alleviating pain, providing psychological and emotional assistance, and facilitating effective communication regarding available treatment alternatives. Palliative care is a comprehensive approach that attends to the physical, emotional, social, and spiritual dimensions of patients with SMA and their families, facilitating their journey with dignity and comfort. Consequently, it enhances the overall well-being and satisfaction of those affected with spinal muscular atrophy (SMA) (Van der Heul et al., 2020).

Social and Emotional Support for Patients and Caregivers

The provision of social and emotional support is of utmost importance for individuals suffering with spinal muscular atrophy (SMA) as well as their careers. Effectively managing a progressive condition necessitates the presence of a robust support system that provides individuals with comprehension, compassion, and a secure environment in which to articulate their emotions. SMA) and their carers can successfully navigate the many emotional dimensions associated with this condition. This fosters a sense of resilience, leading to an overall improvement in their state of well-being and an enhanced capacity to effectively cope with the challenges imposed by SMA (Madruga-Garrido et al., 2021).

Advocacy and Policy Efforts

The advancement of the well-being of individuals with spinal muscular atrophy (SMA) is contingent upon the crucial role played by advocacy and policy actions. Advocacy groups engage in activities aimed at increasing public knowledge, obtaining financial resources for research endeavours,' and advocating for legislative modifications that enhance the availability of therapies, support services, and insurance benefits. Furthermore, advocacy endeavours' foster partnerships among researchers, healthcare practitioners, and patient populations (Mercuri et al., 2019).

Conclusion

The disease spinal muscular atrophy which affects both nerves and muscles causing muscles to become increasingly weak. It mostly affects infants and children but also develops in adult persons.

Recapitulation of Key Points

Spinal Muscular Therapy, Understanding the Pathophysiology, Diagnosis and classification, Disease Modifying therapies, Adjunctive therapies, Gene Therapies.

The Road Ahead: A Vision for the Future

The standard of care for SMA will soon be an early diagnosis utilising newborn screening, followed by an immediate start to treatment with new medications. However, since there are instances where the new medications are insufficiently effective, it is vital to keep developing SMA therapy options.

References

Adami, R., & Bottai, D. (2019). Spinal muscular atrophy modeling and treatment advances by induced pluripotent stem cells studies. *Stem Cell Reviews and Reports*, 15(6), 795-813.

Aksaralikitsunti, M., & Sanmaneechai, O. (2022). Health-related quality of life in Thai children with spinal muscular atrophy. *Pediatrics & Neonatology*, 63(3), 291-297.

Ando, S., Funato, M., Ohuchi, K., Kameyama, T., Inagaki, S., Seki, J., Kawase, C., Tsuruma, K., Shimazawa, M., & Kaneko, H. (2017). Edaravone is a candidate agent for spinal muscular atrophy: *In vitro* analysis using a human induced pluripotent stem cells-derived disease model. *European journal of pharmacology*, 814, 161-168.

Angilletta I, Ferrante R, Giansante R, Lombardi L, Babore A, Dell'Elice A, Alessandrelli E, Notarangelo S, Ranaudo M, Palmarini C, De Laurenzi V, Stuppia L, Rossi C. (2023). Spinal Muscular Atrophy: An Evolving Scenario through New Perspectives in Diagnosis and Advances in Therapies . *Int J Mol Sci.*;24(19):14873.

Arnold, E. S., & Fischbeck, K. H. (2018). Spinal muscular atrophy. *Handbook of clinical neurology,* 148, 591-601.

Baranello, G., Darras, B. T., Day, J. W., Deconinck, N., Klein, A., Masson, R., Mercuri, E., Rose, K., El-Khairi, M., & Gerber, M. (2021). Risdiplam in type 1 spinal muscular atrophy. *New England Journal of Medicine,* 384(10), 915-923.

Burgart, A. M., Magnus, D., Tabor, H. K., Paquette, E. D.-T., Frader, J., Glover, J. J., Jackson, B. M., Harrison, C. H., Urion, D. K., & Graham, R. J. (2018). Ethical challenges confronted when providing nusinersen treatment for spinal muscular atrophy. *JAMA pediatrics*, 172(2), 188-192.

Burglen, L., Lefebvre S., Clermont O., et al., (1996) Structure and organization of the human survival motor neurone (SMN) gene. *Genomics.* 32(3):479–482.

Chiriboga, C. A., Mercuri E., Fischer D., et al., (2019) P.363JEWELFISH: safety and pharmacodynamic data in patients with spinal muscular atrophy (SMA) receiving treatment with risdiplam (RG7916) that have previously been treated with nusinersen. *Neuromuscul Disord.* 29:S187.

Darras, B. T., Monani, U. R., & Darryl, C. (2017). Genetic disorders affecting the motor neuron: spinal muscular atrophy. In *Swaiman's pediatric neurology*, 3(11),1057-1064

Darras, B. T., Farrar M. A., Mercuri E., et al., (2019) An integrated safety analysis of infants and children with symptomatic Spinal Muscular Atrophy (SMA) treated with nusinersen in seven clinical trials. *CNS Drugs*. 33(9):919–932.

Darryl, C., Bertini, E., Swoboda, K. J., Hwu, W. L., Crawford, T. O., Finkel, R. S., ... & NURTURE Study Group. (2019). Nusinersen initiated in infants during the presymptomatic stage of spinal muscular atrophy: Interim efficacy and safety results from the Phase 2 NURTURE study. *Neuromuscular Disorders,* 29(11), 842-856.

DiDonato, C. J., Ingraham S. E., Mendell J. R., et al., (1997) Deletion and conversion in spinal muscular atrophy patients: is there a relationship to severity? *Ann Neurol.* 41(2):230–237.

Dubowitz V., (1999) Very severe spinal muscular atrophy (SMA type 0): an expanding clinical phenotype. *Eur J Paediatr Neurol.* 3(2):49–51.

D'Amico, A., Mercuri, E., Tiziano, F. D., & Bertini, E. (2011). Spinal muscular atrophy. *Orphanet journal of rare diseases,* 6, 1-10.

Farrar, M. A., Park, S. B., Vucic, S., Carey, K. A., Turner, B. J., Gillingwater, T. H., Swoboda, K. J., & Kiernan, M. C. (2017). Emerging therapies and challenges in spinal muscular atrophy. *Annals of neurology,* 81(3), 355-368.

Fujak A, Forst R, Forst J. (2010). Current strategies of conservative and operative treatment of the most frequent muscular disorders. *Orthopade.* 39(1), 38–52.

Govoni, A., Gagliardi, D., Comi, G. P., & Corti, S. (2018). Time is motor neuron: therapeutic window and its correlation with pathogenetic mechanisms in spinal muscular atrophy. *Molecular neurobiology,* 55, 6307-6318.

Groen, E. J., Talbot, K., & Gillingwater, T. H. (2018). Advances in therapy for spinal muscular atrophy: promises and challenges. *Nature Reviews Neurology,* 14(4), 214-224.

Han, F., Ebrahimi-Barough, S., Abolghasemi, R., Ai, J., & Liu, Y. (2020). Cell-based therapy for spinal muscular atrophy. *Stem Cell-based Therapy for Neurodegenerative Diseases,* 117-125.

Iftikhar, M., Frey, J., Shohan, M. J., Malek, S., & Mousa, S. A. (2021). Current and emerging therapies for Duchenne muscular dystrophy and spinal muscular atrophy. *Pharmacology & Therapeutics,* 220, 107719.

Issa, S. S., Shaimardanova, A. A., Solovyeva, V. V., & Rizvanov, A. A. (2023). Various AAV serotypes and their applications in gene therapy: an overview. *Cells,* 12(5), 785.

Jedrzejowska, M., Borkowska J, Zimowski J, et al., (2008) Unaffected patients with a homozygous absence of the SMN1 gene. *Eur J Hum Genet.* 16(8):930–934.

Lefebvre, S., Bürglen, L., Reboullet, S., Clermont, O., Burlet, P., Viollet, L., ... & Melki, J. (1995). Identification and characterization of a spinal muscular atrophy-determining gene. *Cell,* 80(1), 155-165.

Li, J. J., Lin, X., Tang, C., Lu, Y. Q., Hu, X., Zuo, E., Li, H., Ying, W., Sun, Y., & Lai, L. L. (2020). Disruption of splicing-regulatory elements using CRISPR/Cas9 to rescue spinal muscular atrophy in human iPSCs and mice. *National science review,* 7(1), 92-101.

Lin, X., Li, J. J., Qian, W. J., Zhang, Q.-J., Wang, Z. F., Lu, Y. Q., Dong, E. L., He, J., Wang, N., & Ma, L. X. (2017). Modeling the differential phenotypes of spinal muscular atrophy with high-yield generation of motor neurons from human induced pluripotent stem cells. *Oncotarget,* 8(26), 42030.

Madruga-Garrido, M., Vázquez-Costa, J. F., Medina-Cantillo, J., Brañas, M., Cattinari, M. G., de Lemus, M., ... & Maurino, J. (2021). Design of a non-interventional study to validate a set of patient-and caregiver-oriented measurements to assess health outcomes in spinal muscular atrophy (SMA-TOOL Study). *Neurology and Therapy,* 10, 361-373.

McMillan, H. J., Proud, C. M., Farrar, M. A., Alexander, I. E., Muntoni, F., & Servais, L. (2022). Onasemnogene abeparvovec for the treatment of spinal muscular atrophy. *Expert Opinion on Biological Therapy,* 22(9), 1075-1090.

Mendell, J. R., Al-Zaidy, S., Shell, R., Arnold, W. D., Rodino-Klapac, L. R., Prior, T. W., Lowes, L., Alfano, L., Berry, K., & Church, K. (2017). Single-dose gene-replacement therapy for spinal muscular atrophy. *New England Journal of Medicine,* 377(18), 1713-1722.

Mercuri, E., Finkel, R., Scoto, M., Hall, S., Eaton, S., Rashid, A., Balashkina, J., Coratti, G., Pera, M. C., & Samsuddin, S. (2019). Development of an academic disease registry for spinal muscular atrophy. *Neuromuscular disorders,* 29(10), 794-799.

Mercuri, E., Finkel, R. S., Muntoni, F., Wirth, B., Montes, J., Main, M., Mazzone, E. S., Vitale, M., Snyder, B., & Quijano-Roy, S. (2018). Diagnosis and management of spinal muscular atrophy: Part 1: Recommendations for diagnosis, rehabilitation, orthopedic and nutritional care. *Neuromuscular disorders,* 28(2), 103-115.

Mercuri, E., Pera, M. C., Scoto, M., Finkel, R., & Muntoni, F. (2020). Spinal muscular atrophy - insights and challenges in the treatment era. *Nature Reviews Neurology,* 16(12), 706-715.

Mercuri, E., Sumner, C. J., Muntoni, F., Darras, B. T., & Finkel, R. S. (2022). Spinal muscular atrophy. *Nature Reviews Disease Primers,* 8(1), 52.

Messina, S., & Sframeli, M. (2020). New treatments in spinal muscular atrophy: positive results and new challenges. *Journal of clinical medicine,* 9(7), 2222.

Murrell, D. V., Crawford, C. A., Jackson, C. T., Lotze, T. E., & Wiemann, C. M. (2018). Identifying opportunities to provide family-centered care for families with children with type 1 spinal muscular atrophy. *Journal of pediatric nursing*, 43, 111-119.

Nicolau, S., Waldrop, M. A., Connolly, A. M., & Mendell, J. R. (2021, April). Spinal muscular atrophy. In *Seminars in pediatric neurology* (Vol. 37, p. 100878). WB Saunders.

Ottesen, E. W., Singh, N. N., Luo, D., Kaas, B., Gillette, B. J., Seo, J., ... & Singh, R. N. (2023). Diverse targets of SMN2-directed splicing-modulating small molecule therapeutics for spinal muscular atrophy. *Nucleic Acids Research*, 51(12), 5948-5980.

Parente, V., & Corti, S. (2018). Advances in spinal muscular atrophy therapeutics. *Therapeutic advances in neurological disorders,* 11, 1756285618754501.

Pechmann, A., König, K., Bernert, G., Schachtrup, K., Schara, U., Schorling, D., ... & Kirschner, J. (2019). SMArtCARE-A platform to collect real-life outcome data of patients with spinal muscular atrophy. *Orphanet journal of rare diseases*, 14, 1-6.

Prior, T. W., Leach, M. E., & Finanger, E. (2020). *Spinal muscular atrophy,* 03 (12) 16-20.

Ramdas, S., & Servais, L. (2020). New treatments in spinal muscular atrophy: an overview of currently available data. *Expert opinion on pharmacotherapy*, 21(3), 307-315.

Rao, V. K., Kapp, D., & Schroth, M. (2018). Gene therapy for spinal muscular atrophy: an emerging treatment option for a devastating disease. *Journal of managed care & specialty pharmacy*, 24(12-a Suppl), S3-S16.

Ropars, J., Peudenier, S., Genot, A., Barnerias, C., & Espil, C. (2020). Multidisciplinary approach and psychosocial management of spinal muscular atrophy (SMA). *Archives de Pédiatrie,* 27(7), 7S45-47S49.

Ross, L. F., & Kwon, J. M. (2019). Spinal muscular atrophy: Past, present, and future. *Neoreviews,* 20(8), e437-e451.

Scoto, M., Finkel, R., Mercuri, E., & Muntoni, F. (2017). Therapeutic approaches for spinal muscular atrophy (SMA). *Gene therapy,* 24(9), 514-519.

Sari, D. M., Wijaya, L. C. G., Sitorus, W. D. R., & Dewi, M. M. (2022). Psychological burden in spinal muscular atrophy patients and their families: A systematic review. *The Egyptian Journal of Neurology, Psychiatry and Neurosurgery*, 58(1), 140.

Schmalbruch, H., & Haase, G. (2001). Spinal muscular atrophy: present state. *Brain pathology*, 11(2), 231-247.

Shorrock, H. K., Gillingwater, T. H., & Groen, E. J. (2018). Overview of current drugs and molecules in development for spinal muscular atrophy therapy. *Drugs,* 78(3), 293-305.

Strauss, K. A., Farrar, M. A., Muntoni, F., Saito, K., Mendell, J. R., Servais, L., ... & Macek, T. A. (2022). Onasemnogene abeparvovec for presymptomatic infants with two copies of SMN2 at risk for spinal muscular atrophy type 1: the Phase III SPR1NT trial. *Nature medicine*, 28(7), 1381-1389.

Tisdale, S., & Pellizzoni, L. (2015). Disease mechanisms and therapeutic approaches in spinal muscular atrophy. *Journal of Neuroscience*, 35(23), 8691-8700.

Van der Heul, A., Cuppen, I., Wadman, R., Asselman, F., Schoenmakers, M., van de Woude, D., Gerrits, E., van der Pol, W., & Van den Engel-Hoek, L. (2020). Feeding and swallowing problems in infants with spinal muscular atrophy type 1: an observational study. *Journal of Neuromuscular Diseases*, 7(3), 323-330.

Wan, H. W., Carey, K. A., D'Silva, A., Kasparian, N. A., & Farrar, M. A. (2019). "Getting ready for the adult world": how adults with spinal muscular atrophy perceive and experience healthcare, transition and well-being. *Orphanet journal of rare diseases,* 14(1), 1-13.

Wirth, B. (2021). Spinal muscular atrophy: in the challenge lies a solution. *Trends in neurosciences*, 44(4), 306-322.

Zhou, M., Hu, Z., Qiu, L., Zhou, T., Feng, M., Hu, Q., Zeng, B., Li, Z., Sun, Q., & Wu, Y. (2018). Seamless genetic conversion of SMN2 to SMN1 via CRISPR/Cpf1 and single-stranded oligodeoxynucleotides in spinal muscular atrophy patient-specific induced pluripotent stem cells. *Human gene therapy,* 29(11), 1252-1263.

Chapter 9

Recent Updates in the Chemistry of Alzheimer's Synthetic Molecule

Manish Kumar[1,*], PhD,
Nidhi Arora[2], M.Pharm,
Abhishek Tiwari[3], PhD,
Varsha Tiwari[3], PhD,
Beena Kumari[4], PhD,
and Mohit Agrawal[5]

[1]Department of Pharmaceutics, ISF College of Pharmacy, Moga, Punjab, India
[2]Chandigarh Pharmacy College, Chandigarh group of colleges, Jhanjeri, Mohali, India
[3]Amity Institute of Pharmacy, Lucknow, Amity University Uttar Pradesh, Sector 125, Noida-201313, Uttar Pradesh, India
[4]Deparment of Pharmaceutical Scinces, Indira Gandhi University, Meerpur, Rewari, Haryana, Inida
[5]School of Medical & Allied Sciences, K. R. Mangalam University, Gurugram, Haryana, India

Abstract

Alzheimer's disease (AD) is affecting millions of individual's worldwide, imposing significant socio-economic burdens on families and healthcare systems and thus known as progressive neurodegenerative disorder. The lack of effective treatments has driven extensive research into the development of synthetic molecules targeting various aspects of AD pathology. This abstract presents an overview of recent advancements in the chemistry of synthetic molecules designed to

* Corresponding Author's Email: manish_singh17@rediffmail.com.

In: Neurogenerative Disorders
Editors: Mohit Agrawal, Manmohan Singhal, Amit Kumar Nayak et al.
ISBN: 979-8-89530-143-2

combat Alzheimer's disease. The initial section of this abstract emphasizes the amyloid hypothesis, proposing that the buildup of amyloid-beta (Aβ) peptides significantly contributes to the development and advancement of AD. Scientists have concentrated their efforts on creating artificial compounds capable of disrupting Aβ aggregation, regulating Aβ elimination, or countering Aβ-associated harm. The second part highlights the significance of the tau protein in Alzheimer's disease pathology. When tau undergoes abnormal hyperphosphorylation and aggregation, it gives rise to neurofibrillary tangles, a key characteristic of AD. Lately, researchers have been focusing on chemical strategies to create tau kinase inhibitors, tau aggregation inhibitors, and other compounds that can stabilize tau in its natural form. Inflammation and oxidative stress are also crucial components of AD pathogenesis. Researchers have explored the chemistry of antioxidants, anti-inflammatory agents, and metal chelators as means to counteract the detrimental effects of reactive oxygen species and neuroinflammation, thereby protecting neurons from degeneration. Moreover, the blood-brain barrier (BBB) remains a significant challenge in the treatment of AD, limiting the delivery of therapeutics to the brain. New advancements in medicinal chemistry have led to the design of pro-drug strategies, nanoparticles, and BBB shuttle systems, enabling better drug delivery and enhancing the efficacy of potential AD treatments. Furthermore, the abstract sheds light on multifunctional molecules that target multiple pathological pathways simultaneously. These multi-target-directed ligands (MTDLs) aim to address the complex and multifactorial nature of AD, offering a more comprehensive approach to therapeutic intervention.

Keywords: Alzheimer's, clinical trials, artificial intelligence

Introduction

Overview of Alzheimer's Disease

Alzheimer's disease is a complex neurodegenerative disorder characterized by the accumulation of abnormal protein aggregates in the brain, specifically beta-amyloid plaques and tau tangles. Researchers have been actively working to develop synthetic molecules and compounds that can target these protein aggregates or modulate other key factors involved in the disease's progression. Here are some general trends and recent updates in the chemistry of Alzheimer's synthetic molecules.

The Importance of Synthetic Molecules in Alzheimer's Research

Synthetic molecules play a crucial role in Alzheimer's disease research by enabling scientists to explore potential therapeutic interventions, develop diagnostic tools, and enhance our understanding of the underlying mechanisms of the disease (Knapskog et al., 2021).

Drug Developmentl

Synthetic molecules are essential for the development of novel drug candidates targeting various aspects of Alzheimer's disease, such as amyloid-beta aggregation, tau protein tangles, neuro-inflammation, and oxidative stress (Jack Jr et al., 2018). These molecules can serve as potential leads for drug discovery programs. For instance, small molecules that inhibit the aggregation of amyloid-beta peptides have been investigated as potential therapeutics for Alzheimer's disease (Hardy et al., 2002).

Probe Development

Synthetic molecules are used to create specific probes or ligands that can bind to particular molecular targets, allowing researchers to visualize and study disease-related proteins *in vitro* and *in vivo* (Selkoe et al., 2016).

Biomarker Discovery

Synthetic molecules can be engineered to bind to specific biomarkers associated with Alzheimer's disease, aiding in the development of diagnostic tools for early disease detection (Hampel et al., 2004).

Mechanistic Studies

Synthetic molecules allow researchers to modulate specific pathways and processes in Alzheimer's disease models, helping to uncover the underlying molecular mechanisms (Cummings et al., 2014). This can lead to a deeper understanding of the disease and potential therapeutic targets (Ittner et al., 2011).

Structure-Activity Relationship Studies

Synthetic molecules can be modified to understand the structure-activity relationship, guiding the optimization of drug candidates for improved efficacy, specificity, and safety profiles (Copani et al., 1999).

Target Validation

Synthetic molecules can be used to validate potential drug targets by selectively manipulating their activity and observing the resulting effects on disease-related processes (Ballard et al., 2011).

Neurotransmitter Alterations in Alzheimer's Disease

Some of the key neurotransmitter alterations observed in Alzheimer's disease include:

Acetylcholine: One of the most well-studied neurotransmitter alterations in AD is the reduction of acetylcholine, a neurotransmitter that plays a crucial role in memory and cognitive functions (Bartus et al., 1982).

Glutamate: Glutamate is the brain's primary excitatory neurotransmitter and is essential for synaptic plasticity, learning, and memory. In AD, there is evidence of disrupted glutamate signalling, which can lead to excitotoxicity (excessive neuronal activity) and neuronal damage (Whitehouse et al., 1982).

It's important to note that these neurotransmitter alterations are complex and interconnected, and their interactions can vary among individuals with AD. However, developing effective treatments that can modify the course of the disease remains a challenge due to the multifaceted nature of AD and the complexity of neurotransmitter systems in the brain (Sarter et al., 2005).

Acetylcholine Deficiency and Cognitive Impairment

Cholinergic Hypothesis

The cholinergic hypothesis proposes that the primary cause of cognitive decline and memory deficits in AD is the degeneration of cholinergic neurons and subsequent deficiency of acetylcholine.

Cholinergic Neuron Degeneration

In AD, cholinergic neurons, especially those in the basal forebrain and nucleus basalis of Meynert, are particularly vulnerable and undergo degeneration. This leads to a substantial reduction in acetylcholine production and release.

Impact on Cognition

Acetylcholine plays a critical role in memory formation, learning, attention, and other cognitive functions. Its deficiency disrupts the proper functioning of neural circuits involved in memory consolidation and retrieval, leading to cognitive impairment.

Brain Regions Affected

Reduced acetylcholine levels predominantly affect brain regions associated with memory and cognition, including the hippocampus and neocortex. These areas are vital for forming and retrieving memories (Hardy et al., 2002).

Amyloid-Beta and Tau Proteins

Pathological Hallmarks

Amyloid-Beta (Aβ)

Aβ is a peptide derived from the amyloid precursor protein (APP) through enzymatic cleavage. Abnormal accumulation and aggregation of Aβ lead to the formation of plaques, a hallmark feature of AD.Aβ plaques are composed of aggregated Aβ peptides and are typically found between neurons in the brain, disrupting normal cell-to-cell communication (Grundke-Iqbal et al., 1986).

Tau Proteins

Tau is a microtubule-associated protein that helps stabilize microtubules, which are crucial for intracellular transport and maintaining neuronal structure. In AD, tau proteins become hyperphosphorylated, leading to their aggregation into neurofibrillary tangles (NFTs). NFTs disrupt the integrity of neurons and are strongly associated with cognitive decline.

Relationship Between Aβ and Tau

There is a close interplay between Aβ and tau pathology. Aβ accumulation is thought to trigger tau hyperphosphorylation and subsequent aggregation into NFTs (Jack Jr et al., 2018).

Neurotoxic Effects

Both Aβ and tau aggregates have neurotoxic effects. Aβ oligomers disrupt synapses and impair neural transmission, while tau aggregates destabilize the cytoskeleton and disrupt cellular transport mechanisms.

Biomarker Significance

Aβ and tau levels in cerebrospinal fluid (CSF) and brain imaging scans are used as biomarkers for AD diagnosis and progression. Aβ42/40 ratio in CSF and tau protein levels are commonly used biomarkers for AD pathology (Selkoe et al., 2001).

Current Therapeutic Strategies for the Management of Alzheimer's Disease

Several therapeutic strategies for Alzheimer's disease (AD) have been researched and are used to manage the condition. Keep in mind that the field of AD research is continuously evolving, and new developments may have occurred since then (Birks et al., 2016).

Cholinesterase Inhibitors

Cholinesterase inhibitors, such as donepezil, rivastigmine, and galantamine, are commonly prescribed for mild to moderate AD. These drugs work by increasing the levels of acetylcholine, a neurotransmitter that is reduced in AD, in the brain. These drugs work by increasing the levels of acetylcholine, a neurotransmitter that is reduced in Alzheimer's disease, in the brain (Burns et al., 1999; Rogers et al., 1998).

NMDA Receptor Antagonists

NMDA receptor antagonists are a class of drugs that modulate the activity of N-methyl-D-aspartate (NMDA) receptors in the brain. These receptors are involved in synaptic plasticity, learning, and memory. NMDA receptor antagonists have been explored as potential treatments for various neurological conditions, including Alzheimer's disease and certain types of pain disorders.

NMDA Receptors

NMDA receptors are a subtype of glutamate receptors found in the central nervous system. They play a crucial role in synaptic plasticity, which is essential for learning and memory (Reisberg et al., 2003).

Modulators of Amyloid-Beta Aggregation

Modulators of amyloid-beta (Aβ) aggregation are compounds or molecules that influence the formation and stability of Aβ aggregates, which are a central pathological feature of Alzheimer's disease (AD) (Tjernberg et al., 1996).

Aβ Aggregation in Alzheimer's Disease

Alzheimer's disease is characterized by the accumulation of Aβ peptides, which aggregate and form insoluble deposits called amyloid plaques in the brain (Bieschke et al., 2010).

Modulators of Aβ Aggregation

These compounds can be broadly categorized into two types:

Amyloid Inhibitors

These compounds interfere with the process of Aβ aggregation, preventing or slowing down the formation of toxic aggregates.

Amyloid Disruptors

These compounds destabilize existing Aβ aggregates, potentially promoting their clearance (Yang et al., 2005).

Recent Advances in the Chemistry of Alzheimer's Synthetic Molecules

Novel Approaches to Inhibit Amyloid-Beta Aggregation

Inhibiting amyloid-beta (Aβ) aggregation is a promising avenue of research for Alzheimer's disease treatment. Several novel approaches have been explored to achieve this goal (Habchi et al., 2017).

- Peptide-Based Inhibitors
- Small Molecule Inhibitors
- Natural Compounds and Polyphenols
- Metal Chelators
- RNA-Based Approaches
- Nanoparticles and Nanomaterials
- Antibodies and Immunotherapy
- Peptoid-Based Inhibitors (Alarcon-Esposito et al., 2021).

Small Molecule Tau Protein Inhibitors

Developing small molecule inhibitors for tau protein aggregation is another promising avenue of research for Alzheimer's disease (AD) treatment.

Methylene Blue

Methylene blue is a small molecule that has been investigated for its potential to inhibit tau aggregation. It is believed to work by binding to tau proteins and promoting their assembly into less toxic forms, thereby reducing the formation of tau aggregates (Hosokawa et al., 2012).

Leuco-Methylthioninium Bis (Hydromethanesulfonate) (LMTM)

LMTM, also known as TRx0237, is a tau aggregation inhibitor. It is thought to interact with tau and reduce its aggregation into neurofibrillary tangles (Gauthier et al., 2016).

Enhancing Neurotransmitter Function with Synthetic Compounds

Enhancing neurotransmitter function with synthetic compounds is a potential approach to Alzheimer's disease (AD) treatment, as neurotransmitter imbalances are associated with cognitive impairment in AD (Rosler et al., 1999).

- Cholinesterase Inhibitors
- NMDA Receptor Modulators (Reisberg et al., 2003).

Multi-Target-Directed Ligands for Alzheimer's Therapy

Compounds designed to interact with multiple molecular targets involved in the complex pathophysiology of Alzheimer's disease (AD) are known as Multi-Target-Directed Ligands (MTDLs). Their main aim is to address the heterogeneity of the disease and provide a more comprehensive approach to therapy.

Huprine X

Targets

Huprine X is a cholinesterase inhibitor and a β-amyloid aggregation inhibitor. It targets both cholinergic deficits and amyloid pathology in AD.

Ferulic Acid-Based MTDLs

Targets

Some synthetic compounds based on ferulic acid have been designed to target multiple aspects of AD, including acetylcholinesterase inhibition and antioxidant properties.

Curcumin-Based MTDLs

Targets
Curcumin-derived compounds have been investigated as MTDLs due to their potential to interact with various targets, including amyloid-beta, tau, and inflammation-related pathways (Tumiatti et al., 2010).

Structure-Activity Relationship (SAR) Studies

SAR Studies on Amyloid-Beta Inhibitors

Amyloid-beta (Aβ) inhibitors are compounds that target the aggregation of amyloid-beta peptides, which are thought to play a role in the development of Alzheimer's disease (Armstrong et al., 2011).

Here's a basic outline of SAR studies on amyloid-beta inhibitors.

Peptide-Based Inhibitors
Some inhibitors are based on peptide structures that mimic portions of the amyloid-beta peptide sequence. Modifications in the length, amino acid composition, and secondary structure of these peptides have been studied to determine their effects on inhibiting amyloid-beta aggregation.

Small Molecule Inhibitors
These are non-peptide compounds that have been studied as potential amyloid-beta inhibitors. SAR studies involve modifying functional groups, substituents, and other structural features to optimize the inhibitory activity (Imbimbo et al., 2007).

Natural Products
Some natural products have shown potential as amyloid-beta inhibitors. Researchers have explored the structural elements responsible for their inhibitory effects and used SAR studies to improve their potency and selectivity.

Hybrid Molecules
SAR studies have been conducted on hybrid molecules that combine features of both peptide-based and small molecule inhibitors. This approach aims to

leverage the advantages of both types of molecules to create more potent inhibitors.

Computational Modeling

In addition to experimental studies, computational modeling plays a crucial role in SAR studies. Molecular docking, molecular dynamics simulations, and other computational techniques help predict the binding modes of inhibitors and provide insights into their interactions with amyloid-beta (Yan et al., 2014).

SAR Studies on Tau Protein Inhibitors

Tau protein inhibitors are compounds designed to interfere with the aggregation or misfolding of tau proteins, which are implicated in neurodegenerative diseases like Alzheimer's disease and tauopathies. Tau protein aggregation is a hallmark of several neurodegenerative diseases, including Alzheimer's disease (Barten et al., 2012).

Microtubule Stabilizers

Compounds like paclitaxel and epothilone D act as microtubule stabilizers and indirectly inhibit tau aggregation. SAR studies have focused on improving their binding affinity and BBB penetration (Barten et al., 2012).

Small Molecules

Various small molecules, such as methylene blue derivatives and phenothiazines, have shown potential in inhibiting tau aggregation. SAR studies aim to optimize their structures for enhanced tau-binding specificity and reduced side effects (Crowe et al., 2009).

Peptide-Based Inhibitors

Peptide-based inhibitors, like those derived from the microtubule-binding region of tau, are under investigation. SAR studies explore modifications to increase their binding affinity and tau specificity (Chai et al., 2017; Crowe et al., 2013).

SAR Studies on Neurotransmitter Modulators

Neurotransmitter modulators are compounds designed to interact with and affect the activity of neurotransmitter receptors or transporters in the nervous system. These compounds can act as agonists, antagonists, or allosteric modulators (Owens et al., 2001).

Here's a basic outline of SAR studies on Neurotransmitter modulators.

Selective Serotonin Reuptake Inhibitors (SSRIs)

Compounds like fluoxetine (Prozac) and sertraline (Zoloft) are used to treat depression and anxiety by selectively inhibiting the serotonin transporter (SERT). (Owens et al., 2001).

Dopamine Receptor Agonists

Compounds like pramipexole and ropinirole are used to treat Parkinson's disease and restless legs syndrome by acting as agonists at dopamine receptors. (Wolinsky & Swanson, 2008) (Rang et al., 2011).

GABA Receptor Modulators

Benzodiazepines, such as diazepam (Valium), modulate GABA receptors and are used as anxiolytics and sedatives. (Harris et al., 2005; Li, Shiming 2015).

Advances in Drug Delivery Systems for Alzheimer's Molecules

Drug delivery systems for Alzheimer's disease have been a focus of research to improve the effectiveness of drug therapies while minimizing side effects (Roney et al., 2005).

Nanoparticle-Based Drug Delivery

Nanoparticles have shown promise as drug delivery vehicles for Alzheimer's disease (AD) therapy due to their ability to improve drug stability, enhance drug penetration across the blood-brain barrier, and provide controlled release (Shao et al., 2023).

Liposomes and Micelles in Alzheimer's Drug Delivery

Liposomes and micelles are widely studied as drug delivery systems for Alzheimer's disease due to their ability to encapsulate and deliver therapeutic agents to the brain, including potential drugs for Alzheimer's treatment (Misra et al., 2010).

Computational Approaches in Designing Alzheimer's Synthetic Molecules

Computational approaches have become invaluable in designing synthetic molecules for Alzheimer's disease (AD) treatment. These methods enable the prediction of molecular interactions, drug-receptor binding, and the optimization of compound properties.

Molecular Docking Studies

Molecular docking studies are a computational technique used in drug discovery and molecular biology to predict the binding mode and affinity of a small molecule (ligand) to a target protein or receptor (Morris et al., 1998).

Steps in Molecular Docking:

Preparation

Protein and ligand structures are prepared, including removing water molecules, assigning charges, and defining the binding site (Trott et al., 2010).

Search Space

The region around the binding site is defined as the search space, within which the ligand will be docked.

Conformational Sampling

The ligand is subjected to multiple conformations and orientations within the search space (Kitchen et al., 2004).

Scoring

Scoring functions evaluate the fitness of each ligand pose based on energy calculations and interactions with the protein.

Ranking

Ligand poses are ranked by their binding scores, and the most favorable poses are selected (Shoichet et al., 2004).

QSAR Modelling for Alzheimer's Drug Design

Computational techniques used in drug design, including for Alzheimer's disease (AD) drug discovery is known as Quantitative Structure-Activity Relationship (QSAR) modeling. QSAR models relate the structural features of chemical compounds to their biological activities, enabling the prediction of the activity of novel compounds (Roy et al., 2015).

Steps in QSAR Modeling:

Data Collection

High-quality experimental data on the biological activity of a set of compounds (e.g., IC50 values) and their chemical structures are collected.

Descriptor Calculation

Molecular descriptors, such as physicochemical properties, structural features, or fingerprints, are calculated for each compound in the dataset (Tropsha et al., 2010).

Data Splitting

Training and Test sets are the two typical divisions of the dataset in order to develop and validate the QSAR model, respectively.

Model Development

Various regression or classification techniques like multiple linear regression, support vector machines, random forests etc. are used to build the QSAR model by correlating the descriptors with the activity data (Peter et al., 2019).

Model Validation

The model's predictive power is assessed using the test set to ensure its reliability.

Model Interpretation

Important descriptors and their contributions to the activity prediction are analyzed to gain insights into the structure-activity relationship (Neves et al., 2018).

Artificial Intelligence and Machine Learning Applications

Artificial Intelligence (AI) and Machine Learning (ML) have gained prominence in Alzheimer's disease (AD) research and clinical practice. These technologies offer novel approaches for early diagnosis, drug discovery, prediction, and personalized treatment.

Early Diagnosis and Predictions

AI and ML algorithms can analyze various data sources, such as neuroimaging (MRI, PET scans), cerebrospinal fluid biomarkers, genetic data, and cognitive assessments, to identify early signs of AD or predict disease progression. These technologies can detect subtle patterns and changes that may not be apparent to human observers (Zhang et al., 2020).

Challenges and Future Perspectives

A complex neurodegenerative disorder with significant challenges in diagnosis, treatment, and care is known as Alzheimer's disease (AD). Here are some of the key challenges and future perspectives in Alzheimer's disease research and management (Pardridge et al., 2012).

Blood-Brain Barrier Penetration

Penetrating the blood-brain barrier (BBB) is a significant challenge in Alzheimer's disease (AD) drug development. The BBB acts as a protective barrier that limits the entry of many drugs into the brain (Wong et al., 2012).

Target Selectivity and Safety Concerns

Target selectivity and safety concerns are critical challenges in Alzheimer's disease (AD) drug development. Achieving specificity for pathological targets while minimizing off-target effects is essential for the success and safety of potential therapies (Hardy et al., 2002; Grill et al., 2010).

Combining Therapies for Synergistic Effects

Combining therapies for synergistic effects in Alzheimer's disease (AD) is an emerging approach aimed at addressing the complex and multifactorial nature of the disease (Cummings et al., 2018; Heneka et al., 2007; Winblad et al., 2016).

Case Studies of Promising Alzheimer's Molecules

Mechanism of Action and Preclinical Results

Alzheimer's disease is characterized by the progressive degeneration of brain cells, primarily due to two common mechanisms of action. Firstly, the accumulation of beta-amyloid plaques in the brain disrupts cell communication and triggers inflammation, leading to cell death. Secondly, the formation of neurofibrillary tangles, consisting of abnormal tau protein, disrupts the internal structure of neurons, impairing their function and causing cell death. These two mechanisms ultimately result in the loss of cognitive functions, memory decline, and the debilitating symptoms associated with Alzheimer's disease. Understanding these mechanisms is crucial for developing effective treatments and interventions for this devastating neurodegenerative condition (Figure 1).

Clinical trials are research studies conducted to evaluate the safety and effectiveness of new drugs. These trials are crucial for determining whether a new treatment is safe and effective for a specific medical condition (Soderberg et al., 2023) (Figure 2).

Blarcamesine hydrochloride: Blarcamesine hydrochloride is a drug that is undergoing clinical trials to assess its safety and efficacy for the treatment of a specific medical condition (1).

Valiltramiprosate appears to be another drug undergoing clinical trials. Similarly, specific information about its purpose, the phase of the trial, or the medical condition (2).

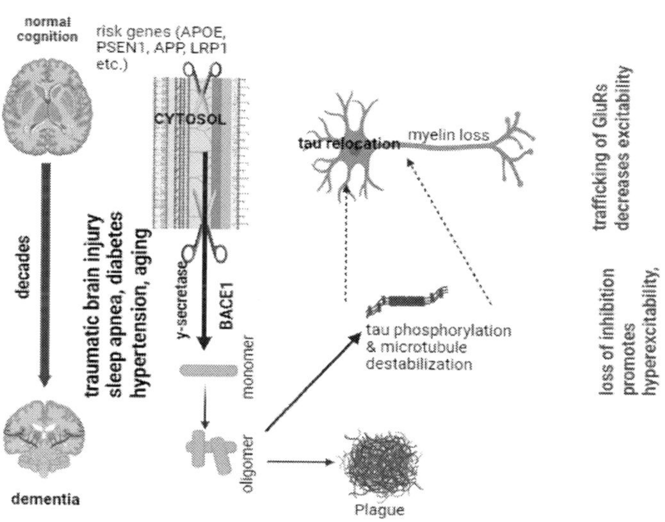

Figure 1. Mechanism of action Alzheimer disease.

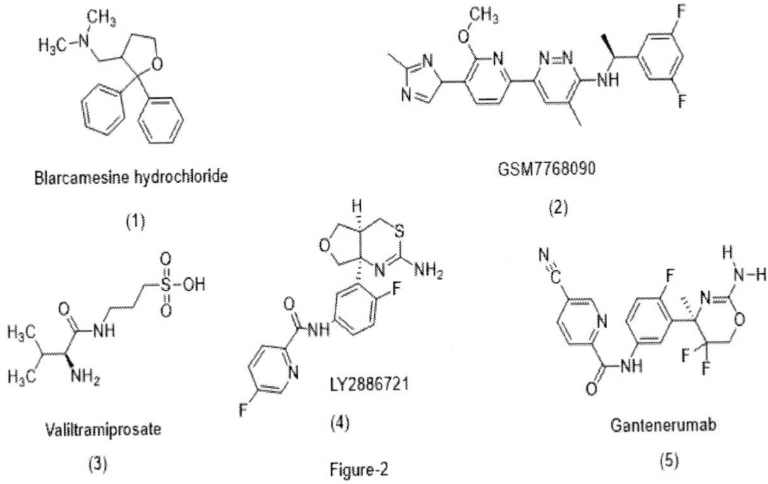

Figure 2. The Chemical structure data of clinical trials molecules.

Gantenerumab is a monoclonal antibody designed to target beta-amyloid plaques in the brain, which are associated with Alzheimer's disease. Clinical trials involving gantenerumab would be focused on testing its efficacy in slowing down or reducing the progression of Alzheimer's disease (3).

LY2886721 is a potential drug candidate developed by Eli Lilly and Company. It's important to note that the status of specific clinical trials may change over time (4).

GSM7768090: Similar to the other compounds, GSM7768090 appears to be a drug candidate undergoing clinical evaluation (5) (Brem et al., 2023).

Clinical Trials and Efficacy Data

This information provides an overview of the ongoing or recently completed clinical trials for various Alzheimer's disease therapeutics, with a focus on the duration of the trials, the number of participants, and the targeted mechanisms (Table 1).

Lecanemab is being investigated for its potential to target and reduce amyloid beta plaques, which are associated with the disease. The Phase III trial aims to evaluate its effectiveness over a 78-week period involving a substantial number of participants.

Table 1. Clinical trials data of Alzheimer drugs

Therapy	Event	Trail Length	Trial Size	Target
Eisai's lecanemab	Phase III results 4Q 2022	78 weeks	1,906 patients	Amyloid beta
Anavex's blarcamesine hydrochloride	Phase III results 4Q 2022	48 weeks	509 patients	Sigma-1 receptor
Alzheon's Valitramiprosate (ALZ-801)	Phase III results May 2021	78 weeks	650 patients	Amyloid beta
Roche's gantenerumab	Two Phase III results November 2022	116 weeks	1,966 patients	Amyloid beta
Eli Lilly's donanemab	Phase III results 2Q 2023	76 weeks	1,800 patients	Amyloid beta

Blarcamesine hydrochloride is being studied for its impact on the Sigma-1 receptor. The Phase III trial, spanning 48 weeks with over 500 participants, seeks to assess the drug's efficacy in the treatment of Alzheimer's disease.

Valitramiprosate (ALZ-801) completed its Phase III trial in May 2021, with a focus on amyloid beta. The trial, lasting 78 weeks and involving 650 participants, aimed to provide insights into the drug's potential in addressing Alzheimer's disease.

Gantenerumab, developed by Roche, is undergoing two Phase III trials, with results expected in November 2022. The trials span 116 weeks and involve a large cohort of 1,966 participants, focusing on the reduction of amyloid beta plaques.

Donanemab, developed by Eli Lilly, is currently in Phase III trials, with results expected in the second quarter of 2023. The trial, lasting 76 weeks and including 1,800 participants, aims to assess the drug's impact on amyloid beta in Alzheimer's disease.

These drugs are undergoing or have recently completed Phase III clinical trials for Alzheimer's disease, with varying trial lengths and participant sizes. The targeted mechanisms primarily focus on addressing amyloid beta or the Sigma-1 receptor.

Addressing Key Challenges and Future Directions

Alzheimer's synthetic molecules are imperative for advancing our understanding and treatment of this devastating neurodegenerative disease. Researchers are actively working to design molecules that can target specific pathological mechanisms underlying Alzheimer's, such as amyloid beta aggregation and tau protein hyperphosphorylation. These synthetic compounds hold promise in modulating disease progression and potentially offering neuroprotective effects. By addressing these challenges, the development of Alzheimer's synthetic molecules may pave the way for more effective therapies in the fight against this devastating condition (Andrews et al., 2023).

Conclusion

The medicinal chemistry of Alzheimer's synthetic molecules has witnessed remarkable progress in recent years. The discovery of new leads, advances in structural elucidation, and the development of multi-target compounds are reshaping the landscape of AD therapeutics. Clinical trials are in progress, and while challenges remain, the future looks promising for the development of effective treatments for Alzheimer's disease.

References

Alarcón-Espósito, Jazmín, Michael Mallea, and Julio Rodríguez-Lavado. "From hybrids to new scaffolds: the latest medicinal chemistry goals in multi-target directed ligands for Alzheimer's disease." *Current neuropharmacology* 19, no. 6 (2021): 832-867.

Andrews, Shea J., Alan E. Renton, Brian Fulton-Howard, Anna Podlesny-Drabiniok, Edoardo Marcora, and Alison M. Goate. "The complex genetic architecture of Alzheimer's disease: novel insights and future directions." *EBioMedicine* 90 (2023).

Armstrong, Anne H., Jermont Chen, Angela Fortner McKoy, and Michael H. Hecht. "Mutations that replace aromatic side chains promote aggregation of the Alzheimer's Aβ peptide." *Biochemistry* 50, no. 19 (2011): 4058-4067.

Ballard, Clive, Serge Gauthier, Anne Corbett, Carol Brayne, Dag Aarsland, and Emma Jones. "Alzheimer's disease." *the Lancet* 377, no. 9770 (2011): 1019-1031.

Barten, Donna M., Patrizia Fanara, Cathy Andorfer, Nina Hoque, PY Anne Wong, Kristofor Husted, Gregory W. Cadelina et al., "Hyperdynamic microtubules, cognitive deficits, and pathology are improved in tau transgenic mice with low doses of the microtubule-stabilizing agent BMS-241027." *Journal of Neuroscience* 32, no. 21 (2012): 7137-7145.

Bartus, Raymond T., Reginald L. Dean III, Bernard Beer, and Arnold S. Lippa. "The cholinergic hypothesis of geriatric memory dysfunction." *Science* 217, no. 4558 (1982): 408-414.

Bieschke, Jan, Jenny Russ, Ralf P. Friedrich, Dagmar E. Ehrnhoefer, Heike Wobst, Katja Neugebauer, and Erich E. Wanker. "EGCG remodels mature α-synuclein and amyloid-β fibrils and reduces cellular toxicity." *Proceedings of the National Academy of Sciences* 107, no. 17 (2010): 7710-7715.

Birks, Jacqueline S., and Cochrane Dementia and Cognitive Improvement Group. "Cholinesterase inhibitors for Alzheimer's disease." *Cochrane database of systematic reviews* 2016, no. 3 (1996).

Brem, Anna-Katharine, Sajini Kuruppu, Casper De Boer, Marijn Muurling, Ana Diaz-Ponce, Dianne Gove, Jelena Curcic et al., "Digital endpoints in clinical trials of Alzheimer's disease and other neurodegenerative diseases: challenges and opportunities." *Frontiers in Neurology* 14 (2023): 1210974.

Burns, A., M. Rossor, J. Hecker, S. Gauthier, H. Petit, H-J. Möller, S. L. Rogers, and L. T. Friedhoff. "The Effects of Donepezil in Alzheimer's Disease–Results from a Multinational Trial1." *Dementia and geriatric cognitive disorders* 10, no. 3 (1999): 237-244.

Copani, A., Fabrizio Condorelli, A. Caruso, C. Vancheri, A. Sala, AM Giuffrida Stella, Pier Luigi Canonico, Ferdinando Nicoletti, and M. A. Sortino. "Mitotic signaling by β-amyloid causes neuronal death." *The FASEB Journal* 13, no. 15 (1999): 2225-2234.

Crowe, Alex, Michael J. James, Virginia M-Y. Lee, Amos B. Smith, John Q. Trojanowski, Carlo Ballatore, and Kurt R. Brunden. "Aminothienopyridazines and methylene blue affect Tau fibrillization via cysteine oxidation." *Journal of Biological Chemistry* 288, no. 16 (2013): 11024-11037.

Cummings, Jeffrey L., Travis Morstorf, and Kate Zhong. "Alzheimer's disease drug-development pipeline: few candidates, frequent failures." *Alzheimer's research & therapy* 6, no. 4 (2014): 1-7.

Cummings, Jeffrey. "Lessons learned from Alzheimer disease: clinical trials with negative outcomes." *Clinical and translational science* 11, no. 2 (2018): 147.

Gauthier, Serge, Howard H. Feldman, Lon S. Schneider, Gordon K. Wilcock, Giovanni B. Frisoni, Jiri H. Hardlund, Hans J. Moebius et al., "Efficacy and safety of tau-aggregation inhibitor therapy in patients with mild or moderate Alzheimer's disease: a randomised, controlled, double-blind, parallel-arm, phase 3 trial." *The Lancet* 388, no. 10062 (2016): 2873-2884.

Grill, Joshua D., and Jeffrey L. Cummings. "Current therapeutic targets for the treatment of Alzheimer's disease." *Expert review of neurotherapeutics* 10, no. 5 (2010): 711-728.

Grundke-Iqbal, Inge, Khalid Iqbal, Yunn-Chyn Tung, Maureen Quinlan, Henryk M. Wisniewski, and Lester I. Binder. "Abnormal phosphorylation of the microtubule-associated protein tau (tau) in Alzheimer cytoskeletal pathology." *Proceedings of the National Academy of Sciences* 83, no. 13 (1986): 4913-4917.

Habchi, Johnny, Sean Chia, Ryan Limbocker, Benedetta Mannini, Minkoo Ahn, Michele Perni, Oskar Hansson et al., "Systematic development of small molecules to inhibit specific microscopic steps of Aβ42 aggregation in Alzheimer's disease." *Proceedings of the National Academy of Sciences* 114, no. 2 (2017): E200-E208.

Hampel, Harald, Stefan J. Teipel, T. Fuchsberger, N. Andreasen, J. Wiltfang, Markus Otto, Y. Shen et al., "Value of CSF β-amyloid1–42 and tau as predictors of Alzheimer's disease in patients with mild cognitive impairment." *Molecular psychiatry* 9, no. 7 (2004): 705-710.

Hardy, John, and Dennis J. Selkoe. "The amyloid hypothesis of Alzheimer's disease: progress and problems on the road to therapeutics." *science* 297, no. 5580 (2002): 353-356.

Heneka, Michael T., and M. Kerry O'Banion. "Inflammatory processes in Alzheimer's disease." *Journal of neuroimmunology* 184, no. 1-2 (2007): 69-91.

Hosokawa, Masato, Tetsuaki Arai, Masami Masuda-Suzukake, Takashi Nonaka, Makiko Yamashita, Haruhiko Akiyama, and Masato Hasegawa. "Methylene blue reduced abnormal tau accumulation in P301L tau transgenic mice." *PloS one* 7, no. 12 (2012): e52389.

Imbimbo, Bruno P., Elda Del Giudice, Davide Colavito, Antonello D'Arrigo, Maurizio Dalle Carbonare, Gino Villetti, Fabrizio Facchinetti et al., "1-(3′, 4′-Dichloro-2-fluoro [1, 1′-biphenyl]-4-yl)-cyclopropanecarboxylic acid (CHF5074), a novel γ-secretase modulator, reduces brain β-amyloid pathology in a transgenic mouse model of Alzheimer's disease without causing peripheral toxicity." *Journal of Pharmacology and Experimental Therapeutics* 323, no. 3 (2007): 822-830.

Ittner, Lars M., and Jürgen Götz. "Amyloid-β and tau—a toxic pas de deux in Alzheimer's disease." *Nature Reviews Neuroscience* 12, no. 2 (2011): 67-72.

Jack Jr, Clifford R., David A. Bennett, Kaj Blennow, Maria C. Carrillo, Billy Dunn, Samantha Budd Haeberlein, David M. Holtzman et al., "NIA-AA research framework: toward a biological definition of Alzheimer's disease." *Alzheimer's & Dementia* 14, no. 4 (2018): 535-562.

Kitchen, Douglas B., Hélène Decornez, John R. Furr, and Jürgen Bajorath. "Docking and scoring in virtual screening for drug discovery: methods and applications." *Nature reviews Drug discovery* 3, no. 11 (2004): 935-949.

Knapskog, Anne-Brita, Knut Engedal, Geir Selbæk, and Anne-Rita Øksengård. "Alzheimer's disease–diagnosis and treatment." *Tidsskrift for den Norske laegeforening: tidsskrift for praktisk medicin, ny raekke* 141, no. 7 (2021).

Li, Shiming. "Synthetic Bioactive Substances 33." *Handbook of Food Chemistry* (2015): 1061.

Misra, Ranjita, Sarbari Acharya, and Sanjeeb K. Sahoo. "Cancer nanotechnology: application of nanotechnology in cancer therapy." *Drug discovery today* 15, no. 19-20 (2010): 842-850.

Morris, Garrett M., David S. Goodsell, Robert S. Halliday, Ruth Huey, William E. Hart, Richard K. Belew, and Arthur J. Olson. "Automated docking using a Lamarckian genetic algorithm and an empirical binding free energy function." *Journal of computational chemistry* 19, no. 14 (1998): 1639-1662.

Neves, Bruno J., Rodolpho C. Braga, Cleber C. Melo-Filho, José Teófilo Moreira-Filho, Eugene N. Muratov, and Carolina Horta Andrade. "QSAR-based virtual screening: advances and applications in drug discovery." *Frontiers in pharmacology* 9 (2018): 1275.

Owens, Michael J., David L. Knight, and Charles B. Nemeroff. "Second-generation SSRIs: human monoamine transporter binding profile of escitalopram and R-fluoxetine." *Biological psychiatry* 50, no. 5 (2001): 345-350.

Pardridge, William M. "Drug transport across the blood–brain barrier." *Journal of cerebral blood flow & metabolism* 32, no. 11 (2012): 1959-1972.

Peter, Swathik Clarancia, Jaspreet Kaur Dhanjal, Vidhi Malik, Navaneethan Radhakrishnan, Mannu Jayakanthan, and Durai Sundar. "Quantitative structure-activity relationship (QSAR): modeling approaches to biological applications." (2019): 661-676.

Rang, Humphrey P., Maureen M. Dale, James M. Ritter, Rod J. Flower, and Graeme Henderson. *Rang & Dale's pharmacology*. Elsevier Health Sciences, 2011.

Reisberg, Barry, Rachelle Doody, Albrecht Stöffler, Frederick Schmitt, Steven Ferris, and Hans Jörg Möbius. "Memantine in moderate-to-severe Alzheimer's disease." *New England Journal of Medicine* 348, no. 14 (2003): 1333-1341.

Rogers, Sharon L., Rachelle S. Doody, Richard C. Mohs, Lawrence T. Friedhoff, and Donepezil Study Group. "Donepezil improves cognition and global function in Alzheimer disease: a 15-week, double-blind, placebo-controlled study." *Archives of internal medicine* 158, no. 9 (1998): 1021-1031.

Roney, Celeste, Padmakar Kulkarni, Veera Arora, Peter Antich, Frederick Bonte, Aimei Wu, N. N. Mallikarjuana et al., "Targeted nanoparticles for drug delivery through the blood–brain barrier for Alzheimer's disease." *Journal of controlled release* 108, no. 2-3 (2005): 193-214.

Rösler, Michael, Tony Bayer, Ravi Anand, Ana Cicin-Sain, Serge Gauthier, Yves Agid, Peter Dal-Bianco, Hannes B. Stähelin, Richard Hartman, and Marguirguis Gharabawi. "Efficacy and safety of rivastigmine in patients with Alzheimer's disease: international randomised controlled trialCommentary: Another piece of the Alzheimer's jigsaw." *Bmj* 318, no. 7184 (1999): 633-640.

Roy, Kunal, Supratik Kar, and Rudra Narayan Das. *A primer on QSAR/QSPR modeling: fundamental concepts*. Springer, 2015.

Sarter, Martin, Michael E. Hasselmo, John P. Bruno, and Ben Givens. "Unraveling the attentional functions of cortical cholinergic inputs: interactions between signal-driven and cognitive modulation of signal detection." *Brain research reviews* 48, no. 1 (2005): 98-111.

Selkoe, Dennis J. "Alzheimer's disease: genes, proteins, and therapy." *Physiological reviews* (2001).

Selkoe, Dennis J., and John Hardy. "The amyloid hypothesis of Alzheimer's disease at 25 years." *EMBO molecular medicine* 8, no. 6 (2016): 595-608.

Shao, Jiang-Yang, Dongmei Li, Jiangjian Shi, Chuang Ma, Yousheng Wang, Xiaomin Liu, Xianyuan Jiang et al., "Recent progress in perovskite solar cells: material science." *Science China Chemistry* 66, no. 1 (2023): 10-64.

Shoichet, Brian K. "Virtual screening of chemical libraries." *Nature* 432, no. 7019 (2004): 862-865.

Söderberg, Linda, Malin Johannesson, Patrik Nygren, Hanna Laudon, Fredrik Eriksson, Gunilla Osswald, Christer Möller, and Lars Lannfelt. "Lecanemab, aducanumab, and gantenerumab—binding profiles to different forms of amyloid-beta might explain efficacy and side effects in clinical trials for Alzheimer's disease." *Neurotherapeutics* 20, no. 1 (2023): 195-206.

Tjernberg, Lars O., Jan Näslund, Fredrik Lindqvist, Jan Johansson, Anders R. Karlström, Johan Thyberg, Lars Terenius, and Christer Nordstedt. "Arrest of-Amyloid Fibril Formation by a Pentapeptide Ligand (∗)." *Journal of Biological Chemistry* 271, no. 15 (1996): 8545-8548.

Tropsha, Alexander. "Best practices for QSAR model development, validation, and exploitation." *Molecular informatics* 29, no. 6-7 (2010): 476-488.

Trott, Oleg, and Arthur J. Olson. "AutoDock Vina: improving the speed and accuracy of docking with a new scoring function, efficient optimization, and multithreading." *Journal of computational chemistry* 31, no. 2 (2010): 455-461.

Tumiatti, Vincenzo, Anna Minarini, MARIA LAURA Bolognesi, Andrea Milelli, Michela Rosini, and Carlo Melchiorre. "Tacrine derivatives and Alzheimer's disease." *Current medicinal chemistry* 17, no. 17 (2010): 1825-1838.

Whitehouse, Peter J., Donald L. Price, Robert G. Struble, Arthur W. Clark, Joseph T. Coyle, and Mahlon R. DeLong. "Alzheimer's disease and senile dementia: loss of neurons in the basal forebrain." *Science* 215, no. 4537 (1982): 1237-1239.

Winblad, Bengt, Philippe Amouyel, Sandrine Andrieu, Clive Ballard, Carol Brayne, Henry Brodaty, Angel Cedazo-Minguez et al., "Defeating Alzheimer's disease and other dementias: a priority for European science and society." *The Lancet Neurology* 15, no. 5 (2016): 455-532.

Wong, Ho Lun, Xiao Yu Wu, and Reina Bendayan. "Nanotechnological advances for the delivery of CNS therapeutics." *Advanced drug delivery reviews* 64, no. 7 (2012): 686-700.

Yan, Riqiang, and Robert Vassar. "Targeting the β secretase BACE1 for Alzheimer's disease therapy." *The Lancet Neurology* 13, no. 3 (2014): 319-329.

Yang, Fusheng, Giselle P. Lim, Aynun N. Begum, Oliver J. Ubeda, Mychica R. Simmons, Surendra S. Ambegaokar, Pingping P. Chen et al., "Curcumin inhibits formation of amyloid β oligomers and fibrils, binds plaques, and reduces amyloid *in vivo*." *Journal of Biological Chemistry* 280, no. 7 (2005): 5892-5901.

Zhang, Li, Mingliang Wang, Mingxia Liu, and Daoqiang Zhang. "A survey on deep learning for neuroimaging-based brain disorder analysis." *Frontiers in neuroscience* 14 (2020): 779.

Chapter 10

Novel Formulation Approaches for Targeting Alzheimer's Disease

Nusrat K. Shaikh[1], PhD,
Jitendra O. Bhangale[2], PhD,
and Mohit Agrawal[3]

[1]Department of Quality Assurance, Smt. N. M. Padalia Pharmacy College, Ahmedabad, Gujarat, India
[2]Department of Pharmacology, Smt. N. M. Padalia Pharmacy College, Ahmedabad, Gujarat, India
[3]School of Medical & Allied Sciences, K.R. Mangalam University, Gurugram, Haryana, India

Abstract

Alzheimer's disease (AD) is a debilitating neuronal malfunction that causes dementia over time. Tragically, the condition is incurable, but it can be prevented from progressing. Tacrine, Donepezil, Galantamine, Rivastigmine, and other cholinesterase inhibitors that are sold on the market have been employed to treat various signs of Alzheimer's disease. This book chapter's goal is to provide light on the disease's cellular and genetic roots, current trends and numerous novel formulation/treatment approaches, such as phytopharmaceuticals and nutritional supplements. To assemble the knowledge on the methods available to treat Alzheimer's disease, a massive literature review was carried out, and published publications from PubMed, Scifinder, Google Scholar, Clinical Trials.org, and Alzheimer Association reports were closely examined. This chapter described several cutting-edge treatments for Alzheimer's disease that bypass the blood-brain barrier, including nanoparticles, in-situ gels, nano-emulsions, hydrogels, liposomes, and

In: Neurogenerative Disorders
Editors: Mohit Agrawal, Manmohan Singhal, Amit Kumar Nayak et al.
ISBN: 979-8-89530-143-2

others. The current section of this chapter addresses the novel remedies for dealing with Alzheimer's disease, possible medical treatments for the illness's therapies, and an archive of innovative treatments in various phases of clinical investigation. The pipeline of innovative therapeutics currently under way in various stages of clinical trials has been given particular attention, as has the study into herbal medicines and cow urine therapy. These topics are also covered in earlier sections of this chapter. The findings imply that the medications undergoing clinical trials may create new avenues for the successful treatment of Alzheimer's patients while enhancing their quality of life. This chapter's conclusion states that both novel and conventional medicines offer hope for a potential future of treating AD.

Keywords: Alzheimer's disease, novel formulation, therapeutic approaches

Introduction

Alzheimer disease (AD) is a neurological condition marked through an ongoing decline of cognitive with motor skills as well as an onset of neuropsychiatric signs. Amyloid-protein (A) plaques, neurofibrillary tangles (NFTs) and loss of neurons are a variety of biological variables that contribute to the development of AD [1]. Inflammation, circulatory alterations, an overproduction of various proteins like synuclein and Transactive response DNA-binding protein 43 (TDP - 43), dysfunctional mitochondria and aberrant synaptic connections are just a few of the additional disorders that are present in addition to the canonical symptoms of AD. A significant risk to the community's health is AD. As the global population generations, more people show signs of gradual cognitive impairment and occupy the age-related risk factor for AD. By 2060, there will cbe 14 million more Americans with dementia from Alzheimer's than the current 5.8 million [2]. A whopping 130 million people will have AD dementia around the world by 2030, up from the current 40 million cases [3, 4]. In recognition of AD's high prevalence and heavy impact, little advance has been made in creating novel treatments. Only 1 new medicine (aducanumab) and 1 additional substance (sodium oligomannate, approved in China in 2019) have been authorised by the Food and Medicine Administration since 2003. Trial design, the findings measurements, relevant populations for trials, biomarkers, and clinical trial conduct have all seen significant advancements with an extensive record of studies that have not revealed any benefit of alternative potential medicines

[5]. These insights serve as the basis for testing ever-narrower predictions in scheduled and ongoing trials.

The National Institute on Ageing and international funders created the Common Alzheimer Disease Research Ontology (CADRO), which lists targets for therapy in AD and related possible mechanisms of action (MOAs) of medications under development. The medications from the CADRO categories that are now or recently in clinical trials are highlighted in this chapter. Biologic treatments, namely monoclonal antibodies (MAbs), and small molecule medicines are the two categories into which the treatments fall. Other research has proposed using tiny compounds, usually able to traverse the blood-brain barrier, as statin-like oral tablets or capsules for the management of AD. One of these is the HMG-CoA reductase inhibitor simvastatin, which the FDA has granted approval for their remedy of hypercholesterolemia and diabetic cardiomyopathy. As a result of simvastatin medication, Retrospective clinical investigations led by Wolozin and colleagues showed a considerable decrease (a minimum of 50 percent) in hazard frequency of developing AD and other neurological disorders [6, 7]. 126 drugs are listed as being in clinical studies on clinicaltrials.gov (accessed January 5, 2023) [8]. 82.5% of these medications are alleged disease-modifying treatments (DMTs). Another 10.3% of pipeline drugs are cognitive-enhancing, and 7.1% of these are drugs being researched to treat behavioural indications of AD. The CADRO categories with the most drugs undergoing trials are those that target A, tau, inflammation, bioenergetics, and synaptic plasticity. The current focus of research is on developing novel disease-modifying medications to decrease the course of disease [9, 10].

Current Treatment Possibilities for AD

A mere two kinds of drug therapy are now available for AD; these are cholinesterase inhibitors, which are used to treat people with mild, moderate, or severe dementia associated with AD as well as cognition brought on by Parkinson's disease [11]. Memantine is also used in people with moderate to severe AD since it functions as both a dopamine agonist and a non-competitive N-methyl-d-aspartate (NMDA) receptor antagonist. The dietary supplement huperzine has been shown to enhance daily activities and memory functions and is utilised in different types of therapy [12]. However, the USFDA does not control it. Individuals who are deficient in vitamin D should take supplements since dementia risk factors have been linked to vitamin D deficiency [13]. In summary, cardiovascular disorders may put individuals at risk in cases of neurological and cerebral conditions [14]. A Mediterranean diet lowers the risk of cognitive deterioration and AD. Additionally, regular aerobic activity is beneficial. It also lessens neuropsychological side effects [15].

Conventional Pharmacotherapy for AD

The following criteria can be implemented to categories the medications currently being administered for AD's treatment: Tacrine, Donepezil, Rivastigmine, Galantamine and Donepezil included as Acetylcholinesterase inhibitors. Memantine is a glutamate inhibitor and an NMDA antagonist.

Acetylcholinesterase Inhibitors

The FDA has approved galantamine for mild and moderate AD correspondingly, donepezil and rivastigmine have been advised for mild, moderate and severe AD [16, 17]. The traditional class of medications used to treat AD is depicted in Figure 1.

Acetylcholinesterase is more active in individuals with AD, which causes more acetylcholine to be broken down and lower levels of acetylcholine in the brain. By inhibiting the acetylcholinesterase enzyme, which is essential for the digestive breakdown of acetylcholine, these drugs increase the amount of the neurotransmitter in the brains of people with mild to moderate AD. Several medication types were found to be generally acceptable among individuals [18]. Rivastigmine is a 'pseudo-irreversible' acetylcholinesterase and butyrylcholinesterase inhibitor, whereas donepezil and galantamine possess the ability to interfere with acetylcholinesterase selectively and reversibly.

Glutamate Inhibitor

Excitotoxicity is a disorder brought on by glutamatergic overstimulation which damages neurons by increasing the calcium burden on them. Memantine is a well-known non-competitive NMDA receptor antagonist that works to mitigate the detrimental consequences of elevated brain glutamate levels [19, 20]. Due to the aforementioned quality, it has established itself as an efficient therapy for treating people with AD. Memantine, a drug approved for the diagnosis and treatment moderate-to-severe AD, has been clinically shown to prove beneficial, improves cognitive abilities and the results for AD patients [21]. The majority of people tolerate the said medication well. There could, however, be modest and temporary negative effects. In accordance with its pharmacological makeup, it could interact with other drugs. Depending on their mode of action, concurrent treatment with levodopa, other dopamine agonists, and anticholinergics may increase their biological activity. Since Memantine and Aches have complementary mechanisms of action, they can be used together. Patients typically experience cumulative benefits from the aforementioned multimodal therapy, with no increase in side effects [22]. Memantine can cause pharmacotoxicity psychosis when combined with other chemically similar NMDA receptor antagonists such amantadine, budipine, ketamine, and dextromethorphan [23, 24].

Novel Formulation for the Treatment of AD

Intranasal drug administration: nose-to-brain transfer favours medications with the lowest oral bioavailability. In comparison to traditional dosage methods, the intranasal route offers an immediate delivery channel through the brain. It also gets rid of the adverse consequences of the barrier between the blood and the brain, resulting in an efficient delivery technique. Different novel drug delivery systems have been developed to address the shortcomings of alternative and classical drug routes for delivery to the brain using nose [25].

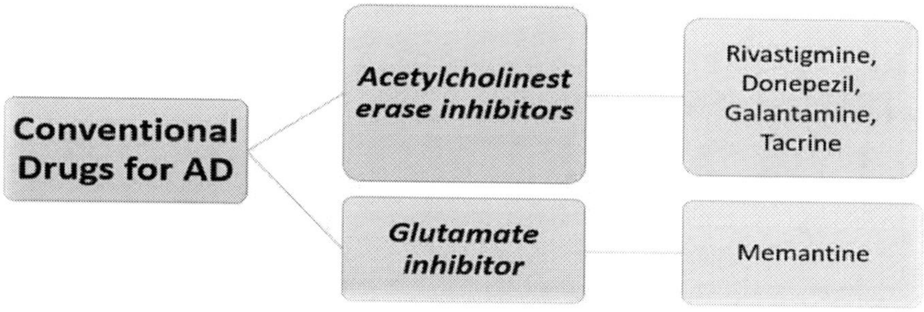

Figure 1. Conventional Class of drugs for AD Treatment.

Nanoparticles

This kind of delivery mechanism is suitable for nasal vaccinations. For instance, miR-132 supports neuron survival and balances neuron shape. The microenvironment of hematoma lesions is improved, cell death after cerebral hemorrhage is reduced, and safeguards are seen after cerebral ischemia. Intranasal administration of nanoparticles (NPs), miR132 in a mouse model with AD and wheat germ agglutinin (WGA) causes a noticeably higher level of synaptic protein expression.

Polymer-Based Nanoparticles

Particle dimensions and poly-dispersibility index were tailored during the development of the interconnected chitosan nanoparticles of memantine-HCl, and the nanoparticle size was discovered to be 129 nm at 4 hours of stirring, 1000 rpm of stirring speed, and a 2:1 concentration ratio of chitosan and tripolyphosphates (TPP) in the finished product. Memantine-loaded nanoparticles of chitosan may be a cutting-edge method of treating Alzheimer's illness when administered intravenously. A different approach polymer used to transport nanomaterials via the intranasal route is poly (lactic-co-glycolic acid, or PLGA). The greatest illustration is olanzapine-loaded PLGA nanoparticles, which are given intravenously to increase the uptake of drugs [26].

Lipid-Based Nanoparticles

Solid lipid nanoparticles (SLNs) and nanostructured lipid carriers (NLCs) are a couple examples of this type of system. In pharmacokinetics and bio-distribution experiments on albino Wistar rats, donepezil-SLNs administered orally had an AUC0- value in the neurological system that was about 2.61 times higher than donepezil-Sol administered intravenously and 2.26 times superior to DPL-Sol administered orally [27].

Liposomes

According to a mouse AD model study, nasal delivery of quercetin liposomes slows the deterioration of cortex and cholinergic nerve cells in brain [28, 29].

Microemulsions

Micro-emulsions administered through the nose are effective at reaching brain tissue. Quick effect onset and a longer action endurance are provided by the hybrid system of clonazepam in a mucosal adhesive agent and a microemulsion composition [30].

Nanogels

Compared to competing technologies, nanogels offer a number of advantages, notably. It can have a soothing and emollient effect, reduce the thickness of postnasal drip, stop anterior formulation leakage, and more. The insulin-loaded nano-gels are administered via nasal route to enhance insulin delivery to the brain.

In-Situ Gelling System

Prior to delivery, the gels remain liquid but go through a soul-to-gel conversion that is caused by any external factor, such as the pH, Heat, ion change, magnetism, or physiological context [31]. In particular, pharmacokinetic analysis showed continuous release of intranasal (IN) and intravenous (IV) NLCs with a noticeably higher area under the curve (AUC) and t-half when compared to rivastigmine solution supplied via the same channel. Furthermore, biological distribution demonstrated that IV NLCs (457.24 38.41.12 ng/mL) and IN NLCs (736.42 34.54 ng/mL) had the capacity to pass the blood-brain barrier, with 4.6 and 5.3-fold larger proportions in the brain, respectively, when compared to IV and IN treatment.

Hydrogels

The 3-dimensional (3D) interconnected networks may absorb a lot of fluid and operate well with biological processes [32, 33]. For instance, the rabbit was used in pharmacokinetic investigation. It was demonstrated that the improved hydrogel enhanced donepezil's mean peak concentration and area under the curve (AUC) by 46% and 39%, respectively, when compared to standard oral tablets.

Nano-Emulsions (NEs)

Nanoscale globules and the mucous membrane in the nose can swallow these highly lipophilic solutions. NEs can be oil-in-water (o/w) or water-in-oil (w/o) emulsion. The main use of oil-in-water (o/w) emulsions is to enclose hydrophobic medications, protect them from enzyme degradation, control drug release, and improve absorption [34, 35]. Like for instance, Rivastigmine-loaded nano-emulsion demonstrated noticeably increased concentrations of drugs in the cerebral cortex in comparison to solution in *ex vivo* diffusion experiments and *in vitro* drug release investigations. Research studies on nasal ciliotoxicity in goat nasal mucosa showed that the optimised formulation was free of the condition.

Novel Formulation Additives for an Anti-Alzheimer's Disease

To increase an anti-Alzheimer drug's solubility in water, formulation additives created specifically for peptide-PEG conjugates are used. The effectiveness of peptide-PEG conjugates as formulation additives has been demonstrated. The oligopeptide segment's structure is unaffected as a result of the drug's non-covalent bonding with it. As a widely used biocompatible polymer, PEG blocks offer medication shielding and water solubility. In order to tweak associations with a medicine, poly (ethylene glycol) (PEG) and oligopeptide segments are combined. This results in an extensive range of formulations ingredients that can produce sequence-dependent dissolution as well as delivery mechanisms. This makes it possible to foresee potential developments for virtually all pertinent polymer-based drug delivery systems that depend on sporadic interactions with host drug molecules [36].

Novel Therapeutic Approaches for Alzheimer's Disease

Anti-Amyloid Therapy

In the biologically induced surroundings, amyloid plaques are made up of Aβ peptides. Aβ aggregation inhibitors and Aβ immunotherapy are two of the three anti-amyloid treatment methods used, and research findings show that both have an impact on AD [37].

Aβ Aggregation Inhibitor

Modern biophysical and structural biologic methods of research are currently concentrated on the examination of chemical features and the discovery of interesting molecules. Tanshinone and uncarinic acid C both have connecting epitopes or planar hydrophobic structures, which enhance A's anti-aggregation properties. Several chemicals interact with the regions of A's N-terminus and 1 turn that control toxicity, including resveratrol and epigallocatechin gallate (EGCG). Several compounds, including quercetin, oleuropein aglycone, and epigallocatechin gallate (EGCG), have the potential to cure AD [38].

Aβ Immunotherapy

Aβ immunotherapy lowers the A burden in an active or passive manner. The United States Food and Drug Administration (FDA) approved acuranumab for the treatment of AD patients in June 2021 [39]. It appears that there is still a disagreement concerning this permission. Next-generation small compounds that target Aβ oligomers, such as PQ912, ALZ-801 and CT1812 additionally remain in development [40].

Anti-Tau Therapy

Microtubules and tau proteins work together to stabilise them in axons and dendrites. Phosphatase modifiers, tau aggregation inhibitors, microtubule stabilisers and kinase inhibitors are some of the anti-tau therapeutic techniques [41].

Phosphatase Modifiers

Phosphatase promoters' lower phosphorylation by stimulating phosphatases like protein phosphatase 2A (PP2A) [42]. Sodium selenate is a key molecule in brain function and a PP2A activator. A supranutritional supplement called sodium selenate enhanced selenium absorption throughout the CNS and was found to be clinically effective treating AD [43].

Kinase Inhibitors

Kinase inhibitors reduce tau hyperphosphorylation and post-translational alterations. It has been discovered that lithium, a mood stabilizer, inhibits glycogen synthase kinase-3β (GSK3 β). Individuals who administered daily dosages of 300 mg of lithium for 15 months saw improvements in their symptoms of AD. According to meta-analyses, lithium had a moderate impact size and slowed the course of cognitive responsiveness in AD patients [44, 45].

Tau Aggregation Inhibitors

A synthetic phenothiazine dye called methylene blue (MB) was the first inhibitor of tau aggregation. *In vitro* polymerization is hindered by MB because it prevents connections between tau molecules [46, 47]. In phase II totally blind clinical trials, a 50-week dosage of MB with 138 mg of MB treatment demonstrated an executive functioning benefit in people with mild to severe AD [48].

Curcumin, A food ingredient and coloring agent, prevents tau from aggregating by reducing tau's -sheet formation and dissolving tau oligomers *in vitro*, it [49]. Working memory was improved in the elderly with cognitive health using an acute and short-term course of treatment of curcumin with enhanced bioavailability (<4 weeks) [50, 51].

Microtubule Stabilizers

A synthetic taxane derivative called TPI-287 (Abeotaxane) is used to treat central nervous system (CNS) cancer or metastases [52, 53]. The creation of neuropeptide having Taxol-binding domain of tubulin has emerged as Additional inventive tactic in conjunction with EpoD, NAP, and TPI-287 [54].

Anti-Neuroinflammatory Therapy

The advanced stage of the disease and the course of AD are both correlated with neuroinflammation [55]. Microglia modulators, astrocyte modulators, glucose resistance management, and microbial treatment are examples of anti-neuroinflammatory tactics.

Microglia Modulators

Selective CSF1R inhibitors like JN-J527, GW2580 and PLX3397 were applied to recombinant AD mice. The safety profile of GW2580 reduced behavioural abnormalities and temporary decline in memory in mice with APP/PS1 mutations by inhibiting neuronal growth [56]. Tau-mediated neurotoxicity and impairment of functioning were reduced when JN-J527 was administered to P301S mice [57].

Astrocyte Modulators

The BBB's ability to remove A is compromised by the astrocyte response. FK506 (Tacrolimus) inhibited the calcineurin/nuclear factor of activated T cells (calcineurin/NFAT) pathway, significantly reduced the cognitive impairment in mice with APP/PS1 mutations [58, 59]. To ascertain its effectiveness in MCI and AD, FK506 is under clinical phase III research.

Microbiome Therapy

Inconsistency in the intestine microflora causes an excess of LPS to be produced there, which raises BBB permeability [60]. A marine-derived oligosaccharide called sodium oligomannate (GV-971) inhibits the intestinal bacteria, destabilizes Aβ aggregates and regulates neuroinflammation [61].

Individuals with mild to moderate AD benefited cognitively from sodium oligomannate, according to phase III double-blind RCTs [62]. For 36 weeks, the subjects took 900 mg of sodium oligomannate. When comparison to the placebo group, the treated group's ADAS-cog performance significantly improved [63]. In November 2019, China approved sodium oligomannate for the management of moderately severe AD [64].

Neuroprotective Agents

The pathophysiology of AD involves neurodegenerative processes. Thus, implementing neuroprotective techniques seeks to postpone both the onset and the progression of AD [65]. Antiepileptic medications, NMDAR modulation, and ω 3 polyunsaturated fatty acid nutritional products are three common choices for neuroprotection.

Antiepileptic Drugs

Epilepsy medications are classified as central nervous system (CNS) depressants and have additionally been proven to have an adverse effect on cognition. In both animal models and human clinical studies, levetiracetam has been found to have neuroprotective benefits in traumatic brain damage [66]. According to recent research [67], it targets the synaptic Vesicle 2A (SV2A) protein to exert its therapeutic effects. Levetiracetam's double-blind crossover RCT in healthy older people revealed that it may be able to enhance mental abilities. Throughout the course of the 5-week treatment period, 1000 mg of levetiracetam were given to each participant. During the levetiracetam treatment phase, the participants showed improved mental agility but also boredom and irritability [68].

Gabapentin, acts as a voltage-gated calcium channel (VGCC) inhibitor and also has an indirect impact on the glutamate system. Treatment with gabapentin demonstrated a protective effect on neurons and reduced brain damage in a dose-responsive way in cerebral ischemia-reperfusion mice [69]. Healthy individuals received a single dose of 50–400 mg of gabapentin, which resulted in a mild cognitive boost [70]. According to preliminary study, gabapentin medication may be beneficial for treating AD in people suffering from dementia who also have BPSD. A single daily gabapentin dose of 200–3600 mg decreased agitation and improved cognition. Weak evidence was used to corroborate the findings [71]. In a double-blinded phase IV RCT, the therapeutic efficacy of gabapentin enacarbil remains to be studied. The effectiveness of gabapentin enacarbil in treating overnight disturbance and syndrome of restless legs among individuals with intermediate to serious AD is still being studied in a double-blinded phase IV RCT [72].

NMDAR Modification

MCI and moderate AD patients tolerated sodium benzoate well. The patients had a 24-week benzoate treatment, with daily dosages varying between 250 to 750 mg. The treated population showed more improvement on the ADAS-Cog than the untreated group [73].

The drug Riluzole is used to treat amyotrophic lateral sclerosis and is categorised as a glutamate modulator. Presynaptic glutamate release is indirectly decreased by riluzole's modification of the postsynaptic N-Methyl D-Aspartate Receptor (NMDAR) stimulation. A phase II double-blind RCT on riluzole was completed to assess the metabolism of neurons and mental abilities in moderate AD patients [74].

A phase II completely blind RCT using the riluzole derivative troriluzole (BHV-4157) is now being finished to evaluate changes in brain function in people with intermediate moderate to severe AD [75].

Omega-3 Polyunsaturated Fatty Acid Supplements

Medications containing eicosapentaenoic acid (EPA) or docosahexaenoic acid (DHA) have been linked to improved memory and learning as well as neuroprotective effects in AD mouse models [76]. According to numerous controlled trials [77, 78], omega-3 fatty acid treatment from 3 to 12 months significantly enhanced cognitive performance in MCI patients as compared to the placebo. In APOE4 carriers, phospholipid DHA dietary supplements may be able to delay the onset of AD [79]. According to a current meta-analysis and systematic review study, only supplementation combining DHA and EPA proved to enhance multiple facets of brain function in individuals with Alzheimer's [80]. An ethyl ester of EPA known as Icosapent ethyl is currently undergoing a phase III RCT to assess its effects on cognitive function and cerebrovascular function in cognitively healthy individuals with AD [81].

The Impact of Anti-Diabetic Agents on the Treatment of Alzheimer's Disease

Insulin treatment is used while addressing AD with an intranasal device. Intranasal insulin delivery reduced memory impairment in MCI and AD, according to a double-blinded RCT. For four months, the subjects experienced 40 IU per day of conventional intranasal insulin [82]. After receiving insulin therapy, individuals with MCI and AD showed better verbal memory, according to a comprehensive analysis of RCTs. Patients who did not carry the APOE4 gene experienced greater regularity in mental gains [83]. Intranasal insulin injections are a safe approach to therapy because there were no noticeable adverse reactions in those who received treatment [84]. In animal models of AD and Parkinson's illness, Liraglutide, lixisenatide, exendin-4, semaglutide, peptides 17, 18, and 20 as well as DA-CIB and DA-JC4, all showed potential therapeutic benefits [85]. Liraglutide was examined in AD treatment, and it showed beneficial effect [86].

The first-line treatment for diabetic mellitus is metformin. Metformin revealed a protective impact on the brain and decreased the incidence of cognition in individuals with diabetes [87, 88]. Individuals with MCI and early AD who were non-diabetic and non-obese underwent a preliminary crossover RCT with metformin. A drug of choice, an 8-month metformin regimen was given a chance to each person. Up to 2000 mg of metformin were taken each day. The outcomes demonstrated that metformin treatment enhanced cognitive abilities in the group receiving treatment and decreased recall memory in the treating group [89]. WY-14643, GW7647, fenofibrate, and gemfibrozil are four Peroxisome proliferator activator receptors (PPARs) agonists that have demonstrated therapeutic promise in AD animal studies. PPAR- γ agonist Pioglitazone is suggested as a diabetes therapy. Among diabetics experiencing a mild amount of AD, an open-label phase II RCT of this drug demonstrated brain improvements. For six months, the subjects took pioglitazone daily doses of 15 to 30 mg [90].

Innovative Formulations for Alzheimer's Disease

The existing circumstance broadens the potential for unique formulation to increase a drug's concentration upon entering the brain. Research on valacyclovir for therapy of Alzheimer's illness can proceed because it had activity that was comparable to donepezil. It has been demonstrated through clinical trials that Valacylovir is just as effective as the antiviral medication valacyclovir (Valtrex) in treating persons having mild to advanced cognitive impairment with HSV-1 or HSV-2 positivity. Scientists have already assessed changes in cognitive performance and daily life skills using evaluations and examinations, as well as amyloid deposition on positron emission tomography (PET) scans in various brain regions. Individuals having consented to lumbar puncture provided measurements of beta-amyloid and tau in cerebrospinal fluid for the researchers. Therefore, we can give Valacyclovir nanotherapeutics for brain targets via nasal delivery to patients which will be safe for individuals.

Citing a conclusion that a confirmatory trial demonstrated clinical effectiveness, the U.S. Food and Drug Administration transformed Leqembi (lecanemab-irmb), intended to treat older individuals with Alzheimer's Disease, to conventional authorization. Leqembi, amyloid beta-directed antibody is the initial medication to go through an expedited authorization to an ordinary certification for the cure of Alzheimer's illness. The medication functions by lessening amyloid plaques, which are a neurological hallmark of the disease that develops in the brain. Leqembi (lecanemab-irmb) was given conventional approval in the US earlier this month for use as a biweekly intravenous (IV) infusion in individuals with moderate dementia or early-stage Alzheimer's disease. A potential remedy for brain disorders may lie in the development of nanoparticle (NP)-based techniques using liposomes, chitosan, dendrimers, quantum dots, micelles and gold nanoparticles.

Herbal medicines is growing with its popuarity due to their reported efficacy, safety, and cost. Centella asiatica, Bacopa monnieri, Curcuma longa, Clitoria ternatea, Withania somnifera, Celastrus paniculatus, Evolvulus alsinoides, Desmodium gangeticum, Eclipta alba, Moringa oleifera, and Convolvulus pluricaulis are a few Indian herbal remedies that have shown promise in treating cognitive impairment. A few natural treatments for memory loss that are readily available in India were also examined.

The Ginkgoaceae family of plants includes the well-known and frequently used Ginkgo biloba (Maidenhair tree). The main components of Ginkgo biloba leaf extracts have been identified as their flavonoids and terpenes phytochemical elements. Its medicinal qualities, such as its neuroprotective, anti-dementia, antioxidant, anti-inflammatory, vasoactive, anti-psychotic, anti-neoplastic, and anti-platelet action, have led to its widespread use. Niosomes are an oral administration technique for GbE that has promise, and individuals can also use Nano Suspension, which contains *Ginkgo biloba L. extract*, to control their Alzheimer's disease.

Smilax china ethanolic bark extract has neuroprotective effects in relation to Alzheimer's disease.

From *in vitro, ex vivo* and *in vivo* investigation it was proved that Naringin loaded PLGA nanoparticles have potential therapeutic effects for management of Alzheimer's Disease. Naringin loaded PLGA nanoparticles have been shown to offer possible beneficial effects for the prevention and treatment of Alzheimer's disease through *in vitro, ex vivo*, and *in vivo* research. As Naringin Nanosuspension shown substantial neuroprotective and anti-neuroinflammatory action, this discovery opens up new possibilities to utilise naringin for various therapeutic and restorative objectives.

Promising innovative remedy using cow urine rehabilitation: A number of herbs can restore bodily faults (Vata, bile, and phlegm) that correspond with the therapy of cow urine; nevertheless, if the body's distribution is unbalanced, it can result in Alzheimer's disease. Many helpful elements are included in some Ayurvedic medications to treat them. Certain Core Herbs, which include *Brahmi, Ashwagandha, Baheda, Shankhpushpi, Mulethi, Shatavari, Shilajit and Gojala,* are employed in cow-urine treatment. Essentially, this indicates that the key ingredient in medicine is cow-urine extract. This extract is created using the local cow breeds' urine. Cow urine with these herbs made the treatment more effective for Alzheimer's disease with an increase in quality of life and complication prevention.

Future Research

Researching prospective agents for pharmaceutical therapies is still difficult. AD is a complex condition that involves a number of pathogenic mechanisms, including insulin dysregulation, misfolded protein aggregation, neuroinflammatory processes, and neurodegeneration. Repositioning medications could be a useful strategy. Anti-inflammatory, neuroprotective, and diabetic medications are some of the prospective choices. The pathogenic processes of A and tau are being discovered as experimental techniques in biophysical and structural biology advance. Understanding the pathophysiology of AD enables us to develop new immunotherapies or locate suitable drugs. The present difficulty in non-pharmacological therapies is standardising the protocol's settings. For instance, the criteria for choosing the rTMS protocol include the locations that will be targeted, the number of times, the length of each session, and the timetable.

Individuals with varying degrees of AD may respond inconsistently to the same rTMS regimen. Future plans may include creating various standardised protocols based on the severity of the condition. Both pharmaceutical and non-pharmacological therapies require careful consideration when choosing susceptible subgroups. A patient's attributes, such as age, gender, genetic variables, medical conditions, environmental influences, and lifestyles, are taken into consideration while establishing a course of therapy. With the help of machine learning advancements, we can now deal with complex factors and create models that foretell the best treatment plans for AD patients. To determine the connection amongst a patient's traits and therapy response, more investigation is necessary. Personalised medicine is a practice that is both predicted and attainable with more research efforts. We firmly believe that plants with medicinal properties and plant-based compounds, either alone or in conjunction with additional substances, would be better treatments for dementia than those currently in use, with fewer adverse effects.

Conclusion

Many individuals today are affected by neurodegenerative disorders, and their prevalence is rising as the population ages. There are currently only symptomatic therapies available. To stop or halt the evolution of these illnesses, novel therapeutic techniques and formulation are urgently needed. Here, we looked over Current treatment possibilities, conventinal pharmacotherapy, Novel formulation, Novel therapeutic strategies for AD. The impact of anti-diabetic agents with innovative formulation for treatment of Alzheimer's disease. These findings may help us develop a single therapy strategy or a combination of strategies to reverse the neurodegeneration that characterises these neurological disorders.

The nose to brain delivery method is beneficial in the diagnosis and treatment of Alzheimer's syndrome since it efficiently hits the brain's neurons through overcoming the Blood-Brain barrier. It also offers better efficacy, efficient accessibility, improved preservation, intake, and bioavailability, at a considerably lower chance of adverse consequences than conventional methods of drug delivery. Given the increasing curiosity in breathing drug administration and its potential advantages, it is predicted that novel nasal products, such as drugs for persistent illnesses, nasal vaccines, and medicinal products that focus on Nervous System and assure favourable effects on the CNS with fewer negative reactions will continue entering the marketplace.

Development of Naringin loaded PLGA nanoparticles, nanoparticle (NP)-based techniques using liposomes, chitosan, dendrimers, quantum dots, micelles and gold nanoparticles for Leqembi (lecanemab-irmb), Valacylovir and other herbal formulations containing *Ginkgo biloba L. extract, Smilax china ethanolic bark extract,* have shown promise in treating cognitive impairment to control their Alzheimer's disease. Cow-urine treatment with certain core herbs like *Brahmi, Ashwagandha, Baheda, Shankhpushpi, Mulethi, Shatavari, Shilajit and Gojala* were employed which have substantial neuroprotective and anti-neuroinflammatory action. Cow urine therapy with these herbs made the treatment more effective for Alzheimer's disease. As a result, this growing business will conduct a lot of investigations and create novel innovations in the decades to come.

References

[1] Aderibigbe, B. A., & Buyana, B. (2018). Alginate in wound dressings. *Pharmaceutics,* 10(2), 42. doi:10.3390/pharmaceutics10020042.

[2] Alsarra, I. A., Hamed, AY., & Alanazi, FK. (2008) Acyclovir liposomes for intranasal systemic delivery: development and pharmacokinetics evaluation. *Drug Deliv,* 15(5), 313-321. doi:10.1080/10717540802035251.

[3] Pfisterer, A. Novel Formulation Additives for an Anti-Alzheimer's Disease Drug. *Advanced Science News.* 2017; 1-8. John Wiley & Sons, Inc. https://www.advancedsciencenews.com/novel-formulation-additives-anti-alzheimers-disease-drug/.

[4] Araya-Quintanilla, F., Gutiérrez-Espinoza, H., Sanchez-Montoya, U., Munoz-Yanez, M. J., Baeza-Vergara, H., Petersen-yanjari, M., & Fernandez-Lecaros, L., (2020). Effectiveness of omega-3 fatty acid supplementation in patients with Alzheimer disease: A systematic review and meta-analysis. *Neurologia,* 35(2), 105-114. doi:10.1016/j.nrl.2017.07.009.

[5] Atri, A., (2019)). Current and future treatments in Alzheimer's disease. *Semin Neurol,* 39(2), 227-240. https://doi.org/10.1055/s-0039-1678581. doi: 10.1055/s-0039-1678581.

[6] Avgerinos, K. I., Kalaitzidis, G., Malli, A., Kalaitzoglou, D., Gr Myserlis, P., & Vasileios-Arsenois, L., (2018). Intranasal insulin in Alzheimer's dementia or mild cognitive impairment: A systematic review. *J. Neurol*, 265(7), 1497–1510. doi: 10.1007/s00415-018-8768-0.

[7] Bansal, D., Yadav, K., Pandey, V., Ganeshpurkar, A., Agnihotri, A., & Dubey, N., (2016). Lactobionic acid coupled liposomes: an innovative strategy for targeting hepatocellular carcinoma. *Drug Deliv,* 23(1), 140-146. doi: 10.3109/10717544.2014.907373.

[8] Bhatt, D. L., Hull, M.A., Song, M., Hulle, C.V., Carlsson, C., John Chapman, M., & Peter, P.T., (2020). Beyond cardiovascular medicine: Potential future uses of icosapent ethyl. *Eur. Heart J. Suppl.,* 22(Suppl. J), J54–J64. doi: 10.1093/eurheartj/suaa119.

[9] Briggs, R., Kennelly, SP., & Neill, D., (2016). Drug treatments in Alzheimer's disease. *Clin. Med (Lond),* 16(3), 247-253. doi: 10.7861/clinmedicine.16-3-247.

[10] Brookmeyer R., Nada, A., Claudia, H.K., & María, M.C., (2018). Forecasting the prevalence of preclinical and clinical Alzheimer's disease in the United States. *Alzheimer's & Dement,* 14(2), 121-129. doi: 10.1016/j.jalz.2017.10.009.

[11] Calvo-Perxas, L., Turro-Garriga, O., Vilalta-Franch, J., Lozano-Gallego, M., Eugenio, R., Marquez, F., Carmona, O., Gich, J., Manzano, A., Vinas, M., Roig, AM., & Garreolmo, J., (2017). Trends in the prescription and long-term utilization of antidementia drugs among patients with Alzheimer's disease in Spain: a cohort study using the registry of dementias of girona. registry of dementias of girona. *Drugs Aging,* 34(4), 303-310. doi: 10.1007/s40266-017-0446-x.

[12] Campbell, J. M., Stephenson, M.D., Courten, B., Chapman, I., Bellman, S.M., Aromataris, E., (2018). Metformin Use Associated with Reduced Risk of Dementia in Patients with Diabetes: A Systematic Review and Meta-Analysis. *J. Alzheimers Dis,* 65, 1225–1236. doi: 10.3233/JAD-180263.

[13] Cardoso, B. R., Roberts, B.R., Malpas, C.B., Vivash, L., Genc, S., Saling, M.M., Desmond, P., Steward, C., Hicks, R.J., Callahan, J., Amy, B., Collins, S., Macfarlane, S., Corcoran, N.M., Hovens, C.M., Velakoulis, D., Brien, T.J., Hare, D.J., & Bush, A.I., (2019). Supranutritional Sodium Selenate Supplementation Delivers Selenium to the Central Nervous System: Results from a Randomized Controlled Pilot Trial in Alzheimer's Disease. *Neurotherapeutics,* 16(1), 192–202. doi: 10.1007/s13311-018-0662-z.

[14] *ClinicalTrials.gov.* Nighttime Agitation and Restless Legs Syndrome in People with Alzheimer's Disease. NCT03082755. Available online: https://ClinicalTrials.gov/show/NCT03082755 (accessed on 1 May 2021).

[15] *ClinicalTrials.gov.* Riluzole in Mild Alzheimer's Disease. NCT01703117. Available online: https://ClinicalTrials.gov/show/ NCT01703117 (accessed on 28 April 2021).

[16] *ClinicalTrials.gov.* Study of BHV-4157 in Alzheimer's Disease. NCT03605667. Available online: https://ClinicalTrials.gov/show/ NCT03605667 (accessed on 28 April 2021).

[17] Cortes-Altamirano, J. L., Olmos-Hernández, A., Bonilla-jaime, H., Bandala, C., Gonzalez-Maciel, A., & Alfaro-Rodriguez, A., (2016). Levetiracetam as an antiepileptic, neuroprotective, and hyperalgesic drug. *Neurol. India,* 64(6), 1266–1275. doi: 10.4103/0028-3886.193801.

[18] Cox, K. H., Pipingas, A., & Scholey, A.B., (2015). Investigation of the effects of solid lipid curcumin on cognition and mood in a healthy older population. *J. Psychopharmacol,* 29(5), 642–651. doi: 10.1177/0269881114552744.

[19] Craft, S., Claxton, A., Baker, L.D., Hanson, A.J., Cholerton, B., Trittschuh, E.H., Dahl, D., Caulder, E., Neth, B., Montine, T.J., Jung, Y., Maldjian, J., Whitlow, C., & Friedman, S., (2017). Effects of Regular and Long-Acting Insulin on Cognition and Alzheimer's Disease Biomarkers: A Pilot Clinical Trial. *J. Alzheimers Dis,* 57(4), 1325–1334. doi: 10.3233/JAD-161256.

[20] Craft, S., Raman, R., Chow, T.W., Rafii, M.S., chung-kai, S., Rissman, R.A., Donohue, M.C., Brewer, J.B., Jenkins, C., harless, K., Gessert, D., & Aisen, P.S., (2020). Safety, Efficacy, and Feasibility of Intranasal Insulin for the Treatment of Mild Cognitive Impairment and Alzheimer Disease Dementia: A Randomized Clinical Trial. *JAMA Neurol,* 77(9), 1099–1109. doi: 10.1001/jamaneurol.2020.1840.

[21] Cummings, J., Lee, G., Zhong, K., Fonseca, J., & Taghva, K., (2012). Alzheimer's disease drug development pipeline: 2021. *Alzheimer's Dement,* 7(1), e12179. doi: 10.1002/trc2.12179.

[22] Cummings, J., Ritter, A., & Zhong, K., (2018). Clinical trials for disease-modifying therapies in Alzheimer's disease: a primer, lessons learned, and a blueprint for the future. *J Alzheimers Dis,* 64(s1), S3-S22. doi: 10.3233/JAD-179901.

[23] Daniels, V., Wood, M., Leclercq, K., Kaminski, M., & Gillard, M., (2013). Modulation of the conformational state of the SV2A protein by an allosteric mechanism as evidenced by ligand binding assays. *Br. J. Pharmacol,* 169(5), 1091–1101. doi: 10.1111/bph.12192.

[24] Dregan, A., & Gulliford, MC., (2013). Leisure-time physical activity over the life course and cognitive functioning in late mid-adult years: a cohort-based investigation. *Psychol Med,* 43(11), 2447-58. doi: 10.1017/S0033291713000305.

[25] Dyall, S. C., (2015). Long-chain omega-3 fatty acids and the brain: A review of the independent and shared effects of EPA, DPA and DHA. Front. *Aging Neurosci,* 7, 52. doi: 10.3389/fnagi.2015.00052.

[26] Eggink, E., Eric, P., Moll, C., Willem, AG., & Edo, R., (2019). A population perspective on prevention of dementia. *J. Clin medicine,* 8(6), 834. doi: 10.3390/jcm 8060834.

[27] Fitzgerald, D. P., Emerson, D.L., Qian, Y., Anwar, T., Liewehr, D.J., Steinberg, S.M., Silberman, S., Palmieri, D., & Steeg, P.S., (2012). TPI-287, a new taxane family member, reduces the brain metastatic colonization of breast cancer cells. *Mol Cancer Ther,* 11(9), 1959–1967. doi: 10.1158/1535-7163.MCT-12-0061.

[28] Gejl, M., Gjedde, A., Egefjord, L., Arne, M., Hansen, S. B., Vang, K., Rodell, A., Hans, B., Gottrup, H., Schacht, A., Niels, M., Brock, B., & Rungby, J., (2016). In Alzheimer's Disease, 6-Month Treatment with GLP-1 Analog Prevents Decline of Brain Glucose Metabolism: Randomized, Placebo-Controlled, Double-Blind Clinical Trial. *Front Aging Neurosci,* 8, 108. doi: 10.3389/fnagi.2016.00108.

[29] Gorelick, P. B., Furie, KL., Iadecola, C., Smith, E.E., Waddy, S.P., Lloyd-Jones, D.M., Bae, H.J., Bauman, M.A., Dichgans, M., Duncan, P.W., Girgus, M., Howard, V.J., Lazar, R.M., Sudha, S., Testai, F.D., Gaal, S.V., Yaffe, K., Wasiak, H., & Zerna, C., (2017). Defining optimal brain health in adults: a presidential advisory from the American Heart Association/American Stroke Association. *Stroke,* 48(10), e284-e303. doi: 10.1161/STR.0000000000000148.

[30] Grossberg, G. T., Manes, F., Allegri, RF., Gutierrez-Robledo, LM., Gloger, S., Xie, L., Jia, XD., Pejovic, V., Miller, ML., Perhach, JL., & Graham, SM., (2013). The safety, tolerability, and efficacy of once-daily Memantine (28 mg): a multinational, randomized, double-blind, placebo-controlled trial in patients with moderate-to-severe Alzheimer's disease taking cholinesterase inhibitors. *CNS Drugs,* 27(6), 469-478. doi: 10.1007/s40263-013-0077-7.

[31] Howard, R., McShane, J., Lindesay, C., Ritchie, A.B., Barber, R., Burns, A., Dening, T., Findlay, D., & Holmes, C., Alan, H., Robin, J., Jones, R., Roy, J., Lan, M., Ajay, M., O'Brien, J., Peter, P., Bart, S., Edmund, J., Katona, C., Hills, R., Knapp, M., Clive, B., Brown, R., Sube, B., Caroline, O., Mary, G., Adams, J., Gray, R., Tony, J., Peter, B., & Patrick P., (2012). Donepezil and Memantine for moderate-to-severe Alzheimer's disease. *N. Engl. J. Med,* 366(10), 893-903. doi: 10.1056/NEJMoa1106668.

[32] Hudry, E., Hai-yan, W., Arbel-Ornath, M., Tadafumi, H., Roland, M., Fan, Z., Spires-Jones, T.L., Betensky, R.A., Bacskai, B.J., & Hyman, B.T., (2012). Inhibition of the NFAT pathway alleviates amyloid β neurotoxicity in a mouse model of Alzheimer's disease. *J. Neurosci,* 32(9), 3176–3192. doi: 10.1523/JNEUROSCI.6439-11.2012.

[33] Kishita, N., Backhouse, T., & Mioshi, EJ., (2020). Nonpharmacological interventions to improve depression, anxiety, and quality of life (QoL) in people with Dementia: an overview of systematic reviews. *Geriatr. Psychiatry Neurol,* 33(1), 28-41. doi: 10. 1177/0891988719856690.

[34] Koenig, A., Mechanic-Hamilton, D., Xie, S.X., & Combs, M.F., (2017). Effects of the Insulin Sensitizer Metformin in Alzheimer Disease: Pilot Data From a Randomized Placebo-controlled Crossover Study. *Alzheimer Dis. Assoc. Disord,* 31(2), 107–113. doi: 10.1097/WAD.0000000000000202.

[35] Kreisl, W. C., Lyoo, C.H., Meghan, M., Snow, J., Jenko, K.J., Kimura, N., Corona, W., Morse, C.L., Zoghbi, S.S., Pike, V.W., Mcmahon, F.J., Turner, R.S., & Innis, R.B., (2013). *In vivo* radioligand binding to translocator protein correlates with severity of Alzheimer's disease. *Brain,* 136(Pt 7), 2228–2238. doi: 10.1093/brain/awt145.

[36] Lee, M. S., Wahlqvist, M.L., Yu-Ching, C., Wen-Hui, F., Jiunn-Tay, L., Jen-chun, k., Hsiao-Yu, L., Ting-Mei, L., Xiu, L., Chih-cheng, H., Andrews, Z.B., & Wen-Harn, P., (2014). Turmeric improves post-prandial working memory in pre-diabetes independent of insulin. *Asia Pac. J. Clin. Nutr,* 23(4), 581–591. doi: 10.6133/apjcn.2014.23.4.24.

[37] Lin, C. H., Chen, P.K., Yue-Cine, C., Liang-Jen, C., Yan-Syun, C., Tsai, G.E., & Hsien-Yuan, L., (2014). Benzoate, a D-amino acid oxidase inhibitor, for the treatment of early-phase Alzheimer disease: A randomized, double-blind, placebo-controlled trial. *Biol. Psychiatry,* 75(9), 678–685. doi: 10.1016/j.biopsych.2013.08.010.

[38] Littlejohns, T. J., Henley, WE., Lang, IA., Annweiler, C., Beauchet, O., Chaves, PH., Fried, L., Kestenbaum, BR., Kuller, LH., Langa, KM., Lopez, OL., Kos, K., Soni, M., & Llewellyn, D.J., (2014). Vitamin D and the risk of dementia and Alzheimer disease. *Neurology,* 83(10), 920-928. doi: 10.1212/WNL.0000000000000755.

[39] Longo, F. M., & Massa, S.M., (2004). Neuroprotective strategies in Alzheimer's disease. NeuroRx, 1, 117–127. doi: 10.1602/neurorx.1.1.117 [CrossRef] 235. Eddy, C.M.; Rickards, H.E. The cognitive impact of antiepileptic drugs. *Ther. Adv. Neurol. Disord.* 2011, 4, 385–407.

[40] Sessa, M., Balestrieri, M.L., Ferrari, G., Servillo, L., Castaldo, D., D'Onofrio, N., Donsì, F., & Tsao, R., (2014). Bioavailability of encapsulated resveratrol into nanoemulsion-based delivery systems. *Food Chem,* 147, 42–50. doi: 10.1016/j.foodchem.2013.09.088.

[41] Mahase, E., (2021). Three FDA advisory panel members resign over approval of Alzheimer's drug. *BMJ,* 373, n1503. doi: 10.1136/bmj.n1503.

[42] Mancuso, R., Fryatt, G., Madeleine, C., Juliane, O., Elena, P., Monzon-sandoval, J., Ribe, E., Winchester, L., Webber, C., Nevado, A., Jacobs, T., Austin, N., Theunis, C., Grauwen, K., Ruiz, E.D., Mudher, A., Vicente-Rodriguez, M., Christine, A.P., Simmons, C., cash, D., Jill, R., Consortium, N.I.M.A., Lovestone, S., Gomez-Nicola, D., & Perry, V.H., (2019). CSF1R inhibitor JNJ-40346527 attenuates microglial proliferation and neurodegeneration in P301S mice. *Brain,* 142(10), 3243–3264. doi: 10.1093/brain/awz241.

[43] Matsunaga, S., Fujishiro, H., Takechi, H., (2019). Efficacy and Safety of Glycogen Synthase Kinase 3 Inhibitors for Alzheimer's Disease: A Systematic Review and Meta-Analysis. *J. Alzheimers Dis*, 69(4), 1031–1039. doi: 10.3233/JAD-190256.

[44] Matsunaga, S., Kishi, T., Annas, P., Basun, H., Hampel, H., & Nakao, L., (2015). Lithium as a Treatment for Alzheimer's Disease: A Systematic Review and Meta-Analysis. *J. Alzheimers Dis*, 48(2), 403–410. doi: 10.3233/JAD-150437.

[45] Mazereeuw, G., Lanctôt, K.L., Chau, S.A., Walter, S., & Nathan, H., (2012). Effects of ω-3 fatty acids on cognitive performance: A meta-analysis. *Neurobiol. Aging,* 33(7), 1482.e17–1482.e29. doi: 10.1016/j.neurobiolaging.2011.12.014.

[46] Miyake, M. M., & Bleier, BS., (2015). The blood-brain barrier and nasal drug delivery to the central nervous system. *Am. J. Rhinol Allergy,* 29(2), 124-127. doi: 10.2500/ajra.2015.29.4149.

[47] Molinuevo, J. L., Llado, A., & Rami, L., (2005). Memantine: targeting glutamate excitotoxicity in Alzheimer's disease and other dementias. *Am. J. Alzheimers Dis. Other Demen,* 20(2), 77-85. doi: 10.1177/153331750502000206

[48] Mondal, P., Das, G., Juhee, K., Pradhan, K., & Ghosh, S., (2018). Crafting of Neuroprotective Octapeptide from Taxol-Binding Pocket of β-Tubulin. *ACS Chem. Neurosci,* 9(3), 615–625. doi: 10.1021/acschemneuro.7b00457.

[49] Oertel, W., & Schulz, JB., (2016). Current, and experimental treatments of Parkinson disease: A guide for neuroscientists. *J. Neurochem,* 139(Suppl. 1), 325-337. doi: 10.1111/jnc.13750.

[50] Olmos-Alonso, A., Schetters, S.T., Sri, S., Askew, K., Renzo, M., Vargas-Caballero, M., Holscher, C., Perry, V.H., & Gomez-Nicola, D., (2016). Pharmacological targeting of CSF1R inhibits microglial proliferation and prevents the progression of Alzheimer's-like pathology. *Brain,* 139(Pt 3), 891–907. doi: 10.1093/brain/awv379.
[51] Ortinski, P., &Meador, K.J., (2004). Cognitive side effects of antiepileptic drugs. *Epilepsy Behav,* 5(Suppl. 1), S60–S65. doi: 10.1016/j.yebeh.2003.11.008.
[52] Ostrowitzki, S., Lasser, R.A., Ernest, D., Philip, S., Barkhof, F., Tania, N., Ashford, E., Sylvie, R., Carsten, H., Paul, D., Klein, G., Mirjana, A., Dubois, B., Boada, M., Kaj, B., Luca, S., & Paulo, F., (2017). A phase III randomized trial of gantenerumab in prodromal Alzheimer's disease. *Alzheimers Res. Ther,* 9(1), 95. doi: 10.1186/s 13195-017-0318-y.
[53] Ostrowski, S. M., Johnson, K., Siefert, M., Shank, S., Sironi, L., Wolozin, B., Landreth, GE., & Ziady, AG., (2016). Simvastatin inhibits protein isoprenylation in the brain. *Neuroscience,* 329, 264-274. doi: 10.1016/j.neuroscience.2016.04.053.
[54] Pagano, K., Tomaselli, S., Molinari, H., & Laura, R., (2020). Natural Compounds as Inhibitors of Aβ Peptide Aggregation: Chemical Requirements and Molecular. Mechanisms. *Front Neurosci,* 14, 619667. doi: 10.3389/fnins.2020.619667.
[55] Patrick, R. P., (2019). Role of phosphatidylcholine-DHA in preventing APOE4-associated Alzheimer's disease. *FASEB J,* 33(2), 1554–1564. doi: 10.1096/fj. 201801412R.
[56] Rai, A., Jain, A., Jain, A., Pandey, V., Chashoo, G., Soni, V., & Sharma, PR., (2015). Targeted SLNs for management of HIV-1 associated dementia. *Drug Dev Ind Pharm,* 41(8), 1321-1327. doi: 10.3109/03639045.2014.948453.
[57] Rane, J. S., Bhaumik, P., & Panda, D., (2017). Curcumin Inhibits Tau Aggregation and Disintegrates Preformed Tau Filaments *in vitro*. *J. Alzheimers Dis,* 60(3), 999–1014. doi: 10.3233/JAD-170351.
[58] Reisberg, B., Doody, R., Stoffler, A., Schmitt, F., Ferris, S., & Mobius, HJ., (2003). Memantine in moderate-to-severe Alzheimer's disease. *N. Engl. J. Med,* 348(14), 1333-1341. doi: 10.1056/NEJMoa013128.
[59] Rojanathammanee, L., Floden, A.M., Manocha, G.D., & Combs, C.K., (2015). Attenuation of microglial activation in a mouse model of Alzheimer's disease via NFAT inhibition. *J. Neuroinflamm,* 12, 42. doi: 10.1186/s12974-015-0255-2.
[60] Rountree, S. D., Atri, A., Lopez, OL., & Doody, RS., (2013). Effectiveness of antidementia drugs in delaying Alzheimer's disease progression. *Alzheimers Dement,* 9(3), 338-345. doi: 10.1016/j.jalz.2012.01.002.
[61] Al Harthi, S., Alavi, S.E., Radwan, M.A., El Khatib, M.M., & AlSarra, I.A., (2019). Nasal delivery of donepezil HCl-loaded hydrogels for the treatment of Alzheimer's disease. *Sci. Rep,* 9(1), 1–20. doi: 10.1038/s41598-019-46032-y.
[62] Bahadur, S., Pardhi, D.M., Rautio, J., Rosenholm, J.M., & Pathak, K., (2020). Intranasal Nano emulsions for direct nose-to-brain delivery of actives for CNS disorders. *Pharmaceutics*, 12(12), 1230. doi: 10.3390/pharmaceutics12121230.
[63] Salameh, T. S., Rhea, E.M., Talbot, K., & Banks, W.A., (2020). Brain uptake pharmacokinetics of incretin receptor agonists showing promise as Alzheimer's and Parkinson's disease therapeutics. *Biochem Pharmacol,* 180, 114187. doi: 10.1016/j. bcp.2020.114187.

[64] Samaras, K., Makkar, S., Crawford, J.D., kochan, N.A., Wen, W., Draper, B., Trollor, J.N., Henry, B., & Sachdev, P.S., (2020). Metformin Use Is Associated With Slowed Cognitive Decline and Reduced Incident Dementia in Older Adults With Type 2 Diabetes: The Sydney Memory and Ageing Study. *Diabetes Care,* 43(11), 2691–2701. doi: 10.2337/dc20-0892.

[65] Sato, T., Hanyu, H., Hiroa, K., Kanetaka, H., Sakurai, H., & Toshihiko, L., (2011). Efficacy of PPAR-γ agonist pioglitazone in mild Alzheimer disease. *Neurobiol Aging,* 32(9), 1626–1633. doi: 10.1016/j.neurobiolaging.2009.10.009.

[66] Scheltens, P., Strooper, BD., Miia, K., Henne, H., Gael, C., Charlotte, ET., Jeffrey, C., & Wiesje, MF., (2021). Alzheimer's disease. *Lancet,* 397(10284), 1577-1590. doi: 10.1016/S0140-6736(20)32205-4.

[67] Schoenberg, M. R. Rum, R.S., Osborn, K.E., & Werz, M.A., (2017). A randomized, double-blind, placebo-controlled crossover study of the effects of levetiracetam on cognition, mood, and balance in healthy older adults. *Epilepsia,* 58(9), 1566–1574. doi: 10.1111/epi.13849.

[68] Seju, U., Kumar, A., & Sawant, KK., (2011). Development, and evaluation of olanzapineloaded PLGA nanoparticles for nose-to-brain delivery: *in vitro* and *in vivo* studies. *Acta Biomater*, 7(12), 4169-4176. doi: 10.1016/j.actbio.2011.07.025.

[69] Singh, M., Kaur, M., Kukreja, H., Chugh, R., Silakari, O., & Singh, D., (2013). Acetylcholinesterase inhibitors as Alzheimer therapy: from nerve toxins to neuroprotection. *Eur. J. Med. Chem,* 70, 165-188. doi: 10.1016/j.ejmech.2013.09.050.

[70] Sochocka, M., Donskow-Łysoniewska, K., Diniz, B.S., Kurpas, D., Ewa B., & Jerzy, L., (2019). The Gut Microbiome Alterations and Inflammation-Driven Pathogenesis of Alzheimer's Disease-a Critical Review. *Mol. Neurobiol,* 56(3), 1841–1851. doi: 10.1007/s12035-018-1188-4.

[71] Soeda, Y., & Takashima, A., (2020). New Insights Into Drug Discovery Targeting Tau Protein. *Front. Mol. Neurosci,* 13, 590896. doi: 10.3389/fnmol.2020.590896.

[72] Sosnik, A., & Seremeta, KP., (2017). Polymeric hydrogels as technology platform for drug delivery applications, *Gels,* 3(3), 25. doi: 10.3390/gels3030025.

[73] Supasitthumrong, T., Bolea-Alamanac, B.M., Selim, A., Woo, V.L., Abdool, P.S., & Davies, S.J., (2019). Gabapentin and pregabalin to treat aggressivity in dementia: A systematic review and illustrative case report. *Br. J. Clin. Pharmacol*, 85(4), 690–703. doi: 10.1111/bcp.13844.

[74] Syed, Y. Y., (2020). Sodium Oligomannate: First Approval. *Drugs,* 80(4), 441–444. doi: 10.1007/s40265-020-01268-1.

[75] Tabet, N., (2006). Acetylcholinesterase inhibitors for Alzheimer's disease: antiinflammatories in acetylcholine clothing. *Age Ageing,* 35(4), 336-338. doi: 10. 1093/ageing/afl027.

[76] Taniguchi, S., Suzuki, N., Masuda, M., Shin-ichi, H., Takeshi, I., Michel, G., & Masato, H., (2005). Inhibition of heparin-induced tau filament formation by phenothiazines, polyphenols, and porphyrins. *J. Biol. Chem,* 280(9), 7614–7623. doi: 10.1074/jbc.M408714200.

[77] Thomas, J., Thomas, C.J., Radcliffe, J., & Itsiopoulos, C., (2015). Omega-3 Fatty Acids in Early Prevention of Inflammatory Neurodegenerative Disease: A Focus on Alzheimer's Disease. *Biomed. Res. Int*, 2015, 172801. doi: 10.1155/2015/172801.

[78] Tolar, M., Abushakra, S., Hey, J.A., Anton, P., & Marwan, S., (2020). Aducanumab, gantenerumab, BAN2401, and ALZ-801-the first wave of amyloid-targeting drugs for Alzheimer's disease with potential for near term approval. *Alzheimers Res. Ther,* 12(1), 95. doi: 10.1186/s13195-020-00663-w.

[79] Vyas, T. K., Babbar. AK., Sharma, RZ., Singh, S., Misra, A., (2006). Intranasal mucoadhesive microemulsions of clonazepam: preliminary studies on brain targeting. *J. Pharm. Sci,* 95(3), 570-580, doi: 10.1002/jps.20480.

[80] Wang, H., Amanuel, AA., Kalkidan, HA., Cristiana, A., Kaja, MA., Foad, AA., & Semaw, FA., (2017). Global, regional, and national under-5 mortality, adult mortality, age-specific mortality, and life expectancy, 1970–2016: a systematic analysis for the Global Burden of Disease Study 2016. *Lancet,* 390(10100), 1084-1150. doi: 10.1016/S0140-6736(17)31833-0.

[81] Wang, T., Kuang, W., Wei, C., Xu, W., Zhang, L., Li, Y., Hailin, L., Peng, Y., Chen, Y., Wang, B., Xiao, J., Honghua, L., Yan, C., Du, Y., Tang, M., He, Z., Haibo, C., Wei, L., Lin, H., Shi, S., Jianzhong, B., Zhou, H., Yan, C., Gao, X., Guan, Y., Qiu, H., Kewei, C., Xianliang, X., Ding, J., Meiyu, G., & Xiao, S., (2020). A phase II randomized trial of sodium oligomannate in Alzheimer's dementia. *Alzheimers Res. Ther*, 12(1), 110. doi: 10.1186/s13195-020-00678-3.

[82] Wang, X., Sun, G., Feng, T, Zhang, J., Xun, H., Tao, W., xie, Z., Xingkun, C., Yang, J., Huan, W., Chang, S., Gong, Y., Ruan, L., Zhang, G., Yan, S., Wen, L., Chen, D., Yang, D., Qingli, Z., Lin, F., Jia, L., Haiyan, Z., Ge, C., Xiao, S., Jian, D., & Meiyu, G., (2019). Sodium oligomannate therapeutically remodels gut microbiota and suppresses gut bacterial amino acids-shaped neuroinflammation to inhibit Alzheimer's disease progression. *Cell Res,* 29(10), 787–803. doi: 10.1038/s41422-019-0216-x.

[83] Wischik, C. M., Edwards, P.C., Lai, R.Y., Roth, M., & Harrington, C.R., (1996). Selective inhibition of Alzheimer disease-like tau aggregation by phenothiazines. *Proc. Natl. Acad. Sci. USA,* 93(20), 11213–11218. doi: 10.1073/pnas.93.20.11213.

[84] Wischik, C. M., Staff, R.T., Wischik, D.J., Peter, B., Murray, A.D., Storey, M.D., Kook, K.A., Harrington, C.R., (2015). Tau aggregation inhibitor therapy: An exploratory phase 2 study in mild or moderate Alzheimer's disease. *J. Alzheimers Dis,* 44(2), 705–720. doi: 10.3233/JAD-142874.

[85] Wolozin, B., Wang, SW., Li, NC., Lee, A., Lee, TA., & Kazis, LE., (2007). Simvastatin is associated with a reduced incidence of dementia and Parkinson's disease. *BMC Med*, 5(1), 20. doi: 10.1186/1741-7015-5-20.

[86] Xiao, S., Chan, P., Tao, W., Hong, Z., Wang, S., Kuang, W., He, J., Pan, X., Zhou, Y., Ji, Y., Wang, L., Yan, C., Peng, Y., Ye, Q., Wang, X., Wu, Y., Qu, Q., Chen, S., Li, S., Wei, C., Jun, X., Peng, D., Zhao, Z., Luo, B., Wu, W., Lu, S., Liu, C., Mao, P., Wang, Q., Zhao, Q., Guo, Q., Zhou, Y., Li, Y., Jiang, L., Ren, W., Ouyang, Y., Yan, W., liu, S., Jia, J., Nan, Z., Liu, Z., He, R., Feng, T., Lu W., Tang, H., Gao, P., Zhang, Y., Chen, L., Wang, L., Yin, Y, Qun, X., Xiao, J., Lin, C., Xi, C., Hui, Z., Dan, G., Xia, M., Lian, T., Peng, G., Xu, Z., Bin, J., Hua, H., Chen, X., Guan, Y., Cui, R., Qiu, H., Xin, X., Chen, H., Yu, D., Jing, Z., Feng, T., Marc, C., Chen, K., Cummings, J.L., Ding, J., Geng, M., & Zhang, Z., (2021). A 36-week multicenter, randomized, double-blind, placebo-controlled, parallel-group, phase 3 clinical trial of sodium oligomannate for mild-to-moderate Alzheimer's dementia. *Alzheimers Res. Ther*, 13(1), 62. doi: 10.1186/s13195-021-00795-7.

[87] Yan, B. C., Wang, J., Rui, Y., Cao, J., Xu, P., Dan, J., Zhu, X., Moo-Ho, Won., Ping, B., & Su, P., (2019). Neuroprotective Effects of Gabapentin Against Cerebral Ischemia Reperfusion-Induced Neuronal Autophagic Injury via Regulation of the PI3K/Akt/mTOR Signaling Pathways. *J. Neuropathol. Exp. Neurol*, 78(2), 157–171. doi: 10.1093/jnen/nly119.

[88] Yiannopoulou, K. G., & Papageorgiou, SG., (2020). Current and Future Treatments in Alzheimer Disease: An Update. *J Cent Nerv Syst Dis*, 12,1179573520907397. doi: 10.1177/1179573520907397.

[89] Yu, T. W., Lane, H. Y., & Lin, C. H., (2021). Novel Therapeutic Approaches for Alzheimer's Disease: An Updated Review. *Int. J. Mol. Sci*, 22(15), 8208. doi: 10. 3390/ijms22158208.

[90] Zumbar, C. T., Usubalieva, A., King, P.D., Li, X., Mifsud, C.S., Dalton, H. M., Sak, M., Urio, S., Bryant, W.M., McElroy, J. P., Farmer, G., & Lehman, N.L., (2018). The CNS penetrating taxane TPI 287 and the AURKA inhibitor alisertib induce synergistic apoptosis in glioblastoma cells. *J. Neurooncol*, 137(3), 481–492. doi: 10.1007/s11060-018-2755-2.

Chapter 11

Current Trends and Updates in the Treatment of Parkinson's Disease

Nitu Kumari[1], MSc,
Santosh Anand[1,*], PhD,
Kamal Shah[2], PhD,
and Nagendra Singh Chauhan[3], PhD

[1]Department of Biotechnology, School of Applied Sciences, REVA University, Bengaluru, India
[2]Institute of Pharmaceutical Research, GLA University, Mathura, India
[3]Drug Testing Laboratory, Avam Anusandhan Kendra, Raipur, India

Abstract

Parkinson's disease (PD) is an age-associated neurodegenerative disorder that worsens as time progresses. Its primary neuropathological feature is pars compacta degeneration brought on by an accumulation of Lewy neurites and Lewy bodies that leads to a reduction in dopamine (DA) levels. The scientific community has made significant contributions toward the development of therapeutic interventions for the treatment and management of PD, but so far, no viable remedy or retardation of neurodegeneration has yet been achieved with existing therapeutic modalities. To treat the associated motor symptoms, only pharmacological treatments are available. These treatments include dopamimetic drugs like DA precursor and DA agonists, as well as inhibitors of monoamineoxidase-B (MAO-B), catechol-O-methyl-transferase (COMT) and decarboxylase enzymes. Through binding to the DA receptors, DA agonists may pass easily across the blood-brain barrier

* Corresponding Author's Email: santosh.anand@reva.edu.in; sanand.biotech@gmail.com.

In: Neurogenerative Disorders
Editors: Mohit Agrawal, Manmohan Singhal, Amit Kumar Nayak et al.
ISBN: 979-8-89530-143-2

and imitate DA's effects, thereby lessening dyskinesia. Apokyn, Kynmobi, Mirapex, Requip, and Neupro are the DA agonists that FDA has currently approved for use. In order to gather information, a thorough review of published articles from PubMed, Science Direct, Scifinder, Google Scholar, and Web of Science was conducted on current updates in the treatment of PD. Based on the literature survey, recent techniques like invasive, non-invasive or minimally invasive treatment, nanoparticle-mediated PD management and PD management by using natural products that have been discussed. Further, this chapter provides an evaluation of current therapeutic approaches for PD and the therapeutic drugs in clinical trial pipeline for updating the readers with the recent therapeutic frontiers for the treatment of PD. The current chapter also encompasses the ongoing research mainly aimed at novel targets to identify promising candidates for the treatment and management of PD.

Keywords: parkinson's disease, dopamine, motor symptoms, PD management, current therapeutics

Introduction

Around the world, a substantial unit of the aged population have been severely impacted by Parkinson's disease (PD). PD is regarded as the second-most prevalent neurodegenerative disorder generally noticed between 55 and 65 years of age. A substantial group of the elderly population are becoming disabled and dying from PD when compared to any other neurological disorder. By 2030, it is predicted that the prevalence of PD will increase by more than 30%, having a substantial impact on society and the economy (Nakmode et al., 2023). The progressive damage of dopaminergic neurons, neuronal-synaptic nucleoproteins deposition and the creation of Lewy bodies are the key pathogenic characteristics of PD (Tian et al., 2023). There are currently no treatment options for the cure of PD. Fortunately a number of drugs including dopamine (DA) agonists and levodopa (L-DOPA) can offer relief only to symptoms. Various treatment approaches have been shown effective such as pharmacology, treatment with pharmacotherapy including L-DOPA, DA agonists, and anticholinergics, together with non-drug interventions like surgery and exercise (Prajjwal et al., 2023). Prolonged use of these therapies, however, can have untoward effects and may not completely stop the progression of the disease. Therefore, it necessitates the hunt for novel, safe, and efficient medications for the treatment and management of PD (Pirker et al., 2023). In these investigations, we concentrated on both new therapeutic strategies and ongoing developments in established medications that aid in the management of PD. To effectively conduct novel, curative and/or treatment research, it is essential to have a thorough grasp of the underlying mechanisms, risk factors, and diagnosis as PD is considered to be a complicated disease (Nakmode et al., 2023)., The present review systemically describes the pathophysiology and diagnosis of PD, and the recent approaches in the management of PD including surgical and device aided therapies, nanoparticle-mediated PD management, treatment with natural products, and α-synuclein (α-syn)-targeted therapies.

Pathophysiology

Neurodegeneration is one of the critical challenges that affect millions of elderly population worldwide. Mitochondria has been proven to play a significant role in the pathogenesis of PD. Specific genes such as Parkin, PINK 1, LRRK2, SNCA, and DJ-1 are associated with mitochondrial dysfunction in PD as evidenced from earlier *in vivo* and *in vitro* findings (Figure 1). Mitochondrial DNA also plays a crucial role in PD pathophysiology (Abrishamdar et al., 2022; Qi et el., 2023).

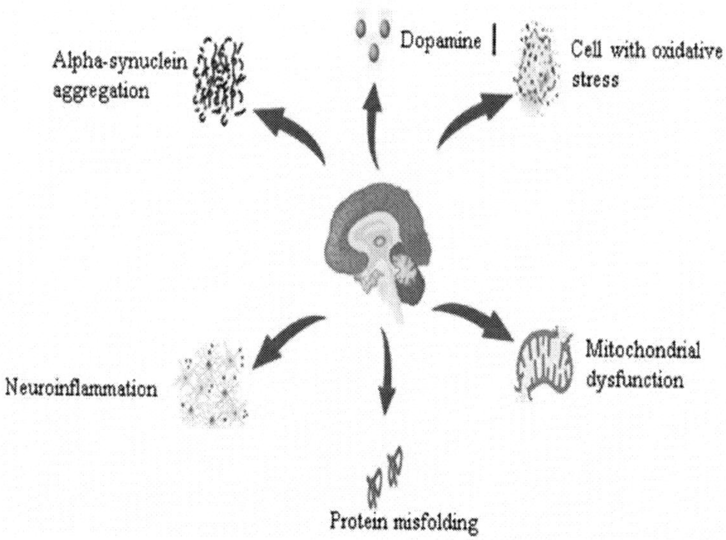

Figure 1. Pathophysiology of Parkinson's Diseases.

Genetic Basis

More than 20 genes and loci have been discovered since the recognition of the very first gene associated with PD in 1997. The estimated percentage of cases attributable to these monogenic causes of PD varies between research and study populations and is thought to be between 5-25% of all cases. It has been demonstrated that PD is attributed to mutations in the gene coding sequence and complete duplications and triplications that change the gene functionality. Major genes linked with PD are *SNCA*, *LRRK2*, *VPS*35, *PRKN*, *PINK 1*, *PARK7* (Xia et al., 2022; Battis et al., 2023; Han and He, 2023; Granek et al., 2023).

SNCA

The SNCA gene, that produces the 16 kilodaltons α-syn protein, was the first gene identified to be associated with PD. The important role of α-syn protein in PD pathogenesis is consistent with the finding that dominant SNCA mutations are accountable for PD and these mutations may have different impacts at the molecular level (Zhou et al., 2023). The N-terminal domain of the α-syn is affected by the mutations p.A53T, p.A30P, and p.E46K. The p.A53T and p.A30P mutations promote the development of protofibrils and progressively bigger aggregates (Gasser, 2023). Mutations in p.E46K have been found to improve C-terminal and N-terminal interactions and raise the N-terminal positive charge, whereas the p.A53T and p.A30P mutations have the reverse effect. A recent study compared dopaminergic neurons in patients with p.A30P mutation in SNCA to gene-corrected clones and found that the patient cells had defective mitochondrial respiration, rotenone sensitivity, and unusual lipid metabolism (Jia et al., 2022).

LRRK2

Leucine-rich repeat kinase 2 (*LRRK2*) is one of the most widely mutated genes in familial PD (Snead et al., 2022). Research findings have demonstrated that the pathogenic LRRK2 mutations universally enhance substrate phosphorylation, and this increase in substrate phosphorylation causes neurodegeneration in LRRK2-associated PD. Rab proteins are most likely the primary substrates, however it is yet unclear how Rab phosphorylation results in neurodegeneration (Ito and Tate., 2023).

VPS35

A crucial part of the retromeric complex that facilitates the retrograde transport of molecules from endosomes to the cell surface and Golgi trans-network, is the gene that codes for the vacuolar protein sorting 35 ortholog (VPS35), which in turn binds mitochondria-associated protein ligase (MAPL) (Ying et al., 2023). The D686N variation (formerly D620N) impairs interaction between VPS35 and MAPL, increasing mitochondrial fragmentation and fission, which affects complex I assembly and activity (Williams et al., 2022). Furthermore, the D686N variant prevents association with the multifunctional protein 2, that interacts with the aminoacyl tRNA synthetase complex and promotes its growth and transport to the nucleus, wherein it stimulates the PARK1 leading to neuroinflammation and neurodegeneration (Rangel et al., 2023).

PRKN and PINK1

The gene product of the PRKN gene, E3 ubiquitin ligase parkin functions in coordination with the neuroprotective PINK1 protein in a pathway of the mitochondrial quality control (MQC) system (Pereira et al., 2023). The MQC performs a variety of tasks, including controlling the continuous and timely turnover of mitochondria as well as the management of mitochondrial morphology, ATP levels, and the regulation of interconnected and dynamic networks of mitochondria through fusion and fission (Cavallieri et al., 2023). Parkin, a protein that is normally found in the cytoplasm is drawn to depolarized outer mitochondrial membrane (OMM) and encourages the ubiquitination of OMM proteins involved in upregulating mitochondrial fusion (Agarwal and Muqit, 2022). It functions downstream of PINK1 in a shared pathway to perform similar roles in the cell. In fact, due to decreased mitochondrial division, missense mutants of parkin and PINK1 showed a loss of mitochondrial integrity, resulting in neurodegeneration (Bhatti et al., 2023).

PARK7

Researchers studied that when compared to wild-type mice, DJ-1-deficient mice exhibit a marked decline in dopaminergic neuronal function, which can be brought on by ageing or neurotoxic injections (Zhang et al., 2023). Dopaminergic neurons are shielded by DJ-1 from oxidative stress (OS) and mitochondrial dysfunction (Lee et al., 2022). Oxidation of DJ-1 protein at the cysteine 106 residue (Cys106) in situations of OS strengthens its neuroprotective properties (Liu et al., 2023). Mutations in the protein PARK7 have been reported in subjects with rare early-onset of PD (Cho et al., 2023).

Dopamine (DA)

DA as a neurotransmitter plays a fundamental role in numerous mental and physical activities including reward, motivation, mood, sleep, voluntary movement and attention. Owing to numerous functions exhibited by DA, its levels should be firmly regulated, as an augmented concentration or its deficiency may be involved in pathological conditions (Chakrabarti and Bisaglia, 2023). Tyrosine hydroxylase and aromatic amino acid decarboxylase are responsible for the production of DA in the cytoplasm, and the vesicular monoamine transporter 2 (VMAT2) sequesters it quickly into synaptic vesicles, where the low pH stabilises it (Hurben and Tretyakova, 2022). Immediately after being released into the synaptic cleft, DA is quickly reabsorbed by the DA transporter. If the concentration of cytosolic DA is higher, it can be metabolised by the enzyme monoamine oxidase (MAO) into the toxic compound 3,4-dihydroxyphenilacetldehyde (DOPAL) and finally to anontoxic metabolite 3,4-dihydroxyphenylacetic acid (DOPAC) by aldehyde dehydrogenase. At cytosolic pH, DA undergoes auto-oxidation producing reactive quinones (DAQs) and ROS in the process. Both DOPAL and DAQs can interact with cytosolic nucleophiles impacting their function and finally resulting in mitochondrial dysfunction. PD neurotoxicity appears to be caused by the interaction between DOPAL and α-syn (Nagatsu et al., 2022; Nam et al., 2022).

Mitochondrial Dysfunction and Oxidative Stress

OS is caused by the imbalance between the levels of reactive oxygen species (ROS) and antioxidant defence system (Betteridge, 2000). Increased OS and mitochondrial dysfunction have been regarded as central events responsible for the progressive decline of the dopaminergic neurons in PD (Vastegani et al., 2023). Huge amounts of ATP-based energy may be supported by the mitochondrial oxidative phosphorylation process that regulates energy-dependent cell activities like cell motility, protein folding, and metabolism (He et al., 2023). Mitophagy is the selective removal of damaged mitochondria through autophagy. Mitochondria strive to preserve a homeostasis between the mitophagy and biogenesis to uphold mitochondrial quality. Additionally, the electron carriers in the mitochondrial electron transport chaincan produce reactive ROS, that are closely associated with OS. ROS weaken and/or blocks oxidative phosphorylation, release caspase-3, decrease ATP synthesis, and cause mitochondrial injury. They also cause protein oxidation and lipid peroxidation in mitochondrial membranes, and damage to mitochondrial membrane structure, mitochondrial DNA, and electron transport chain enzyme complexes (Tian et al., 2020).

Protein Misfolding

Protein aggregation and misfolding associated with almost all neurodegenerative diseases are the precursors of inclusion bodies aggregation in the neuronal cells (Basha et al., 2023). A proteostasis network is an advanced biological system that regulates the entire procedure which results in correctly folded functioning proteins. A quantitative rise in misfolded proteins prone to aggregation acts as the precursor of many neurodegenerative diseases owing to dysregulation of proteostasis. When α-syn loses its original structure during PD pathogenesis, a cascade of polymerizations that result in the creation of toxic inclusions is set off (Mohammed et al., 2023). Ubiquitin (26S proteasome's proteolysis signal) and chaperones helps in refolding misfolded proteins are frequently reported in these aggregates. The recognition of disease-prone genetic mutations that codes for multiple ubiquitin–proteasome cascade proteins in PD has strengthened the association between the neurodegeneration and ubiquitin–proteasome system (Behl et al., 2022).

Neuroinflammation

Chronic neuroinflammation is one of the hallmark of PD wherein innate immunity of the nervous system is overactivated. Overactivation of innate immunity leads to the secretion of inflammatory mediators including nitric oxide, COX-2, and inducible nitric oxide synthase (iNOS) due to OS, infection, aging, and pollution. These inflammatory mediators further lead to activation of MAPK (mitogen-activated protein kinase), NF-κB, and PI3K/AKT pathways triggering neuroinflammation and promoting neuronal damage and cell death (Liu et al., 2021; Bowirrat., 2022).

Recent Therapeutic Approaches to PD Management

Although PD is the second most prevalent neurodegenerative disorder, there is a shortage of efficient treatments, particularly those which modify the pathogenesis of the disease. Instead, other alternatives focus on treating the motor-related symptoms and non-motor-related symptoms independently to provide patients with symptomatic relief (Lamptey et al., 2022) (Figure 2).

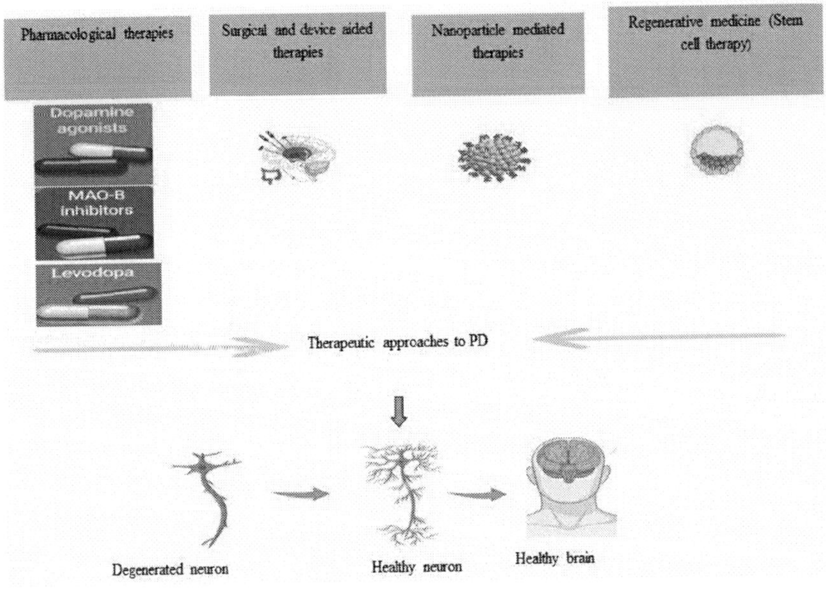

Figure 2. Current Therapeutic approaches in the management of Parkinson's Diseases.

Oral Treatment Options

The main strategy for treating PD is to restore the decreasing DA levels in the substantia nigra region. Various approaches have been adopted to increase DA levels (Wang et al., 2023).

Levodopa

As a direct precursor of DA, L-DOPA aids in the recovery of DA-related motor deficits (Rusch et al., 2023). L-DOPA (3,4-dihydroxy-L-phenylalanine) which is supplemented orally is a precursor of DA and is frequently used during early and late course of PD (Li et al., 2022). In contrast to peripheral DA, L-DOPA delivered through the gastrointestinal tract gets an easy entry to the blood-brain barrier (BBB) and is converted to DA for further use. L-DOPA and carbidopa are typically provided in conjunction to enhance absorption and avoid early peripheral conversion to DA. L-DOPA is coupled with carbidopa to prevent its breakdown in the peripheral areas before reaching the brain (Vliet et al., 2023).

Dopamine Agonists

Dopamine agonists (DAs) have been considered as significant therapeutics in PD treatment. Although DAs have been revealed to be promising candidates in the management of PD, they are constrained by certain side effects. In terms of affinity, selectivity, receptor subtype, receptor occupancy, chemical make-up, and intrinsic activity on the receptor, DAs can differ significantly (Namballa et al., 2023). D2/D3 (D2-like) DA receptors are the primary targets of majority of currently licensed DAs for treating PD. However, selective D1/D5 (D1-like) DA receptor activation may allow for robust motor function activation while preventing adverse effects (AEs) brought on by D2/D3 receptor agonism (Bezard et al., 2023; Issacson et al., 2023).

MAO-B Inhibitors

Inhibitors of MAO-B are frequently employed to treat the symptoms of PD. Early-stage PD has been effectively treated with MAO-B inhibitor monotherapy, whereas in advanced stages PD have been successfully treated with MAO-B inhibitors in the form of adjuvant medications. The MAO-B based therapeutic modalities have been found to be effective in treating patient's non-motor and motor symptoms, reduction of "OFF" time, and potential for delaying or preventing disease progression (Tan et al., 2022).

COMT Inhibitors

The enzyme COMT (catechol-O-methyltransferase) is responsible for O-methylating catechol substrates such as catecholamines, catechol oestrogens, and catechol medicines. For the treatment of motor fluctuations in PD patients, COMT inhibitors are crucial therapeutic drugs (Jost, 2022). Before reaching the brain, 3-O-methyldopa is quickly and extensively metabolised from L-DOPA by the action of COMT in the peripheral tissues, which reduces its effectiveness. Several COMT inhibitors are given as adjuvants to increase the bioavailability of L-DOPA, aiming to circumvent problems caused by the minimal quantity of L-DOPA that reaches the brain. As a result, blocking COMT has gained popularity as a method of raising catecholamine levels (Vicente et al., 2022; Regensburger et al., 2023).

Adenosine A2A Antagonists

To integrate the nigra-striatal DA and cortico-striatal glutamate signaling, and to regulate the cortico-striatal synaptic plasticity and cognition, the adenosine A2A receptors (A2ARs) are upregulated in the striatum (Nagaoka et al., 2023). By co-localizing and building heterodimers with the metabotropic glutamate 5 receptors in the striatum and DA D2 receptors, striatal A2ARs can play a regulatory role in instrumental learning. Inhibitory control over motor activity and certain cognitive processes, including goal-directed behaviour in healthy mice and action sequence learning in PD patients, are exerted by the striatal A2AR activation (Cai et al., 2023). It has been shown that adenosine A2A receptor antagonist/inverse agonist KW-6356 is effective when used alone to treat PD patients (Ohno et al., 2023). Nourianz (istradefylline), a selective adenosine A2A receptor (A2AR) antagonist was recently licenced by the U.S. Food and Drug administration for the treatment of OFF-patients with PD. A2AR antagonists have been demonstrated in preclinical investigations to control neuroprotection and cognitive deficits in subjects with PD or traumatic brain injury (Zhao et al., 2023).

Amantadine

The drug amantadine hydrochloride was formulated as an antiviral substance. PD patient's motor symptoms and the course of their influenza virus infection both improved as a result of one of the first amantadine clinical trials. The Food and Drug Administration in 1973 approved amantadine for treating PD. According to Dutta (2023), amantadine activates the presynaptic DA receptor D2, which inhibits the DA transporter involved in DA reuptake. It inhibited MAO-B in animal trials, which reduced DA breakdown (Chew et al., 2023). Interestingly, Rissardo et al., (2023) showed that amantadine is an σ1 receptor agonist, which is probably associated with the psychostimulant-like attributes of this drug. Akyuz et al., (2023) reported that amantadine successfully blocks alpha-7 nicotinic receptors suggesting its anticholinergic adverse effects namely urinary retention, xerostomia, and constipation. It may further impact serotoninergic cascades, elevating serotonin availability. Also, amantadine has been reported to augment serotonin secretion and prevent serotonin uptake in presynaptic neurons in rat models.

Surgical and Device Aided Therapies

Invasive Treatment

An invasive technique is one that uses instrumentation along with the puncture needle to provide concentrated entry into the body with the help of percutaneous puncture or incision (Cousins et al., 2019).

Deep Brain Stimulation

The primary therapeutic strategy for severe and medically unresponsive movement disorders such as PD, dystonia, and essential tremor is deep brain stimulation (DBS). For PD patients who exhibit motor fluctuations, medication-resistant tremor, and/or dyskinesia, DBS is an effective treatment

(Bhattacharya et al., 2022; Desai et al., 2023). An extension linking the electrode to the implantable pulse generator (IPG) and one or more electrodes are implanted into a specified area of the brain during this invasive, well-established neurosurgical procedure. The battery and circuits that produce the electrical signal and transport it to the desired brain structure are housed inside the IPG. The DBS system enables the administration of electrical pulses to particular brain regions with little impact on surrounding areas (Senevirathne et al., 2023).

Surgical Lesion Therapies

Thermocoagulation can be used in radiofrequency pallidotomy, an ablative treatment to create a localised unilateral lesion in the globus pallidum internum (GPi) (Bouthour et al., 2023). DBS has replaced unilateral posteroventral pallidotomy because it only permits a unilateral regimen owing to safety concerns pertaining to bilateral intervention with no impact on axial symptoms and does not allow patients to spill off antiparkinsonian drugs. However, it is proved to be effective on mitochondria, has a lesser risk of infection, and is unquestionably still a low-cost attractive strategy for patients who cannot have closed follow-up visits for their condition (Fabbri et al., 2023).

Levodopa-Carbidopa Suspension

Suspension of L-DOPA-carbidopa (LC) is a stable gel suspension, which is subjected continuously through a percutaneous gastrojejunostomy and portable pump thus delivering L-DOPA to the jejunumdirectly, bypassing thegastrointestinal(GI)-associated absorption issues (Leta et al., 2023; Chaudhuri et al., 2022). Although LC has consistently shown to be a safe and effective treatment option for sleep disruption, it has already been shown to be useful in lowering dyskinesias and other motor characteristics in advanced PD (Tall et al., 2023).

Subcutaneous Infusion of Apomorphine

Due to its high lipophilic character apomorphine is easily absorbed. Apomorphine is rapidly bioavailable when administered subcutaneously at regular intervals, avoiding problems with GI-transit time and first-pass hepatic metabolism (Fabbri et al., 2023). Despite its effectiveness, it is typically underutilised since people with the Off condition may find it difficult to administer a subcutaneous injection. The formulation is typically a 10 or 20 mg/ml solution of apomorphine hydrochloride, initiating with the lowest dosage ranging from 2 to 6 mg, with up to 5 or 6 injections each day in combination with domperidone (Torres et al., 2023).

Non-Invasive Electrical Stimulation

It was established for the first time that electrical stimulation might alter motor nerve response in an animal model. Roberts Bartholow conducted an electrical stimulation experiment on conscious persons in 1874. Grand epileptic seizures were created during the experiment due to uncertain signal management, proving that electrical stimulation was effective in controlling human cerebral functioning (Zhang et al., 2023). Transcranial magnetic stimulation (TMS) and transcranial electrical stimulation (TES) which use coils or electrodes for the application of electric or magnetic forces to the human scalp, are two non-invasive strategies that are frequently practiced in clinics. These techniques cause neuroplastic and acute changes in cortical excitability (Mosilhy et al., 2022). Epilepsy, stroke, schizophrenia, and depression can all be treated using TES and TMS (Guo et al., 2023). These non-invasive procedures have the benefits of being safe, well-tolerated, affordable, and simple to use (Shahsavari et al., 2022). Overall, it is important and required to create novel neuromodulatory approaches that are non-invasive and have great spatial resolution (Liu et al., 2022). "Temporally interfering" (TI) electrical stimulation, a novel non-invasive brain stimulation approach was proposed by Grossman et al., in 2017. It is important to note that TI electrical stimulation, which has the advantages of both non-invasiveness and spatial targeting, can stimulate targets in deep brain regions without any surgical procedures. All these non-invasive techniques have the potential to cure neuropsychiatric diseases as they can activate deep and interior targets in the brain (Guo et al., 2023).

Organic Nanoparticles

Organic NPs are usually biodegradable and can elicit drug release upon cellular uptake and internalization, leading to long-term therapeutic effects. These can be synthesized using several strategies namely ionic association, chemical reduction in solution, solvent displacement, and photochemical processes (Duan et al., 2023). Organic NPs offer numerous benefits like structural versatility, better biocompatibility, and great scope for chemical alterations. These advantages impart NPs with a variety of applications like stimulus response and targeting, but the complexity of their synthesis and preparation limits their further employability in drug delivery to the brain (Lei et al., 2023).

Inorganic Nanoparticles

According to Dhaka et al., (2023), inorganic particles with different particle sizes ranging from 1 to 100 nm and morphologies make up the class of inorganic-based NPs. Additionally, undergoing various surface alterations, inorganic-based NPs can connect to drug molecules in a variety of ways including electrostatic contacts, hydrophobic interactions, and covalent bonds. Magnetic NPs, carbon NPs, metallic NPs, and nanozymes are the main types of inorganic-based NPs (Rafatmah et al., 2023).

Polymer-Based Nanoparticles

Polymeric NPs are one of the earliest and most effective means as drug delivery systems (DDS). These "colloidal systems that can be conjugated from biodegradable and biocompatible polymers into which drugs are dissolved, encapsulated, entrapped, chemically bounded, or surface-adsorbed" are referred to as nanocarriers (Hernando et al., 2023). Polyesters including polycaprolactone (PCL), polylactide acid (PLA), and poly lactic-co-glycolic acid (PLGA) were among the most often used materials for the formulation of polymeric NPs (Janrao et al., 2023). With this nanotechnology-based strategy, the DA neurotransmitter has been encapsulated in PLGA NPs for administration to 6-OHDA animal model of PD. The outcomes of *in vivo* tests showed that, DDS was suitable for correcting the neurobehavioral and neurochemical impairments seen in PD (Mishra et al., 2023). After administering polymeric NPs intraperitoneally, Monge-Fuentes et al., (2021) verified the results reported above using a comparable nanoformulation. Findings of the study demonstrated that increasing DA levels at the nigrostriatal circuit helped the 6-OHDA-treated mice to ameliorate the motor deficit.

Lipid-Based Nanoparticles

Lipid nanoparticles (LNPs) offer several advantages including the potential for a high loading capacity for hydrophobic drugs, a controlled drug-release profile, biocompatibility, and better stability compared to liposomes (Jacob et al., 2022). Additionally, because of their small size and lipidic nature, LNPs offer a significant potential for drug targeting through surface alterations, enabling simple transport across biological membranes (Singh et al., 2023). For the purpose of potentiating drug delivery to the brain, different methods of modifying nanostructured lipid carriers (NLCs) and solid LNPs have been used. These methods include size manipulation, hydrophilic coating, and surface binding with a molecule that binds to brain receptors enabling the avoidance of rapid removal by the reticuloendothelial system (Desai et al., 2023). As a result, LNPs help achieve therapeutic concentration with lower quantities of therapeutic molecules, minimising the toxicity of integrated pharmaceuticals due to lesser interaction with non-target organs. For the nose-to-brain distribution and intravenous route, a particle size of 200 nm diameter is suitable for straightforward entry into the CNS (Nakmode et al., 2023).

PD Treatment with Natural Products

Marine Products

According to Silva et al., (2023), the marine ecosystem has shown to be a resource for unusual and diversified chemical compounds possessing significant therapeutic promise for the cure of a variety of ailments, including neurological impairments. There have been reports of about 60 chemicals isolated from marine fungi, soft coral, bacteria, seaweed, molluscs, sea cucumbers, sponges, and starfish possessing neuroprotective potential for PD therapy. Among them alkaloids, terpenes, peptides, quinones, polyphenols, lipids, polysaccharides, pigments, and mycotoxins are the major compounds (Carroll et al., 2023). Through the suppression of NF-KB factor translocation, reduction in OS, prevention of mitochondrial dysfunction, blocking of inflammatory pathways and prevention of α-syn aggregation, they can affect a number of PD markers (Barber et al., 2023). Pant and Vasundhara., (2023) reported that Neoechinulin A, an alkaloid derived from various marine fungal species showed the capacity to lessen the neurotoxic effects brought on by rotenone and 1-methyl-4-phenylpyridinium (MPP+) in PC12 cells.

Traditional Herbs

Herbs have been utilised for centuries as traditional treatments for neurodegenerative diseases because they have a natural ability to heal with negligible untoward effects. Numerous herbal formulations with promising antioxidant properties have been found to be effective at protecting neurons, while only a small number have revealed to promote neuronal regeneration (Ezzat et al., 2023). Herbal secondary metabolites like flavonoids and other polyphenolic compounds successfully scavenge the neuronal damage and promote regeneration by identifying the crucial role of ROS and other free radicals (Kumar et al., 2023). Numerous earlier research has shown that herbal medication can successfully reduce motor as well as non-motor symptoms in PDsuggesting the efficacy of herbal medicine as an alternative therapy for PD treatment (Jun et al., 2023).

Regenerative Medicine in PD

Gene, Cell, and Tissue Regenerative Therapies

At present there is no proper treatment regimen for PD that can stop or reverse the disease progression. To combat this problem, the requirement for novel therapeutic approaches like gene therapy has recently attracted the attention of scientists. Adeno-associated virus (AAV), lentivirus, or any non-pathogenic virus can be used as a vector in gene therapy to deliver a therapeutic gene and treat diseases (Ail et al., 2023). The conversion of L-DOPA into DA is orchestrated by the enzyme aromatic L-amino acid decarboxylase (AADC). The dopaminergic nigrostriatal pathway tends to alter with PD progression and thus the expression of AADC decreases. As a result of this, disease symptoms deteriorate and the efficiency of L-DOPA treatment declines (patients need to take steadily higher doses). AADC gene therapy has successfully completed phase 1 of clinical trial for the treatment of PD (conducted between 2013 and 2020) (Kozlowska et al., 2023).

For many years, cell-based treatments for PD that safeguard dopaminergic neurons have been under consideration (Wang et al., 2023). A disease-modifying method of PD called stem cell transplantation has emerged. It employs replacing damaged cells and bystander effects such as the production of neurotrophic and anti-inflammatory factors. According to recent research, transplanted cells target the gut-brain axis by reducing the inflammatory response in the stomach and slowing down the brain neurodegenerative cell death pathways (Lee et al., 2023).

Optogenetic Therapy

Optogenetics is the study of the genetic regulation of cells that express light-sensitive ion channels. The analysis of brain circuits has been made easier by the development of optogenetic methods. With great temporal specificity, individual set of neurons and their projections can be precisely stimulated and inhibited using optogenetics. These methods are particularly well adapted to analysing the brain circuitry causing motor and cognitive impairment in animal models (Parker et al., 2022). Chen et al., (2023) carried out studies on 6-hydroxydopamine (6-OHDA)-induced PD mouse models to examine the function of GABAergic neurons in the zona incerta (ZI). The mice subjected to chemogenetic/optogenetic stimulation showed a reduction in GABA-positive neurons in the ZI, followed by activating or inhibiting GABAergic neurons. Chemogenetic/optogenetic activation of GABAergic neurons greatly enhanced the motor function of PD animals, and repeated rounds of chemogenetic activation of ZI GABAergic neurons was found to elevate the DA levels in the striatum.

Alpha-Synuclein Targeted Therapies

The 140 amino acid soluble protein known as α-syn is composed of three distinct regions: an amino-terminal lipid-binding region, a core hydrophobic non-amyloid region, the non-amyloid component domain, and a disordered carboxy-terminal. Its predicted molecular weight is 14,000 Da. Increased copy number (duplications or triplications) of the SNCA gene and N-terminal point mutations in α-syn results in autosomal dominant types of familial PD (Rodger et al., 2023). Immunisation and inhibition of α-syn aggregation are the two main α-syn targeted therapies. Active immunisation, in which the immune system is prompted to develop antibodies against α-syn, and passive immunisation, in which antibodies are administered directly are the two ways that immunotherapies work (Calabresi et al., 2023). The protein α-syn may result in harmful oligomers by aggregation. Consequently, a potentially effective neuroprotective and/or PD treatment strategy is to decrease α-syn protein synthesis and/or aggregation at the source using gene-silencing techniques (Rodger et al., 2023).

Autophagy Enhancement Treatment Strategy

As autophagy may remove damaged mitochondria and neuronal protein clumps, it is believed to play a neuroprotective role in PD. Fibrillar α-syn aggregation, which is a prominent component of Lewy bodies (LBs), results in intracellular organelle breakdown and dopaminergic neuronal death (Ma et al., 2023). Additionally, these effects are made worse by the inhibition of autophagy caused by chloroquine, while it can be reversed by the activation of autophagy caused by rapamycin (Geng et al., 2023). Dopaminergic neurons are particularly susceptible to mitochondrial dysfunction because of their high metabolic activity and high energy requirements. Due to ROS overproduction and OS brought on by mitophagy dysfunction, the timely turnover of damaged mitochondria must be maintained in order to prevent the advancement of PD. Autophagy plays a valuable role in PD by eliminating damaged mitochondria and aggregated α-syn as a crucial degradation mechanism (Zhang et al., 2023; Lu et al., 2023). α-syn overabundance and mutations in PD-linked genes (PINK1, LRRK2, PRKN, and GBA) weaken autophagy, leading to augmented α-syn aggregation and other neuromodulatory proteins in the PD brain, worsening neuronal degeneration and inflammation and creating a vicious cycle in the PD pathogenesis (Ma et al., 2023).

Supplementary Therapies for the Treatment and Prevention of PD

Music Therapy, Diet and Phytotherapy

A growing body of research on PD management is documented and it has been found that music therapy can promote health and wellness. Especially for motor symptoms, rhythm has been found to be very helpful (Hersh et al., 2023). It has been suggested that the rhythms in music can cause the motor neurons to work, which causes the muscles to contract and the body to move in time with the beat. In particular, the auditory processing area interacts with the nearby motor area upon music stimulation exhibiting commensurate motor performance (Fan et al., 2023). A possible management plan can involve dietary adjustments and lifestyle changes. Numerous studies have demonstrated that nutrition may be used to modify fatigue and depression in PD (Lawrie et al., 2022).

Both synthetic and natural antioxidant-rich plant materials have been found to be potent therapeutics for neurodegenerative diseases (NDDs) (Vijay et al., 2023). Recent studies have demonstrated the neuroprotective properties of natural compounds and also their potential to lower inflammation and OS.

Natural antioxidants like carotenoids, polyphenols, and vitamins C and E are widely distributed in vegetables, fruits, herbs, and nuts. Polyphenols from green tea, resveratrol from grapes, curcumin from turmeric, and other plant-based antioxidants are some examples of compounds that have undergone substantial research (Mittal et al., 2023). Even though they appear promising, more study is necessary to completely comprehend and validate their function for considering them as a potential therapeutic intervention in NDDs (Pilipovic et al., 2023).

Table 1. Some FDA approved therapies for PD

Name	Therapeutic Mechanism	Approval Year	Mechanism of action	References
Symmetrel (Indopharma ceuticals)	Anti-excitotoxicity	2003	NMDA Glutamate Receptor antagonist	Muller et al., 2023
Artane (Witeh-ayers research)	Neurotransmitter system	2003	Anticholinergic	Chopade et al., 2023
Parcopa (Schwarz pharma)	Neurotransmitter system	2004	Combination of Carbidopa and L-DOPA	Lewis et al., 2023
Zelapar (Valeant pharmaceuticals)	Neurotransmitter system	2006	MAO inhibitor	Chew et al., 2023
Requipxl (Glaxosmith kline)	Neurotransmitter system	2008	DA agonist	Hall et al., 2020
Sinemet (MERCK)	Neurotransmitter system	2014	Combination of Carbidopa and L-DOPA	Chopade et al., 2023
Rytary (Impax)	Neurotransmitter system	2015	Combination of Carbidopa and L-DOPA	Lenka et al., 2022
Duopa (Abbvie)	Neurotransmitter system	2015	Combination of Carbidopa and L-DOPA and COMT inhibitor	Chopade et al., 2023
Ongentys (Neurocrine biosciences)	Neurotransmitter system	2020	COMT inhibitor	Berger et al., 2022
Kynmobi (Sunovion)	Neurotransmitter system	2020	DA agonist	Chopade et al., 2023

Table 2. PD therapy in recent clinical trials

Compounds	Action	Id	Trial Phase	References
Quercetin	Reduces brain injuries through anti-apoptosis, autophagy enhancement and significant metabolic regulation	NCT 01376011 NCT 01376611	I	Xu et al., 2023
Cannabidiol	Motor/Tremor improvement	NCT 03582137 NCT 02818777	II	Bahji et al., 2022
Ginsenoside Rd	Helpful in Neuroprotection	NCT 00591084 NCT 00815763	III	Mittal et al., 2023

Table 3. NPs under treatment trials for PD

NPs	Diseases	Mechanism	Effects	References
Magnetic ironoxide NPS + reduced radiotherapy	Glioblastomia multiformie	Increased Caspase-3, heats of protein, and programmed death ligand 1 levels suppress tumour growth	Enhanced the overall survival rate of patient	Roque et al., 2023
Ultrasmall magnetic iron oxide	Ischemic stroke	Activates macrophages	Targeted inflammatory cytokines more effectively	Parra et al., 2023
Nano-curcumin	Migraine	Intercellular adhesion molecule 1, TNF-α gene expression suppressed	Relieved Headache	Guo et al., 2023

FDA Approved Drugs for PD Treatment

Numerous drugs including donepezil, galantamine, memantine, and riluzole have received FDA approval for the treatment of neurological disorders (Mittal et al., 2023) (Table 1). However, these medications have limited effectiveness in delaying the progression of disease and originated with side effects including headaches, gastrointestinal problems, and different functional issues. To improve the local therapeutic efficacy of these medications and lessen their side effects, innovative drug delivery mechanisms are warranted (Duan et al., 2023).

Therapies in Clinical Trials for PD Treatment

To date there are numerous treatment options for PD which are already approved and some of them are under different phases of clinical trial (Table 2). Clinical trials on humans (acccpted on 21st March 2023) have documented the therapeutic efficacy of anthocyanins on memory-related ailments and dementia patients (Sadowska et al., 2023).

Nanomedicine for PD Treatment under Clinical Trial

The fact that there are currently over 250 US FDA-approved nano-based drugs in the market is proof of the effectiveness of NPs in biomedical studies. The most widely used nanodrugs have been found as liposomal formulations, which make up about 33% of the drugs currently in the market. Recent studies have demonstrated that omega-3 fatty acids and curcumin NPs significantly reduced inflammation by reducing the production of ICAM-1, TNF-α, and COX-2/iNOS in subjects with migraine (Guo et al., 2023) (Table 3).

Conclusion

PD is a devastating age-linked neurological disorder. Clinical signs of PD include motor abnormalities such as dyskinesia, rest tremor, and disorder of fast eye movement behaviour. PD modifying drugs are not yet available. There are only a few symptomatic relief treatments available. Pharmacotherapy is the most used form of PD treatment. The usual course of treatment does not heal or reverse the illness. Some of the most frequently prescribed conventional drugs for PD include DA precursors, COMT inhibitors, MAO-B inhibitors, and central anticholinergics. Each of these drugs has a distinct set of therapeutic benefits and drawbacks. There are numerous drugs currently undergoing clinical investigations that are part of the developing trends in PD treatment that are efficient and continually changing. It has been demonstrated that early use of DA agonists, either alone or in combination with L-DOPA, can halt or delay the onset of motor issues. A lot of preclinical studies have also demonstrated that DA agonists have protective effects in a variety of *in vitro* and *in vivo* circumstances. The current chapter focuses on the ongoing therapeutic strategies in the management of PD with the limitations of the existing one. Furrther, it also covers the therapeutic strategies under clinical trials which may be accepted for PD management in the near future.

Acknowledgments

The authors acknowledge the Department of Biotechnology, School of Applied Sciences, REVA University for providing the necessary facilities.

Disclaimer

None.

References

Abhishek, K., Saksham, R., Deepti, K., Rao, N. G, Surya, P., Vinay, K., Vidhu, S., & Priya B. (2023). Medicinal Plants and Herbal Formulations Ameliorating Neurodegeneration: Remedies Combating Parkinson's and Alzheimer's Disease. *Journal of Young Pharmacists,* 15(2), 194-200.

Abrishamdar, M., Jalali, M. S., & Farbood, Y. (2023). Targeting Mitochondria as a Therapeutic Approach for Parkinson's Disease. *Cellular and Molecular Neurobiology*, 43(4), 1499-1518.

Agarwal, S., & Muqit, M. M. K. (2022). PTEN-induced kinase 1 (PINK1) and Parkin: Unlocking a mitochondrial quality control pathway linked to Parkinson's disease. *Current Opinion in Neurobiology,* 72, 111-119.

Ail, D., Malki, H., Zin, E. A., & Dalkara, D. (2023). Adeno-Associated Virus (AAV) - Based Gene Therapies for Retinal Diseases: Where are We? *The Application of Clinical Genetics*, 16, 111-130.

Akyuz, E., Celik, B. R., Aslan, F. S., Sahin, H., & Angelopoulou, E. (2023). Exploring the Role of Neurotransmitters in Multiple Sclerosis: An Expanded Review. *ACS Chemical Neuroscience,* 14(4), 527-553.

Bahji, A., Breward, N., Duff, W., Absher, N., Patten, S. B., Alcorn, J., & Mousseau, D. D. (2022). Cannabinoids in the management of behavioral, psychological, and motor symptoms of neurocognitive disorders: a mixed studies systematic review. *Journal of Cannabis Research*, 4(1), 11.

Barber, K., Mendonca, P., & Soliman, K. F. A. (2023). The Neuroprotective Effects and Therapeutic Potential of the Chalcone Cardamonin for Alzheimer's Disease. *Brain Sciences,* 13(1), 145.

Basha, S., Mukunda, D. C., Rodrigues, J., Gail D'Souza, M., Gangadharan, G., Pai, A. R., & Mahato, K. K. (2023). A comprehensive review of protein misfolding disorders, underlying mechanism, clinical diagnosis, and therapeutic strategies. *Ageing Research Reviews,* 90, 102017.

Battis, K., Xiang, W., & Winkler, J. (2023). The Bidirectional Interplay of α-Synuclein with Lipids in the Central Nervous System and Its Implications for the Pathogenesis of Parkinson's Disease. *International Journal of Molecular Sciences*, 24(17), 13270.

Behl, T., Kumar, S., Althafar, Z. M., Sehgal, A., Singh, S., Sharma, N., Badavath, V. N., Yadav, S., Bhatia, S., Al-Harrasi, A., Almoshari, Y., Almikhlafi, M. A., & Bungau, S. (2022). Exploring the Role of Ubiquitin-Proteasome System in Parkinson's Disease. *Molecular Neurobiology*, 59(7), 4257-4273.

Berger, A. A., Winnick, A., Izygon, J., Jacob, B. M., Kaye, J. S., Kaye, R. J., Neuchat, E. E., Kaye, A. M., Alpaugh, E. S., Cornett, E. M., Han, A. H., & Kaye, A. D. (2022). Opicapone, a Novel Catechol-O-methyl Transferase Inhibitor, for Treatment of Parkinson's Disease "Off" Episodes. *Health Psychology Research,* 10(3), 36074.

Betteridge, D. J. (2000). What is oxidative stress? *Metabolism,* 49, 3-8.

Bezard, E., Gray, D., Kozak, R., Leoni, M., Combs, C., & Duvvuri, S. (2024). Rationale and Development of Tavapadon, a D1/D5-Selective Partial Dopamine Agonist for the Treatment of Parkinson's Disease. *CNS & Neurological Disorders Drug Targets* (23(4), 476-487.

Bhattacharya, A., Mrudula, K., Sreepada, S. S., Sathyaprabha, T. N., Pal, P. K., Chen, R., & Udupa, K. (2022). An Overview of Noninvasive Brain Stimulation: Basic Principles and Clinical Applications. *Canadian Journal of Neurological Sciences*, 49(4), 479-492.

Bhatti, J. S., Kaur, S., Mishra, J., Dibbanti, H., Singh, A., Reddy, A. P., Bhatti, G. K., & Reddy, P. H. (2023). Targeting dynamin-related protein-1 as a potential therapeutic approach for mitochondrial dysfunction in Alzheimer's disease. *Biochimica et Biophysica Acta (BBA) Molecular Basis of Disease,* 1869(7), 166798.

Bouthour, W., Newman, N. J., & Biousse, V. (2023). Focused Ultrasound Ablation in Parkinson's Disease. *The New England Journal of Medicine,* 388(19), 1822.

Bowirrat, A. (2022). Immunosenescence and Aging: Neuroinflammation Is a Prominent Feature of Alzheimer's Disease and Is a Likely Contributor to Neurodegenerative Disease Pathogenesis. *Journal of Personalized Medicine,* 12(11), 1817.

Cai, Q., Xu, N., He, Y., Zhu, J., Ye, F., Luo, Z., Lu, R., Huang, L., Zhang, F., Chen, J. F., & Li, Y. (2023). α-Synuclein Aggregates in the Nigro-Striatal Dopaminergic Pathway Impair Fine Movement: Partial Reversal by the Adenosine A_{2A} Receptor Antagonist. *International Journal of Molecular Sciences,* 24(2), 1365.

Calabresi, P., Mechelli, A., Natale, G., Volpicelli-Daley, L., Di Lazzaro, G., & Ghiglieri, V. (2023). Alpha-synuclein in Parkinson's disease and other synucleinopathies: from overt neurodegeneration back to early synaptic dysfunction. *Cell Death & Disease*, 14(3), 176.

Carroll, A. R., Copp, B. R., Davis, R. A., Keyzers, R. A., & Prinsep, M. R. (2022). Marine natural products. *Natural Products Reports*, 39(6), 1122-1171.

Castillo-Rangel, C., Marin, G., Hernández-Contreras, K. A., Vichi-Ramírez, M. M., Zarate-Calderon, C., Torres-Pineda, O., Diaz-Chiguer, D. L., De la Mora González, D., Gómez Apo, E., Teco-Cortes, J. A., Santos-Paez, F. M., Coello-Torres, M. L. Á., Baldoncini, M., Reyes Soto, G., Aranda-Abreu, G. E., & García, L. I. (2023). Neuroinflammation in Parkinson's Disease: From Gene to Clinic: A Systematic Review. *International Journal of Molecular Sciences,* 24(6), 5792.

Castillo-Torres, S. A., Lees, A. J., & Merello, M. (2022). Intermittent Apomorphine Use for off Period Rescue in Parkinson's Disease: A Pragmatic Review of over Three Decades of Clinical Experience. *Movement Disorders Clinical Practice,* 10(2), 190-208.

Cavallieri, F., Cury, R. G., Guimarães, T., Fioravanti, V., Grisanti, S., Rossi, J., Monfrini, E., Zedde, M., Di Fonzo, A., Valzania, F., & Moro, E. (2023). Recent Advances in the Treatment of Genetic Forms of Parkinson's Disease: Hype or Hope? *Cells*, 12(5), 764.

Chakrabarti, S., & Bisaglia, M. (2023). Oxidative Stress and Neuroinflammation in Parkinson's Disease: The Role of Dopamine Oxidation Products. *Antioxidants (Basel)*, 12(4), 955.

Chaudhuri, K. R., Antonini, A., Pahwa, R., Odin, P., Titova, N., Thakkar, S., Snedecor, S. J., Hegde, S., Alobaidi, A., Parra, J. C., Zadikoff, C., Bergmann, L., & Standaert, D. G. (2022). Effects of Levodopa-Carbidopa Intestinal Gel on Dyskinesia and Non-Motor Symptoms Including Sleep: Results from a Meta-Analysis with 24-Month Follow-Up. *Journal of Parkinson's Disease,* 12(7), 2071-2083.

Chen, F., Qian, J., Cao, Z., Li, A., Cui, J., Shi, L., & Xie, J. (2023). Chemogenetic and optogenetic stimulation of zona incerta GABAergic neurons ameliorates motor impairment in Parkinson's disease. *iScience,* 26(7), 107149.

Chew, Z. X., Lim, C. L., Ng, K. Y., Chye, S. M., Ling, A. P. K., & Koh, R. Y. (2023). The Role of Monoamine Oxidase B Inhibitors in the Treatment of Parkinson's Disease - An Update. *CNS & Neurological Disorders Drug Targets*, 22(3), 329-352.

Cho, N., Joo, J., Choi, S., Kang, B. G., Lee, A. J., Youn, S. Y., Park, S. H., Kim, E. M., Masliah, E., Ko, Y., Cha, S. S., Jung, I., & Kim, K. K. A novel splicing variant of DJ-1 in Parkinson's disease induces mitochondrial dysfunction. *Heliyon,* 9(3), 14039.

Cousins, S., Blencowe, N. S., Blazeby, J. M. (2019). What is an invasive procedure? A definition to inform study design, evidence synthesis and research tracking. *BMJ Open,* 9(7), 028576.

Cruz-Vicente, P., Gonçalves, A. M., Barroca-Ferreira, J., Silvestre, S. M., Romão, M. J., Queiroz, J. A., Gallardo, E., & Passarinha, L. A. (2022). Unveiling the biopathway for the design of novel COMT inhibitors. *Drug Discovery Today,* 27(10), 103328.

Desai Kapadia, N., Marquez-Chin, C., & Chen, R. (2023). Editorial: Non-invasive stimulation: role in neurorehabilitation. *Frontiers in Rehabilitation Sciences,* 4, 1263530.

Desai, N., Rana, D., Salave, S., Gupta, R., Patel, P., Karunakaran, B., Sharma, A., Giri, J., Benival, D., & Kommineni, N. (2023). Chitosan: A Potential Biopolymer in Drug Delivery and Biomedical Applications. *Pharmaceutics*, 15(4):1313.

Dhaka, A., Mali, S. C., Sharma, S., & Trivedi, R. (2023). A review on biological synthesis of silver nanoparticles and their potential applications. *Results in Chemistry,* 6, 101108.

Duan, L., Li, X., Ji, R., Hao, Z., Kong, M., Wen, X., Guan, F., & Ma, S. (2023). Nanoparticle-Based Drug Delivery Systems: An Inspiring Therapeutic Strategy for Neurodegenerative Diseases. *Polymers (Basel),* 15(9), 2196.

Dutta, R. (2023). Psychosis in Parkinson's Disease and Current Management Trends-An Updated Review of Literature. *Journal of Neuroscience and Neurological Disorders,* 7, 27-56.

Ezzat, S. M., Marghany, R., El Mahdi, N., & Salem, M. A. (2023). Brain Function, Stroke, and Medicinal Herbs. In C. Egbuna & M. Rudrapal (Eds.), *Phytochemical Drug Discovery for Central Nervous System Disorders: Biochemistry and Therapeutic Effects* (pp. 161-180). Wiley Online Library. https://doi.org/10.1002/9781119794127.ch6.

Fabbri, M., Barbosa, R., & Rascol, O. (2023). Off-time Treatment Options for Parkinson's Disease. *Neurology and Therapy*, 12(2), 391-424.

Fan, L., Hu, E. Y., Hey, G. E., & Hu, W. (2023). Music Therapy for Gait and Speech Deficits in Parkinson's Disease: A Mini-Review. *Brain Sciences,* 13(7), 993.

Gasser, T. (2023). Genetic testing for Parkinson's disease in clinical practice. *Journal of Neural Transmission*, 130(6), 777-782.

Geng, X., Zou, Y., Li, S., Qi, R., Yu, H., & Li, J. (2023). MALAT1 Mediates α-Synuclein Expression through miR-23b-3p to Induce Autophagic Impairment and the Inflammatory Response in Microglia to Promote Apoptosis in Dopaminergic Neuronal Cells. *Mediators of Inflammation*, 2023:4477492.

Granek, Z., Barczuk, J., Siwecka, N., Rozpędek-Kamińska, W., Kucharska, E., & Majsterek, I. (2023). *GBA1* Gene Mutations in α-Synucleinopathies-Molecular Mechanisms Underlying Pathology and Their Clinical Significance. *International Journal of Molecular Sciences,* 24(3), 2044.

Guo, W., He, Y., Zhang, W., Sun, Y., Wang, J., Liu, S., & Ming, D. (2023). A novel non-invasive brain stimulation technique: "Temporally interfering electrical stimulation." *Frontiers in Neuroscience,* 17, 1092539.

Guo, Z. H., Khattak, S., Rauf, M. A., Ansari, M. A., Alomary, M. N., Razak, S., Yang, C. Y., Wu, D. D., & Ji, X. Y. (2023). Role of Nanomedicine-Based Therapeutics in the Treatment of CNS Disorders. *Molecules,* 28(3), 1283.

Hall, M. F., & Church, F. C. (2020). Integrative medicine and health therapy for Parkinson disease. *Topics in Geriatric Rehabilitation,* 36(3), 176-186.

Han, Y., & He, Z. (2023). Concomitant protein pathogenesis in Parkinson's disease and perspective mechanisms. *Frontiers in Aging Neuroscience*, 15, 1189809.

He, T., Lin, X., Su, A., Zhang, Y., Xing, Z., Mi, L., Wei, T., Li, Z., & Wu, W. (2023). Mitochondrial dysfunction-targeting therapeutics of natural products in Parkinson's disease. *Frontiers in Pharmacology,* 14, 1117337.

Hernando, S., Santos-Vizcaíno, E., Igartua, M., & Hernandez, R. M. (2023). Targeting the central nervous system: From synthetic nanoparticles to extracellular vesicles-Focus on Alzheimer's and Parkinson's disease. *WIREs Nanomedicine and Nanobiotechnology,* 15(5), 1898.

Hersh, D., Kong, S. J., & Smith, J. (2023). It's quite good fun: A qualitative study of a singing/songwriting programme for people with Parkinson's disease and their spouses. *International Journal of Language & Communication Disorders,* 58(6), 2103-2116.

Hurben, A. K., & Tretyakova, N. Y. (2022). Role of Protein Damage Inflicted by Dopamine Metabolites in Parkinson's Disease: Evidence, Tools, and Outlook. *Chemical Research in Toxicology,* 35(10), 1789-1804.

Isaacson, S. H., Hauser, R. A., Pahwa, R., Gray, D., & Duvvuri, S. (2023). Dopamine agonists in Parkinson's disease: Impact of D1-like or D2-like dopamine receptor subtype selectivity and avenues for future treatment. *Clinical Parkinsonism & Related Disorders,* 9, 100212.

Ito, G., & Utsunomiya-Tate N. (2023). Overview of the Impact of Pathogenic LRRK2 Mutations in Parkinson's Disease. *Biomolecules*, 13(5), 845.

Jacob, S., Nair, A. B., Shah, J., Gupta, S., Boddu, S. H. S., Sreeharsha, N., Joseph, A., Shinu, P., & Morsy, M. A. (2022). Lipid Nanoparticles as a Promising Drug Delivery Carrier for Topical Ocular Therapy-An Overview on Recent Advances. *Pharmaceutics,* 14(3), 533.

Janrao, C., Khopade, S., Bavaskar, A., Gomte, S. S., Agnihotri, T. G., & Jain, A. (2023). Recent advances of polymer based nanosystems in cancer management. *Journal of Biomaterial Science Polymer Edition,* 34(9), 1274-1335.

Jia, F., Fellner, A., & Kumar, K. R. (2022). Monogenic Parkinson's Disease: Genotype, Phenotype, Pathophysiology, and Genetic Testing. *Genes (Basel),* 13(3), 471.

Jost, W. H. (2022). Evaluating Opicapone as Add-on Treatment to Levodopa/DDCI in Patients with Parkinson's Disease. *Neuropsychiatric Disease and Treatment*, 18, 1603-1618.

Jun, P., Zhao, H., Jung, I. C., Kwon, O., Han, C. H., Won, J., & Jang, J. H. (2023). Efficacy of herbal medicine treatment based on syndrome differentiation for Parkinson's disease: A systematic review and meta-analysis of randomized placebo-controlled clinical trials. *Frontiers in Pharmacology*, 14:1108407.

Kozłowska, M., Kotarba, S., Tambor, J., Winiarski, M., Moczulska, H., Pietrusiński, M., & Borowiec, M. (2023). Parkinson's disease gene therapy: a comparative effectiveness review of completed clinical trials in terms of their possible implementation in treatment. *Medical Science Pulse,* 17(1), 24-31.

Lamptey, R. N. L., Chaulagain, B., Trivedi, R., Gothwal, A., Layek, B., & Singh, J. (2022). A Review of the Common Neurodegenerative Disorders: Current Therapeutic Approaches and the Potential Role of Nanotherapeutics. *International Journal of Molecular Sciences*, 23(3), 1851.

Lawrie, S., Coe, S., Mansoubi, M., Welch, J., Razzaque, J., Hu, M. T., & Dawes, H. (2023). Dietary Patterns and Nonmotor Symptoms in Parkinson's Disease: A Cross-Sectional Analysis. *Journal of the American Nutrition Association,* 42(4), 393-402.

Lee, J. Y., Castelli, V., Sanberg, P. R., & Borlongan, C. V. (2023). Probing Gut Participation in Parkinson's Disease Pathology and Treatment via Stem Cell Therapy. *International Journal of Molecular Sciences*, 24(13), 10600.

Lee, Y., Kim, J., Kim, H., Han, J. E., Kim, S., Kang, K. H., Kim, D., Kim, J. M., & Koh, H. (2022). Pyruvate Dehydrogenase Kinase Protects Dopaminergic Neurons from Oxidative Stress in *Drosophila DJ-1* Null Mutants. *Molecules and Cells,* 45(7), 454-464.

Lei, L., Tu, Q., Zhang, X., Xiang, S., Xiao, B., Zhai, S., Yu, H., Tang, L., Guo, B., Chen, X., & Zhang, C. (2023). Stimulus-responsive curcumin-based polydopamine nanoparticles for targeting Parkinson's disease by modulating α-synuclein aggregation and reactive oxygen species. *Chemical Engineering Journal*, 461, 141606.

Lenka, A., Di Maria, G., Lamotte, G., Bahroo, L., & Jankovic, J. (2022). Practical pearls to improve the efficacy and tolerability of levodopa in Parkinson's disease. *Expert Review of Neurotherapeutics,* 22(6), 489-498.

Leta, V., Klingelhoefer, L., Longardner, K., Campagnolo, M., Levent, H. Ç., Aureli, F., Metta, V., Bhidayasiri, R., Chung-Faye, G., Falup-Pecurariu, C., Stocchi, F., Jenner, P., Warnecke, T., & Ray Chaudhuri, K. (2023). International Parkinson and Movement Disorders Society Non-Motor Parkinson's Disease Study Group. Gastrointestinal barriers to levodopa transport and absorption in Parkinson's disease. *European Journal of Neurology,* 30(5), 1465-1480.

Lewis, M. M., Van Scoy, L. J., De Jesus, S., Hakun, J. G., Eslinger, P. J., Fernandez-Mendoza, J., Kong, L., Yang, Y., Snyder, B. L., Loktionova, N., Duvvuri, S., Gray, D. L., Huang, X., & Mailman, R. B. (2023). Dopamine D_1 Agonists: First Potential Treatment for Late-Stage Parkinson's Disease. *Biomolecules*, 13(5), 829.

Li, J., Li, N., Wei, J., Feng, C., Chen, Y., Chen, T., Ai, Z., Zhu, X., Ji, W., & Li, T. (2022). Genetically engineered mesenchymal stem cells with dopamine synthesis for Parkinson's disease in animal models. *npj Parkinsons Disease*, 8(1), 175.

Liu, B., Zhang, Y., Yang, Z., Liu, M., Zhang, C., Zhao, Y., & Song, C. (2021). ω-3 DPA Protected Neurons from Neuroinflammation by Balancing Microglia M1/M2

Polarizations through Inhibiting NF-κB/MAPK p38 Signaling and Activating Neuron-BDNF-PI3K/AKT Pathways. *Marine Drugs,* 19(11), 587.

Liu, S., Xu, S., Liu, S., & Chen, H. (2023). Importance of DJ-1 in autophagy regulation and disease. *Archives of Biochemistry and Biophysics*, 743, 109672.

Liu, X., Qiu, F., Hou, L., & Wang, X. (2022). Review of Noninvasive or Minimally Invasive Deep Brain Stimulation. *Frontiers in Behavioral Neuroscience*, 15, 820017.

Lu, Y., Li, Z., Zhang, S., Zhang, T., Liu, Y., & Zhang, L. (2023). Cellular mitophagy: Mechanism, roles in diseases and small molecule pharmacological regulation. *Theranostics,* 13(2), 736-766.

Ma, Z., Liang, H., Hu, B., Cai, S., & Yan, D. (2023). Autophagy-regulating miRNAs: Novel therapeutic targets for Parkinson's disease (Review). *International Journal of Molecular Medicine,* 51(6), 50.

Martínez-Parra, L., Piñol-Cancer, M., Sanchez-Cano, C., Miguel-Coello, A. B., Di Silvio, D., Gomez, A. M., Uriel, C., Plaza-García, S., Gallego, M., Pazos, R., & Groult, H. (2023). A Comparative Study of Ultrasmall Calcium Carbonate Nanoparticles for Targeting and Imaging Atherosclerotic Plaque. *ACS Nano,* 17(14), 13811-13825.

Merecz-Sadowska, A., Sitarek, P., Kowalczyk, T., Zajdel, K., Jęcek, M., Nowak, P., & Zajdel, R. (2023). Food Anthocyanins: Malvidin and Its Glycosides as Promising Antioxidant and Anti-Inflammatory Agents with Potential Health Benefits. *Nutrients,* 15(13), 3016.

Mishra, S., Sharma, V., & Kushwaha, S. (2023). A Study of the Impulse Control Behaviours in Persons with Parkinson's Disease. *Indian Journal of Clinical Psychology*, 50(1).

Mittal, P., Dhankhar, S., Chauhan, S., Garg, N., Bhattacharya, T., Ali, M., Chaudhary, A. A., Rudayni, H. A., Al-Zharani, M., Ahmad, W., Khan, S. U., Singh, T. G., & Mujwar, S. (2023). A Review on Natural Antioxidants for Their Role in the Treatment of Parkinson's Disease. *Pharmaceuticals,* 16(7), 908.

Mohammed, S., Russo, I., & Ramazzina, I. (2023). Uncovering the Role of Natural and Synthetic Small Molecules in Counteracting the Burden of α-Synuclein Aggregates and Related Toxicity in Different Models of Parkinson's Disease. *International Journal of Molecular Sciences*, 24(17), 13370.

Monge-Fuentes, V., Biolchi Mayer, A., Lima, M. R., Geraldes, L. R., Zanotto, L. N., Moreira, K. G., Martins, O. P., Piva, H. L., Felipe, M. S. S., Amaral, A. C., Bocca, A. L., Tedesco, A. C., & Mortari, M. R. (2021). Dopamine-loaded nanoparticle systems circumvent the blood-brain barrier restoring motor function in mouse model for Parkinson's Disease. *Scientific Reports,* 11(1), 15185.

Moradi Vastegani, S., Nasrolahi, A., Ghaderi, S., Belali, R., Rashno, M., Farzaneh, M., & Khoshnam, S. E. (2023). Mitochondrial Dysfunction and Parkinson's Disease: Pathogenesis and Therapeutic Strategies. *Neurochemical Research,* 48(8), 2285-2308.

Mosilhy, E. A., Alshial, E. E., Eltaras, M. M., Rahman, M. M. A., Helmy, H. I., Elazoul, A. H., Hamdy, O., & Mohammed, H. S. (2022). Non-invasive transcranial brain modulation for neurological disorders treatment: A narrative review. *Life Sciences,* 307, 120869.

Muller, T., Riederer, P., & Kuhn, W. (2023). Aminoadamantanes: from treatment of Parkinson's and Alzheimer's disease to symptom amelioration of long COVID-19 syndrome? *Expert Review of Clinical Pharmacology*, 16(2), 101-107.

Nagaoka, K., Asaoka, N., Nagayasu, K., Shirakawa, H., & Kaneko, S. (2023). Enhancement of adenosine A_{2A} signaling improves dopamine D_2 receptor antagonist-induced dyskinesia *via* β-arrestin signaling. *Frontiers in Neuroscience,* 16, 1082375.

Nagatsu, T., Nakashima, A., Watanabe, H., Ito, S., & Wakamatsu, K. (2022). Neuromelanin in Parkinson's Disease: Tyrosine Hydroxylase and Tyrosinase. *International Journal of Molecular Sciences,* 23(8), 4176.

Nakmode, D. D., Day, C. M., Song, Y., & Garg, S. (2023). The Management of Parkinson's Disease: An Overview of the Current Advancements in Drug Delivery Systems. *Pharmaceutics*, 15(5), 1503.

Nam, M. H., Sa, M., Ju, Y. H., Park, M. G., & Lee, C. J. (2022). Revisiting the Role of Astrocytic MAOB in Parkinson's Disease. *International Journal of Molecular Sciences,* 23(8), 4453.

Namballa, H. K., Dorogan, M., Gudipally, A. R., Okafor, S., Gadhiya, S., & Harding, W. W. (2023). Discovery of Selective Dopamine Receptor Ligands Derived from (-)-Stepholidine via C-3 Alkoxylation and C-3/C-9 Dialkoxylation. *Journal of Medicinal Chemistry,* 66(14), 10060-10079.

Ohno, Y., Suzuki, M., Asada, H., Kanda, T., Saki, M., Miyagi, H., Yasunaga, M., Suno, C., Iwata, S., Saito, J. I., & Uchida, S. (2023). *In Vitro* Pharmacological Profile of KW-6356, a Novel Adenosine A_{2A} Receptor Antagonist/Inverse Agonist. *Molecular Pharmacology,* 103(6), 311-324.

Pant, A., & Vasundhara, M. (2023). Endophytic fungi: a potential source for drugs against central nervous system disorders. *Brazilian Journal of Microbiology*, 54(3), 1479-1499.

Parker, K. L., Kim, Y., Alberico, S. L., Emmons, E. B., & Narayanan, N. S. (2016). Optogenetic approaches to evaluate striatal function in animal models of Parkinson disease. *Dialogues in Clinical Neuroscience*, 18(1), 99-107.

Pereira, S. L., Grossmann, D., Delcambre, S., Hermann, A., & Grünewald, A. (2023). Novel insights into Parkin-mediated mitochondrial dysfunction and neuroinflammation in Parkinson's disease. *Current Opinion in Neurobiology*, 80, 102720.

Pilipovic, K., Jurisic Grubesic, R., Dolenec, P., Kucic, N., Juretić, L., & Mrsic-Pelcic, J. (2023). Plant-Based Antioxidants for Prevention and Treatment of Neurodegenerative Diseases: Phytotherapeutic Potential of *Laurus nobilis*, *Aronia melanocarpa*, and Celastrol. *Antioxidants (Basel),* 12(3), 746.

Pirker, W., Katzenschlager, R., Hallett, M., & Poewe, W. (2023). Pharmacological Treatment of Tremor in Parkinson's Disease Revisited. *Journal of Parkinson's Disease,* 13(2), 127-144.

Prajjwal, P., Sanga, H. S., Acharya, K., Tango, T., John, J., Rodriguez, R. S., Marsool, M. D., Sulaimanov, M., Ahmed, A., & Hussin, O. A. 2023). Parkinson's disease updates: Addressing the pathophysiology, risk factors, genetics, diagnosis, medical and surgical treatment. *Annals of Medicine and Surgery*, 85(10), 4887-4902.

Qi, R., Sammler, E., Gonzalez-Hunt, C. P., Barraza, I., Pena, N., Rouanet, J. P., Naaldijk, Y., Goodson, S., Fuzzati, M., Blandini, F., Erickson, K. I., Weinstein, A. M., Lutz, M.

W., Kwok, J. B., Halliday, G. M., Dzamko, N., Padmanabhan, S., Alcalay, R. N., Waters, C., Hogarth, P., Simuni, T., Smith, D., Marras, C., Tonelli, F., Alessi, D. R., West, A. B., Shiva, S., Hilfiker, S., & Sanders, L. H. (2023). A blood-based marker of mitochondrial DNA damage in Parkinson's disease. *Science Translational Medicine*, 15(711), 1557.

Rafatmah, E., & Hemmateenejad, B. (2023). Metal nanoparticles for sensing applications. In A. Barhoum & Z. Altintas (Eds.), *Fundamentals of Sensor Technology*. (pp. 311-366). Woodhead Publishing. https://doi.org/10.1016/B978-0-323-88431-0.00019-3.

Regensburger, M., Ip, C. W., Kohl, Z., Schrader, C., Urban, P. P., Kassubek, J., & Jost, W. H. (2023). Clinical benefit of MAO-B and COMT inhibition in Parkinson's disease: practical considerations. *Journal of Neural Transmission,* 130(6), 847-861.

Rissardo, J. P., & Fornari Caprara, A. L. (2023). Myoclonus Secondary to Amantadine: Case Report and Literature Review. *Clinics and Practice,* 13(4), 830-837.

Rodger, A. T., ALNasser, M., & Carter, W. G. (2023). Are Therapies That Target α-Synuclein Effective at Halting Parkinson's Disease Progression? A Systematic Review. *International Journal of Molecular Sciences,* 24(13), 11022.

Roque, D., Cruz, N., Ferreira, H. A., Reis, C. P., Matela, N., Herculano-Carvalho, M., Cascao, R., & Faria, C. C. (2023). Nanoparticle-Based Treatment in Glioblastoma. *Journal of Personalized Medicine,* 13(9), 1328.

Rusch, C., Flanagan, R., Suh, H., & Subramanian, I. (2023). To restrict or not to restrict? Practical considerations for optimizing dietary protein interactions on levodopa absorption in Parkinson's disease. *npj Parkinson's Disease*, 9(1), 98.

Senevirathne, D. K. L., Mahboob, A., Zhai, K., Paul, P., Kammen, A., Lee, D. J., Yousef, M. S., & Chaari, A. (2023). Deep Brain Stimulation beyond the Clinic: Navigating the Future of Parkinson's and Alzheimer's Disease Therapy. *Cells,* 12(11), 1478.

Shabani, L., Abbasi, M., Azarnew, Z., Amani, A. M., & Vaez, A. (2023). Neuro-nanotechnology: diagnostic and therapeutic nano-based strategies in applied neuroscience. *Biomedical Engineering Online,* 22(1),1.

Shahsavari, D., Kudaravalli, P., Yap, J. E. L., & Vega, K. J. (2022). Expanding beyond endoscopy: A review of non-invasive modalities in Barrett's esophagus screening and surveillance. *World Journal of Gastroenterology,* 28(32), 4516-4526.

Silva, J., Alves, C., Soledade, F., Martins, A., Pinteus, S., Gaspar, H., Alfonso, A., & Pedrosa, R. (2023). Marine-Derived Components: Can They Be a Potential Therapeutic Approach to Parkinson's Disease? *Marine Drugs, 21*(8), 451.

Singh, S., Khurana, K., Chauhan, S. B., & Singh, I. (2023). Emulsomes: new lipidic carriers for drug delivery with special mention to brain drug transport. *Future Journal of Pharmaceutical Sciences,* 9(1), 1-17.

Snead, D. M., Matyszewski, M., Dickey, A. M., Lin, Y. X., Leschziner, A. E., & Reck-Peterson, S. L. (2022). Structural basis for Parkinson's disease-linked LRRK2's binding to microtubules. *Nature Structural & Molecular Biology,* 29(12), 1196-1207.

Tall, P., Qamar, M. A., Batzu, L., Leta, V., Falup-Pecurariu, C., & Ray Chaudhuri, K. (2023). Non-oral continuous drug delivery-based therapies and sleep dysfunction in Parkinson's disease. *Journal of Neural Transmission,* 130(11), 1443-1449.

Tan, Y. Y., Jenner, P., & Chen, S. D. (2022). Monoamine Oxidase-B Inhibitors for the Treatment of Parkinson's Disease: Past, Present, and Future. *Journal of Parkinsons Disease,* 12(2), 477-493.

Tchekalarova, J., & Tzoneva, R. (2023). Oxidative Stress and Aging as Risk Factors for Alzheimer's Disease and Parkinson's Disease: The Role of the Antioxidant Melatonin. *International Journal of Molecular Sciences*, 24(3), 3022.

Tian, Y., Lu, J., Hao, X., Li, H., Zhang, G., Liu, X., Li, X., Zhao, C., Kuang, W., Chen, D., & Zhu, M. (2020). FTH1 Inhibits Ferroptosis Through Ferritinophagy in the 6-OHDA Model of Parkinson's Disease. *Neurotherapeutics,* 17(4), 1796-1812.

Tian, Y., Xian, J., Tian, Y., & Gao, X. (2023). Establishment of a staging model for Parkinson's disease in mice. *Cellular and Molecular Biology* (Noisy-le-grand), 69(4), 141-146.

van Vliet, E. F., Knol, M. J., Schiffelers, R. M., Caiazzo, M., Fens, M. H. A. M. (2023). Levodopa-loaded nanoparticles for the treatment of Parkinson's disease. *Journal of Controlled Release,* 360, 212-224.

Vijay, A., & Balakrishnan, A. (2023). Plant-Derived Natural Products Targeting Multiple Pathways as Potential Therapeutics in the Treatment of Parkinson's Disease. In S. Pathak, A. Banerjee, A., & A. K. Duttaroy (Eds.), (pp. 263-280) *Evidence-based Functional Foods for Prevention of Age-related Diseases.* Springer, Singapore. https://doi.org/10.1007/978-981-99-0534-8_14.

Wang, F., Sun, Z., Peng, D., Gianchandani, S., Le, W., Boltze, J., & Li, S. (2023). Cell-therapy for Parkinson's disease: a systematic review and meta-analysis. *Journal of Translational Medicine*, 21(1), 601.

Wang, Y., Xia, Y., Kou, L., Yin, S., Chi, X., Li, J., Sun, Y., Wu, J., Zhou, Q., Zou, W., Jin, Z., Huang, J., Xiong, N., & Wang, T. (2023). Astrocyte-to-neuron reprogramming and crosstalk in the treatment of Parkinson's disease. *Neurobiology of Disease*, 184, 106224.

Williams, E. T., Chen, X., Otero, P. A., & Moore, D. J. (2022). Understanding the contributions of VPS35 and the retromer in neurodegenerative disease. *Neurobiology of Disease*, 170, 105768.

Xia, N., Cabin, D. E., Fang, F., & Reijo Pera, R. A. (2022). Parkinson's Disease: Overview of Transcription Factor Regulation, Genetics, and Cellular and Animal Models. *Frontiers in Neuroscience*, 16, 894620.

Xu, H., Wang, E., Chen, F., Xiao, J., & Wang, M. (2021). Neuroprotective Phytochemicals in Experimental Ischemic Stroke: Mechanisms and Potential Clinical Applications. *Oxidative Medicine and Cellular Longevity,* 2021, 6687386.

Ying, Z., Ye, N., Ma, Q., Chen, F., Li, N., & Zhen, X. (2023). Targeted to neuronal organelles for CNS drug development. *Advanced Drug Delivery Reviews,* 200, 115025.

Zhang, L., Wu, J., Zhu, Z., He, Y., & Fang, R. (2023). Mitochondrion: A bridge linking aging and degenerative diseases. *Life Sciences,* 322, 121666.

Zhang, S., Qin, Y., Wang, J., Yu, Y., Wu, L., & Zhang, T. (2023). Noninvasive Electrical Stimulation Neuromodulation and Digital Brain Technology: A Review. *Biomedicines,* 11(6), 1513.

Zhang, S., Yan, H., Ding, J., Wang, R., Feng, Y., Zhang, X., Kong, X., Gong, H., Lu, X., Ma, A., Hua, Y., Liu, H., Guo, J., Gao, H., Zhou, Z., Wang, R., Chen, P., Liu, T., & Kong, X. (2023). Skeletal muscle-specific DJ-1 ablation-induced atrogenes expression and mitochondrial dysfunction contributing to muscular atrophy. *Journal of Cachexia Sarcopenia and Muscle,* 14(5), 2126-2142.

Zhao, Y., Zhou, Y. G., & Chen, J. F. (2024). Targeting the adenosine A_{2A} receptor for neuroprotection and cognitive improvement in traumatic brain injury and Parkinson's disease. *Chinese Journal of Traumatology,* 27(3), 125-133.

Zhou, Y., Li, Z., Chi, C., Li, C., Yang, M., & Liu, B. (2023). Identification of Hub Genes and Potential Molecular Pathogenesis in Substantia Nigra in Parkinson's Disease via Bioinformatics Analysis. *Parkinsons Disease,* 2023, 6755569.

Chapter 12

Traumatic Brain Injury: Pathophysiology and Treatment Approaches

Ravina Kumari[1], M.Pharm,
Ajay Singh Kushwah[1,*], PhD,
Roopal Mittal[2], M.Pharm,
and Shailesh Sharma[1], PhD
[1]Amar Shaheed Baba Ajit Singh Jujhar Singh Memorial College of Pharmacy, Bela (An Autonomous College) Ropar, Punjab, India
[2]RKSD College of Pharmacy, Kaithal, Haryana, India

Abstract

Traumatic brain injury (TBI) can be caused by a vigorous strike, propulsion, or jerk to the cranium or body, or by any object penetrating the skull and damaging the brain internally. Traumatic brain injury will overtake many ailments as the most ubiquitous health concern and cause of disability, predicting that the World Health Organization's yearly TBI affects around 10 million people globally, which includes both the young and old segments of the population. Further makes it a major public issue having a grave impact on society. TBI represents the leading cause of morbidity and mortality in young adults worldwide. Other causes of TBI are everyday accidents, assaults, and sports injuries; in all of these cases, TBI can range in severity from a concussion to a coma. The pathophysiology of brain injury involves a complex event that leads to brain damage, including oxidative stress, inflammation, and apoptosis. The initial injury caused by mechanical force disrupts the release of neurotransmitters via the blood-brain barrier (BBB), inflammatory

* Corresponding Author's Email: kushwah_ph05@yahoo.co.in.

In: Neurogenerative Disorders
Editors: Mohit Agrawal, Manmohan Singhal, Amit Kumar Nayak et al.
ISBN: 979-8-89530-143-2

mediators, oxidative stress, and neuronal death. Consequently, it causes a secondary cascade of neuroinflammation, excitotoxicity, and apoptosis, further exacerbating the primary injury. There have been no specific treatments for traumatic brain injuries until now. But the development of various current neuroprotective drugs has been driven primarily by secondary brain injuries, with many serving as direct targets. The chapter intends to emphasize the crucial facts from the pathophysiological study and the prospect of treatment, and it also focuses on recent areas of relevant future research directions.

Keywords: traumatic brain injury, pathophysiology, brain damage, neuroinflammation, oxidative stress, exocytotoxicity, apoptosis, neuroprotective drugs

Introduction

An intracranial injury, sometimes referred to as a traumatic brain injury (TBI), is neuronal damage brought on by an outside strike. Mild traumatic brain injury (mTBI/concussion) and severe traumatic brain injury are two different categories of TBI that may be distinguished depending on severity (Acabchuk et al., 2021; Pearson et al., 2012). TBI can be classified as mild, moderate, or severe, with mild instances accounting for roughly 80% of cases (Temkin et al., 2022). But even a minor traumatic brain injury can cause crippling manifestations (McMahon et al., 2014; Ganti et al., 2019). The brain is a semi-solid organ that weighs 1400 g and occupies 80% of the cerebral vault (Rockswold et al., 2019). It uses about 20% of the total volume of oxygen that the body receives. The brain receives roughly 15% of the heart's total demand to support this high metabolic rate. Maintaining proper CPP is essential for optimal brain function (Heegaard and Biros, 2007). Vessels can constrict and dilate according to changing physiological situations, which promotes desirable CBF. Direct tissue damage and impaired CBF modulation result from traumatic brain injury (Zwienenberg and Muizelaar 2001).

The pathophysiology of brain injury involves a complex event that results in brain damage, including oxidative stress, inflammation, and apoptosis (Freire et al., 2023). Initial injury caused by mechanical force disrupts the blood-cerebrospinal fluid barrier, leading to the primary initiation of inflammatory mediator release, oxidative stress, and neuronal death. This causes a secondary cascade of neuroinflammation, exocitotoxicity, and apoptosis, further exacerbating the primary injury (Hoffe and Holahan 2022; Raghupathi 2004; Akamatsu and Hanafy 2020).

Oxidative Stress and Trauma-Related Brain Damage

Oxidative stress is one of the key pathophysiologic pathways for brain incapacitation. As a consequence of brain injury, reactive oxygen species (ROS) and reactive nitrogen species (RNS) are released, resulting in oxidative damage to lipids, proteins, and DNA. This subsequently activates pro-inflammatory signaling pathways and exacerbates brain damage by promoting neuronal apoptosis.

Brain injury pathophysiology involves several crucial pathways, one of which is oxidative stress. According to several studies (Hall 1997; Marklund et al., 2001; Ismail et al., 2020), ROS are produced in TBI by mitochondrial leakage, the arachidonic acid cascade phenomenon, mediator release, and acetylcholine (Ach) oxidation. A key source of ROS generation is neutrophil migration, which pierces the brain after a TBI and largely creates these molecules through the action of the enzymes nicotinamide, adenine dinucleotide phosphate (NADPH), and oxidase $(NOX)_2$ (Liu et al., 2017; Temkin et al., 2022).

Traumatic Brain Injury and Neurotoxicity

Neuroinflammation is a decisive mechanism in the focalization of neuronal damage. Production of pro-inflammatory cytokines, chemokines, and other inflammatory mediators increases after traumatic brain damage increases and activates the immune system, including microglia and astrocytes. This, in turn, promotes neuronal death and worsens brain damage.

Epidemiology of Traumatic Brain Injury

TBI, one of the main roots of mortality and morbidity, has a high prevalence worldwide and constitutes a significant social, economic, and health issue for the whole world (Maas et al., 2017). According to WHO statistics, it is the third-leading cause of death in poor countries. TBI also mainly affects people between the ages of 15 and 24, with another peak occurring in those 75 or older. According to epidemiology, falls and violence-related incidents are the leading causes of moderate-to-severe TBI. Other causes include motor vehicles, bicycles, and pedestrian collisions with vehicles. Comprehensive epidemiological investigations of traumatic brain injury are still lacking in India. 60–70% of traumatic brain injuries in India are the result of traffic accidents. According to studies, India has the highest global rate of fatal traffic accidents, and TBI alone causes neurological damage in 1.5–1.7 million people (Das, Mohapatra, and Mohapatra 2012). In the United States, TBI is responsible for nearly 40% of all acute injury deaths. Each year, 20,000 patients suffering from TBI require hospitalization, while 1.74 million people suffer from mild TBI (Gururaj 2002).

The census of 2001 shows that India's disability rate increased from 1.9% in 1991 to 2.1% in 2001. A traumatic brain injury (TBI) can cause dysfunction and intellectual disability in various domains, including physiological, emotional, cognitive, and communal, which can significantly decrease the health-related quality of life (HRQL) of the sufferers. A thorough epidemiological study of TBI is still lacking in India. According to research done in the 1990s, it was predicted that every year in India, TBI affects up to 1 million individuals, which is probably an underestimation of the actual situation (Ingebrigtsen et al., 1998).

Mechanisms of Traumatic Brain Injury

Primary Brain Injury

The initial impact on the skull is referred to as the "primary injury." This damage to tissues and cells in the brain is irreversible and incurable. The different classifications of primary traumatic brain injuries are.

Focal Brain Injury

The circumstances of injury influence the relative degree of focused or diffuse trauma, and primary damage in brain tissue can be either diffuse or localized (Albert-Weissenberger and Sirén 2010).

a. Skull Fractures: Two different kinds of skull fractures are basilar and vault fractures. Vault fractures frequently have linear patterns and can even affect the sinuses. Scattered forces lead to basilar fractures, which can damage cranial nerves (Cernak 2005).

b. Intracranial hemorrhage: consists of epidural and subdural hematomas. Epidural hematoma develops when the skull is affected and dural arteries and veins are damaged, often by bone fractures, while subdural hematoma is caused by damage to a cortical vein or pial artery and is responsible for high mortality (Cernak 2005).
c. Coup and Counter-Coup Contusion: The phrase "coup and counter-coup injury" describes cerebral contusions that originate from the impacted site on the contrasting cranial site and were brought on by a hard blow to the head (Laurer, Lenzlinger, and McIntosh 2000).
d. Concussions: Widespread neurological damage is caused by concussions caused by malformation of the deep brain structure. A direct bruise to the head could result in impulsive force being transferred to the upper thoracic region or other parts of the body (Len and Neary 2011).

Diffuse Brain Injury

This is a type of injury induced by acceleration or deceleration forces that results in morphological and diffuse degeneration of cerebral white matter resulting from functional injury to the brainstem and axons (Albert-Weissenberger and Sirén 2010).

Secondary Brain Injury

Begins with a traumatic injury, develops over the following hours to days until it becomes clinically apparent, and then for a period of days or months. Its nexus of anatomical and physiological changes is complex and poorly understood (Graham et al., 1995). The different types are as follows.

Intracranial Secondary Injury

a. Neurotoxic cascades: They arise from edema, neuronal death, and the release of chemicals that disrupt the BBB due to direct trauma and ischemia, as well as from reperfusion injury that occurs when vascular flow is restored. Release of excitatory amino acids, platelet-activating factor, and ROS are the three most damaging pathways, with the ubiquitous nitric oxide radical just entering the picture.

b. Calcium channel disorder: excitatory amino acids are thought to be released by local tissue damage, which stimulates N-methyl-D-aspartate (NMDA) glutamate receptors in nearby cells. Cells subsequently experience a massive influx of calcium ions, causing cellular edema and metabolic failure.
c. Production of oxygen-free radicals: Oxygen-free radicals can be produced by several processes. Free radicals are created when cells fail metabolically. Vascular injury and ischemia can activate the arachidonic acid cascade, releasing prostaglandins, prostacyclins, and leukotrienes that produce free radicals. Platelet-activating stimuli can significantly stimulate free radical generation and SOD degradation. Free radical production may also be influenced by nitric oxide (NO), and the outcome is improved by inhibiting nitric oxide synthase. Additional vascular damage caused by free radicals results in increased vascular permeability and vasogenic edema. This results in greater global ischemia, which further triggers brain edema.
d. Hematoma formation: Meningeal vascular rupture often occurs in conjunction with a skull fracture. Compression of the brain by this hematoma will result in local ischemia, movement of central structures, and potentially fatal damage to the brainstem. Traumatic rupture of cerebral vessels results in subdural or subarachnoid hemorrhage, which causes a hematoma within the brain or between the duramater and the surface of the brain. A problem with subdural and subarachnoid hemorrhage can lead to further cerebral ischemia and vasospasm due to blood in the subarachnoid space, localized compression and swelling of brain material, and increased intracranial pressure.

Extracranial Secondary Injury

a. Respiratory failure: When a head injury causes loss of consciousness, there may be a brief period of central apnea that may cause severe hypoxia. Any hypoxia will increase cerebral ischemia, volume, CBF, and ICP. Therefore, the head trauma patient is particularly susceptible to respiratory failure.

b. Blood loss: The difference between the pressure within the skull and the pressure in the arteries, known as cerebral perfusion pressure (CPP), plays a role in defining cerebral perfusion (ICP). With increased ICP, a decrease in MAP can lead to cerebral ischemia. Blood loss from multiple traumas often leads to hypotension, which must be carefully avoided and treated. Anemia can result from blood loss, which increases the risk of cerebral ischemia. The physiological impacts of traumatic brain injury are presented schematically in Figure 1.

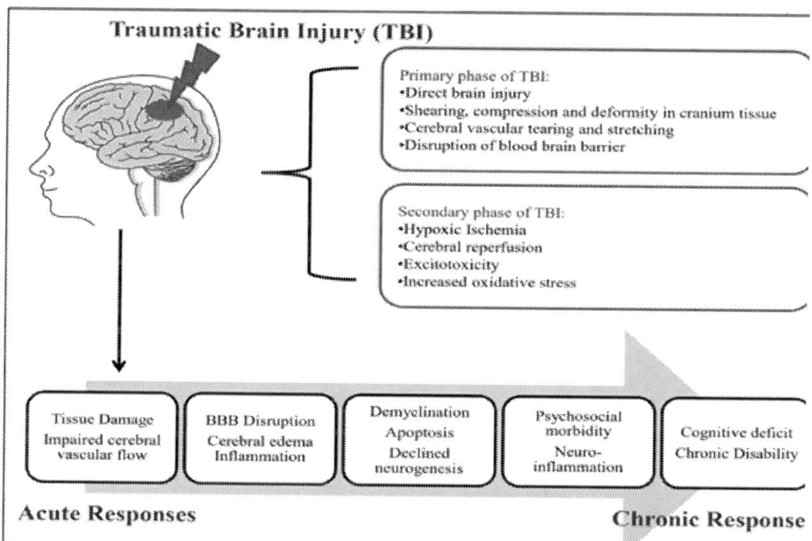

Figure 1. Physiological impacts of traumatic brain injury.

Diagnostic Evaluation of Traumatic Brain Injury

Clinical evidence, most notably a neurological examination, is used to support the diagnosis, which is supposed to be based on the circumstantial lesion and anecdotal evidence. For example, the Glasgow Coma Scale and pin point pupil in reflex to light are two such clinical indicators (Valadka, Andrews, and Bullock 2001). The diagnosis, prognosis, and therapy options are all determined with the use of neuroimaging (Zink 2001). TBI and its psychological consequences can be identified using the DSM-5 (Wortzel and Arciniegas 2014; Simpson 2014).

Computed Tomography (CT) Imaging Techniques

It is the ideal radiologic test in an emergency situation because it is rapid, precise, and widely available. To ascertain whether the damage has advanced, subsequent CT scans may be conducted (Maas et al., 2017). Regarding the benefit of imaging for imperative categorization, it is generally acknowledged that CT scans are the initial test of choice for the majority of injury types, particularly at severe levels of injury.

This is brought on by its widespread accessibility and excellent accuracy in detecting hemorrhages, contusions, and mass effects, which direct acute therapy and have established prognostic importance. To handle heterogeneity in the size, distribution, and number of lesions as well as findings like swelling, gray-white matter differentiation lack, possible confirmation of cisterns and sulcus, tissue drifts, and fissure effects, more complicated Schematic categorization, such as the Rotterdam scale and others, is necessary (Saatman et al., 2008).

Magnetic Resonance Imaging (MRI) Imaging Techniques

For the detection and classification of certain illnesses, MRI provides superior sensitivity and specificity, particularly for DAI and more subtle imaging symptoms observed in "concussive" type head injuries. As a first imaging modality, MRI is preferred for specific study questions. FLAIR and T2 sequences are effective in detecting non-hemorrhagic white matter lesions within the diffuse white matter injury range, while gradient echo and susceptibility-weighted imaging are sensitive to blood products. Like ischemia, diffusion-weighted imaging is sensitive to DAI only in an acute environment. Even though major advancements have been made (Gallagher, Hutchinson, and Pickard 2007), it is still unclear whether DTI or other new approaches will offer superior sensitivity in identifying axonal damage or the ability to track or predict functional recovery or treatment response.

In addition to providing more information than CT, magnetic resonance imaging (MRI) can also reveal information on the long-term results anticipated. Longer-term damage features, such as diffuse axonal injury, can be detected more effectively than with CT. However, MRI is not employed in emergency situations due to a variety of factors, such as its relative ineffectiveness in identifying bleeding and fractures, the time it takes to acquire pictures, the difficulty in accessing the patient within the scanner, and the incompatibility of the technology with metal devices used in emergency treatment. High-definition fiber tracking (HDFT), an MRI variation since 2012, is a technology.

Positron Emission Tomography (PET) Imaging Techniques

Currently, patients with TBI can benefit from isotope- or metabolite-based methods such as xenon CT, single photon emission CT, or positron emission tomography (PET), which have provided an approach to the nuanced interplay between nervosity and metabolism. While these imaging techniques have the primary benefit of giving region-specific information, neuroimaging approaches have the major drawback of reflecting just one moment in time. The prominent bedside cranial monitoring methods, on the other hand, can give continuous measures of cerebral vascular flow, oxygen perfusion, and other physiological parameters, but they only represent a single location in the extremely vast and frequently diverse intracranial compartment. Because of this, it was anticipated that neuroimaging would continue to be utilized more frequently in research concerns concerning hemodynamics and metabolism in the brain (Saatman et al., 2008).

A specific diagnosis may be supported by additional methods. Although there is still evidence to support their utility, head injuries are either so minor as not to require imaging or serious enough to warrant a more precise CT scan. When risk factors like penetrating head trauma are present, angiography may be used to identify blood vessel disease (Maas, Stocchetti, and Bullock 2008). By measuring cerebral blood flow or metabolism, functional imaging can infer neural activity in certain locations and perhaps aid in outcome prediction. To determine the severe cognitive effects and help with the management of the therapy, neuropsychological testing might be done. There are many different types of instruments, ranging from quick assessments of broad mental function to full requisites consisting of several domain-classified examinations (Zink 2001).

Treatment of Traumatic Brain Injury

Starting emergency care within the "golden hour" after an accident is crucial. Patients with moderate-to-severe injuries are often treated in intensive care units and neurosurgery wards. The treatment plan is determined by the patient's level of recovery. During the acute stage, the primary objectives are to stabilize the patient and focus on preventing any further harm. Since the initial damage caused by trauma cannot be reversed, the focus is on preventing any additional harm. During the sub-acute and chronic phases of recovery, rehabilitation is the primary form of care. Authoritative reviews of recent research have been conducted to influence treatment choices for TBI, leading to the development of international clinical recommendations. These recommendations aim to provide clear guidance on the most effective treatment options for individuals in the sub-acute and chronic phases of recovery.

Pre-Hospital Care and Early Management

The approach, length, and lead team of a doctor or paramedic are also proven to have an impact on the outcome in patients with traumatic brain injuries. According to the analysis of data from two randomized trials of Pre-hospital hypertonic resuscitation involving 2049 patients, those transported by air had a higher rate of pre-hospital intubation (81% vs. 36%), received more intravenous fluids (with a mean of 1.3 L compared to 0.8 L for ground transport), and experienced longer pre-hospital times (with a mean of 76.1 min compared to 43.5 min for ground transport) (Bulger et al., 2012). A study showed that the mode of transportation did not significantly impact survival or neurologic outcomes after 6 months. Similarly, a retrospective analysis of 194 patients found that air-based emergency medical services were associated with lower rates of both death (21% vs. 25%) and neurological impairments (25% vs. 31%) (Berlot et al., 2009).

Early Management of TBI

Hypoxemia

The preservation of a clean and unobstructed airway is the first and most crucial factor in TBI. The most significant risk connected to a poorer prognosis is hypoxemia, which requires immediate care (Chi et al., 2006). Skilled clinicians must quickly induce intubation in patients with severe TBI. Securing the airway while protecting the cervical spine, which should always be treated as though it has been hurt, a recent retrospective cohort study of 101 individual patients found that lidocaine can be safely used without causing negative hemodynamic alterations (Lin, Hou, and Jouvet 1996).

Hypercarbia/hypocarbia

Normocarbia (PaCO2 between 35 and 40 mmHg) should be maintained in intubated patients. In order to prevent hypoxemia or changes in breathing that might not be seen, monitoring of oxygen supply and capnography are advised in patients who have had serious head injuries. End-tidal capnography, which typically measures EtCO2 at 30-35 mmHg, is the method that evaluates this the best (Badjatia et al., 2008). If there are other serious wounds, notably chest wounds, stomach aspiration, or severe pulmonary edema, oxygenation and breathing may become challenging. It is necessary to apply the proper positive end expiratory pressure (PEEP). There is no evidence to support the claims that 10 mmHg PEEP reduces cerebral vascular flow or increases intracraniam pressure (ICP), and ICP may even decrease with better oxygenation (Mascia et al., 2007).

Hypotension/Hypertension

Studies have shown that even one episode of hypotension significantly affects the result since it is such a significant secondary brain injury (Pearson et al., 2012). In order to maintain optimal blood pressure, vasopressors may be employed in the case of hypotension in addition to fluid resuscitation for euvolaemia. BTF advises that a MAP of at least 80 mmHg be present before inserting an ICP monitor. A disturbed cerebral perfusion may be indicated by hypertension, a physiological reaction that may result from a sympathetic surge. A short-acting beta blocker infusion, which keeps blood pressure stable, is highly helpful for the management of hypertension to attain CPP objectives. In contrast to systemic nitrate vasodilators and anti-arrhythmic calcium channel blockers, these substances do not produce cerebral vasodilatation, which prevents them from raising ICP and cerebral blood volume (Haddad and Arabi 2012).

Fluid Resuscitation

It is also crucial to maintaining adequate CPP through the quick administration of fluids. There is still a lot of disagreement around the choice of fluids, though. Hypertonic fluids may decrease TBI biomarkers and are associated with improved outcomes, according to certain research. Multiple studies have suggested that colloids should not be used as the first choice of fluid in patients with severe TBI. Isotonic crystalloids, on the other hand, are a safer and more cost-effective alternative. However, the present research on the role of colloids in mild to moderately severe brain damage is inconclusive. Therefore, well-designed randomized controlled trials are needed to establish the efficacy of colloids in such cases.

pH value: By lowering ICP, reducing the metabolic demands on the brain, minimizing intervention of the blood-brain barrier, and minimizing inflammatory mediator release, hypothermia has some protective benefits in TBI. The efficiency of induced hypothermia in treating traumatic brain injury (TBI) is currently unknown, despite the fact that it is already a widely established method for enhancing outcomes after anoxic brain damage linked to cardiac arrest (Fox et al., 2010). The onset of hypothermia upon ICU admission was also observed to be correlated with piercing injury, Injury Severity Score (ISS) > 25, and exploratory laparotomy (Bukur et al., 2012). Further research is desirable to determine the sway of safety measures taken to avoid the onset of hypothermia and the efficacy of remedies employed to bring temperatures back to normal.

Surgery and Surgical Interventions

Mass lesions can be surgically removed, as can brain-penetrating objects. Surgery is used to remove urgent mass lesions, such as contusions or hematomas, that significantly alter the cerebral structures. Blood that has accumulated inside cerebral hematomas can be suctioned, extracted with forceps, or floated away with water. The goal of surgery is to stop bleeding by identifying bleeding blood vessels.

A craniotomy may be required in cases of penetrating brain injury to remove affected tissue surgically. To expel out fragments of shattered cranium or things lodged in the brain, a craniotomy, which involves cutting into the skull, may be required.

In the very short time after a TBI, de-compressive craniectomy (DC) is frequently carried out during procedures to repair hematomas; a temporary portion of the skull is removed (primary DC) (Cooper et al., 2011). The Glasgow Coma Scale (GCS) scores of patients who undergo secondary DC, which is performed hours or days after a traumatic brain injury to control persistently high intracranial pressures, are worse than those who receive standard medical treatments. They also have higher risks of death, vegetative state, or severe disability (Carney et al., 2017).

Medications and Pharmacological Approaches

Psychostimulants

Methylphenidate is commonly used to treat ADHD, which shares symptoms and neurotransmitter aberrations with brain damage. Executive functioning difficulties characterize ADHD (Writer and Schillerstrom, 2009). The pathophysiological mediators and neuronal targets in traumatic brain injury (TBI) are shown in Figure 2. A recent review study found that "at present there is insufficient evidence to support routine use of methylphenidate or other amphetamines to promote recovery from TBI (Forsyth and Jayamoni 2003), while at least 10 clinical trials have shown that methylphenidate can help adult and pediatric patients with neurocognitive deficits due to brain injury, particularly in attention seeking, memory impact, cognition processing, and vocal coordination (Siddall 2005). We consider methylphenidate to be beneficial since it acts quickly and has a low risk of negative effects.

Antidepressants

Post-TBI mental disorders are underdiagnosed and undertreated, despite the fact that they might have serious effects. The positive news is that current research indicates that antidepressants can be used to treat both neuropsychiatric and extra neurological abnormalities resulting from brain damage.

Especially in sub-acute recovery (Meythaler et al., 2001) but also in chronic situations, selective serotonin reuptake inhibitors (SSRIs) have been proven to be effective in managing behavioral disorders in TBI patients. Near the frontal lobes, the most typical location of traumatic contusion, there is a large concentration of 5-HT and Adr fibers (DeMarchi et al., 2005). Since both fibers are frequently damaged in TBI, it is possible that newer antidepressants like mirtazapine and venlafaxine, which have effects on both norepinephrine (norEpi) and serotonin (5-HT), are also beneficial in treating TBI aftereffects. However, there is a dearth of clinical research on these medications' effectiveness in treating TBI. Similar to other drugs, bupropion raises levels of both dopamine and norepinephrine while weakly inhibiting serotonin reuptake. This drug has been successful in treating restlessness when taken 150 mg daily (Teng et al., 2001).

Anti-Parkinson Drugs

Amantadine, rimatidine, bromocriptine, and L-dopa with carbidopa (e.g., Sinemet), which are antiparkinsonian medications, all work by different processes but eventually raise dopamine levels in the brain. Amantadine can operate post-synaptically to enhance the number of or change the shape of dopamine receptors. It also acts presynaptically to promote dopamine release or block its absorption (Schneider, 1999). Amantadine, a noncompetitive NMDA receptor antagonist, may provide defense against potential glutamate-mediated excitotoxicity in the context of traumatic brain injury (TBI). Patients who received amantadine also showed improvements in arousal and level of consciousness (LOC) as assessed by the Glasgow Coma Scale, both of which were changes in the outcome LOC. Interestingly, one study also found a decrease in mortality (Saniova et al., 2004). No research has, to date, indicated that memory has improved.

Anticonvulsants

Treatment of TBI symptoms with anticonvulsants has had mixed outcomes. Valproic acid, for instance, improves the inhibitory control brought about by the neurotransmitter GABA, supporting the stabilization of the central nervous system as a whole; however, results have been conflicting. Studies have demonstrated that administering daily doses of 600 to 2250 mg of valproic acid (resulting in serum levels of 40 to 100 g/mL) can have positive neuro-cognitive effects. These effects include improvement in recent memory and problem-solving abilities, as well as the amelioration of neuropsychiatric and neurobehavioral symptoms such as depression, mania, destructive and aggressive behavior, restless inability, impulsivity, labiality, and attentiveness (Wroblewski et al., 1997). In contrast, a controlled experiment revealed that valproic acid had a detrimental influence on decision-making speed, while another study suggested that valproic acid usage was associated with a higher death risk (Kim and Humaran 2002).

Other Drugs

Modafinil is a medication that helps to increase alertness, and it is often used to treat conditions like narcolepsy and idiopathic hypersomnia. These conditions can cause symptoms similar to those of traumatic brain injury (TBI), such as excessive daytime sleepiness, lack of focus, and decreased ability to socially interact. Although the particular mechanism of action is yet unknown, modafinil is thought to be able to reduce GABA (γ-amino butyric acid) or raise glutamate levels in the nondeterministic anterior hypothalamus, hippocampus, and amygdala (Lin, Hou, and Jouvet, 1996; Ferraro et al., 1999).

Beta-blockers such as propranolol and pindolol have been shown in four randomized control studies to have positive effects on neurobehavioral symptoms of aggression and agitation during both chronic and sub-acute phases. For the treatment of TBI-related neuropsychiatric and neurobehavioral complications, this family of medications merits additional study (Fleminger et al., 1996). In an effort to help the brain rebalance its neurotransmitter levels, neuroleptics are being used more often in the context of delirium. It should nevertheless be emphasized that there is some data suggesting that dopamine blocking may harm recovery (Failla, Conley, and Wagner 2016; Goldstein 1995).

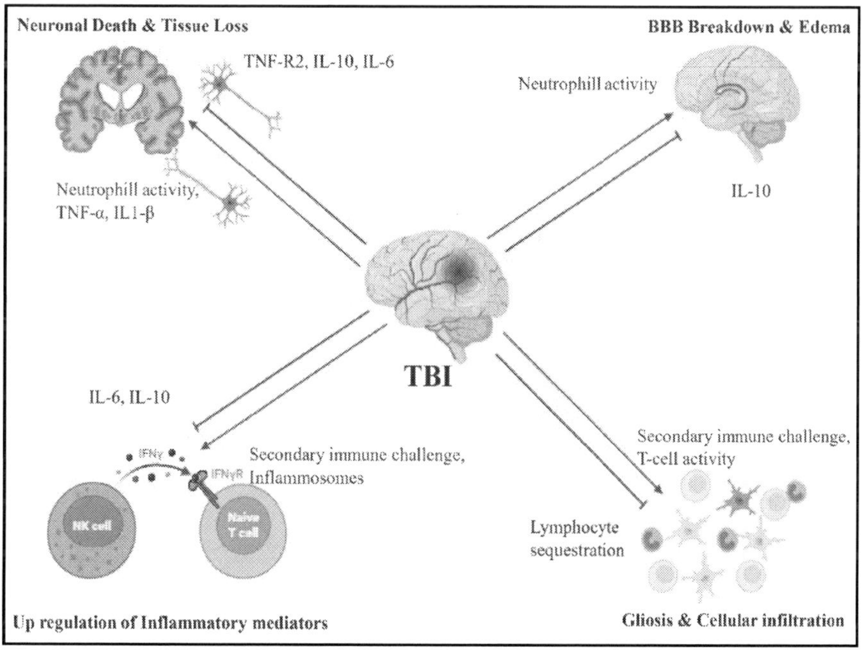

Figure 2. Pathophysiological mediators and neuronal targets in traumatic brain injury (TBI).

Neuroprotective Strategies

Numerous single-targeted damage mechanisms, including excitotoxicity caused by ionotropic glutamate receptors, were the focus of the majority of unsuccessful clinical trials. Combination pharmacological therapy for TBI may be costly and less effective than single-agent treatment, as unexpected drug interactions may occur.

Hypothermia and Brain Cooling

In a number of animals TBI models, neuroprotection was achieved by inducing hypothermia, which is achieved by reducing body temperature to between 32 and 35°C (Busto et al., 1989; Vitarbo et al., 2004). The amount of histopathological damage brought on by a brain injury can be significantly impacted by even small changes in brain temperature. Mild hypothermia shields the brain from ischemia and traumatic brain injury, but mild hyperthermia worsens neurological results (Dietrich et al., 1994). Selective brain cooling may thus be helpful in reducing the negative effects of brain damage. A considerable decrease in the quantity of necrotic cortical neurons and the extent of contusions was also brought about by post-traumatic hypothermia in rats following experimental TBI. Clinical investigations have demonstrated that hypothermia lowers intracranial pressure (Zhi, Zhang, and Lin 2003), increases brain and jugular vein oxygenation, and decreases cerebral metabolic rate. Contradictory findings have been found in clinical studies, and a randomized multi-center investigation found no appreciable differences between normothermia and hypothermia in terms of neurological recovery or fatalities in patients (Clifton et al., 2001). Several researchers have suggested that modifying experimental setups, such as administering treatment to specific subpopulations, beginning treatment earlier or continuing it for a longer duration, varying the temperature, and altering warming techniques, may lead to improved results. Others have proposed that combining hypothermia with pharmaceutical neuroprotection could enhance the efficacy of medication or broaden the therapeutic window. However, the use of hypothermia as a neuroprotective treatment for clinical TBI should be approached with caution if there is no compelling clinical research to support it.

Antioxidant Therapies

Endogenous antioxidants, both non-enzymatic (such as GSH, melatonin, and coenzyme Q10) and enzymatic (such as SOD, CAT, and GPx), maintain free radical levels under regulation in healthy individuals (Mirończuk-Chodakowska, Witkowska, and Zujko 2018). In order to prevent or cure the elevated oxidative stress associated with disease states, antioxidant supplementation - whether through food or medication - plays a crucial role in health management.

Ascorbic Acid (Vitamin C)

In mammalian tissues, ascorbic acid (AA) is a prevalent water-soluble antioxidant. It serves as a reducing cofactor in enzymatic processes (Roof, Hoffman, and Stein, 1997). A lack of ascorbic acid (AA) can cause problems with the integrity of connective tissue since it helps recycle oxidized tocopherol (Vitamin E), which is important for the redox state of tocopherol in biological membranes. AA is an essential nutrient that cannot be synthesized by most animals, including humans. It is particularly prevalent in the brain and interacts with a variety of ROS and RNS, including peroxynitrile and hydroxyl radicals, through one or two electron processes. Although only one preclinical and one clinical study have looked at the effects of AA in traumatic brain injury (TBI), it has been shown that the level of AA in cerebral tissue decreases rapidly after experimental TBI. Hence, the body depends on foods that are high in vitamin C to maintain adequate levels of AA (Xiao et al., 2008). After severe TBI, it remains significantly below control values for a longer time, while in moderately wounded animals, it returns to pre-impact concentrations within 72 hours (Tavazzi et al., 2005; Tyurin et al., 2000). The comparatively weak effects of AA seen in this study might be attributed to the SVCT2 (Sodium-Dependent Vitamin C Transporter 2) transporter's dysfunction, which is typically responsible for ensuring the transfer of electrogenic AA into cells.

N-Acetyl-Cysteine

The low-molecular-weight antioxidant that mammals may turn out to be GSH (Limongi et al., 2019). High quantities of this amino acid are necessary to provide appropriate GSH tissue levels since cysteine is the source of the SH group that GSH needs. In situations of oxidative and nitrosative stress, increased availability of cysteine is necessary due to the critical role of GSH in detoxification processes. This is required to scavenge ROS and RNS and eliminate xenobiotics. The antioxidant GSH is a significant reducing agent for protein SH groups and has been shown to play a role in controlling inflammation (Steullet et al., 2006). GSH appears to function as an ionotropic receptor activator, which raises the possibility that it plays a part in cerebral neuro transmission (Ansari, Roberts, and Scheff 2008). In another study, individuals with moderate closed-head traumatic brain injury (TBI) were treated with oral doses of 150 mg/kg of N-acetylcysteine (NAC) through gastric gavage at 1, 24, 48, and 72 hours after the injury. The results of the study showed that NAC improved the values of brain cortex IL-4, GSH, TAS, vitamin A, AA, and α-tocopherols and increased erythrocyte GSHPx levels while decreasing plasma lipid peroxidation and IL-1β levels (Santos-Buelga and Feliciano 2017).

Flavonoids

The group of more than 5000 naturally occurring chemicals known as flavonoids is mostly found in fungi and plants (Izzi et al., 2012). An extremely low oxidoreductive potential is a flavanol-defining trait, making it possible for it to operate as a strong antioxidant against any sort of ROS and RNS (Theadom et al., 2013). Comparing research looking at the efficacy of flavanoids-based medicines is challenging since it is challenging to locate two studies looking at the same flavanoids. In modest pilot clinical research, oral enzogenol (1 g/die) was given for 6 weeks to 60 patients with minor traumatic brain injuries who began exhibiting symptoms 3 to 12 months after the accident. Before and after the therapy, cognitive functioning was examined.

Resveratrol

Resveratrol, an antioxidant, is predominantly hydrophobic in nature, with a small yet considerable solubility in water and excellent solubility in organic solvents. It consists of two 6-carbon aromatic rings, one with two OH groups and the other with only one, which are connected by a carbon double bond (C = C) bridge, allowing the presence of both cis- and trans-resveratrol. Red grape skin contains a significant amount of this type of polyphenol. Red wine, on the other hand, has the highest concentration of resveratrol among all meals. The "French paradox," which refers to the low incidence of cardiovascular diseases in the French population despite their high consumption of a diet rich in saturated fats, was first suggested as a possible explanation for the beneficial effects of resveratrol (Tsai, Ho, and Chen 2017). This paradox refers to the apparent low resveratrol intake caused by high red wine consumption.

α-Tocopherol (Vitamin E)

Known for their exceptional antioxidant activity, tocopherols are a class of fat-soluble chemicals that are concentrated in a wide range of vegetable oils. Four tocopherols and four tocotrienols are tocopherol congeners with vitamin E activity; the former has a side chain harbored by a saturated hydrocarbon, while the latter has a side chain harbored by an unsaturated hydrocarbon made up of three isoprene units (Comitato, Ambra, and Virgili 2017). During the study, rats were fed a regular diet for four weeks, with some being given 500 IU/kg of tocopherols while others were not. After four weeks, all the rats were subjected to a fluid percussion injury, which caused mild TBI. The results showed that rats that had been given an α-tocopherol-rich diet experienced fewer decreases in SOD, Sir2 (NAD+-dependent protein deacetylase), and BDNF (brain-derived neurotrophic factor), as well as fewer impairments in motor function caused by TBI (Artuch et al., 2009). A study has shown that a diet rich in alpha-tocopherol can help reduce the negative effects of mild traumatic brain injury (TBI) on motor function, synaptic plasticity, and cognitive skills. The study found that the diet helped prevent decreases in SOD, Sir2, and BDNF levels induced by TBI. Based on these findings, the researchers suggest that dietary tocopherol supplementation might be an effective way to mitigate the negative effects of mild TBI.

Carotenoids

A group of pigments known as carotenoids, which have a total of 8 isoprene units and 40 carbon atoms, are produced by plants, algae, and photosynthetic bacteria (Cho et al., 2018). Carotenoids are organic pigments that are commonly found in plants. There are over 1100 known carotenoids, which can be divided into two main groups: xanthophyll-class carotenoids, which contain oxygen, and carotenes-class carotenoids, which are solely composed of hydrocarbons. When it comes to testing carotenoids in the human brain, several types can be identified, including α-carotene, β-carotene, γ-carotene, β-cryptoxanthin, lutein, and zeaxanthin. Carotenoids are generally known to have anti-inflammatory, antioxidant, and autophagy-moderating actions. Numerous studies have been conducted on the possible therapeutic benefits of different carotenoids for a range of conditions, including neurodegenerative disorders (Zhang et al., 2017). The effects of other carotenoids on TBI animal models have been studied, along with their impact on molecular pathways. One of these carotenoids, Fucoxanthin has demonstrated neuroprotective benefits by controlling the Nrf2-ARE and Nrf2-autophagy pathways. Additionally, bexarotene has been found to reduce apoptosis and inflammation by up regulating the long non-coding RNA Neat1 (Zhong et al., 2017) and enhancing the neurological recovery of mice following TBI (Wang et al., 2015). Crocin administration has demonstrated neuroprotective benefits that are only partially reliant on Notch signaling activity (Tan et al., 2017). The last powerful antioxidant, lutein, which can penetrate the blood-brain barrier and has anti-inflammatory and anti-apoptotic properties, demonstrated protective benefits by reducing the production of interleukin (IL), IL-1, and IL-6, as well as monocyte chemoattractant protein (MCP) 1 (Lauritzen et al., 2001).

Omega-3 Fatty Acids

Omega-3 fatty acids are a type of polyunsaturated fatty acids that have 18–22 carbon atoms and three to six double bonds in their carbon chains. All of these PUFAs have one double bond on the third carbon atom, which is distant from the -atom when counting the last carbon atom as the -atom. For humans, omega-3 fatty acids are either semi-essential (eicosapentaenoic acid, docosahexaenoic acid) or essential (linolenic acid). Linolenic acid is the precursor to the other omega-3 fatty acids, but it cannot be produced by our body and must be consumed through food in sufficient proportions.

In a recent clinical case, an older patient with traumatic head trauma who was taking warfarin and supplementing it with fish oil (rich in omega-3 fatty acids) developed irreversible, fatal warfarin-induced anti coagulation. This study highlights the synergistic effect of the two treatments (warfarin and omega-3 fatty acids) in inhibiting platelet aggregation and promoting uncontrollable bleeding, even though it only reports one case (McCrory 2003).

Conclusion

Traumatic brain injury (TBI) can be spawned by a vigorous strike, propulsion, or jerk to the cranium or body or from any object piercing the skull and damaging the brain internally. The pathophysiology of brain injury involves a complex event that leads to brain damage, including oxidative stress, inflammation, and apoptosis. The initial injury caused by mechanical force disrupts the release of neurotransmitters via the blood-brain barrier (BBB), inflammatory mediators, oxidative damage, and neuronal death. This causes a secondary cascade of neuroinflammation, excitcytotoxicity, and apoptosis, further exacerbating the primary injury. Drugs used largely for other purposes are also included in novel pharmacological therapies for TBI. Only a few clinical trials have looked at whether cutting-edge pharmaceutical treatments might lessen TBI-related subsequent brain damage. According to a recent comprehensive review, several innovative treatment approaches (statins, N-acetyl cysteine, enzogenol, cerebrolysin, and nitric-oxide synthase inhibitors) may improve functional results, while other medications failed to show any neuroprotective benefits. Vehicle accidents are a major contributor to traumatic brain injuries (TBI); thus, preventing them or lessening their effects can lessen both the frequency and severity of TBI. By using seat belts, kid safety seats, motorcycle helmets, roll bars, and airbags, together with other safety features, damage in accidents can be minimized.

Continuous efforts have been made over several decades to develop therapeutic strategies for TBI recovery, despite the lack of effective treatment options available today. Standard medical and surgical interventions are crucial for the acute management of TBI patients. Due to the improvement in critical management guidelines during the acute phase, there has been an enhancement in the number of TBI survivors with different disabilities. This research calls for a shift towards neuronal restoration and neuronal rehabilitation for TBI.

A distinctive set of approaches used by healthcare workers in this scheme enabled them to comprehend and associate with the individual, build a connection, and work together to find direction. The emanated social leisure activity was, therefore, personally influential and leveled in the person's insight into themselves. This sense of self was further enhanced through social participation in leisure and recreational activities, which were tailored to match their individual characteristics and goals.

Disclaimer

None.

References

Acabchuk, R. L., Brisson, J. M., Park, C. L., Babbott-Bryan, N., Parmelee, O. A., & Johnson, B. T. (2021). Therapeutic effects of meditation, yoga, and mindfulness-based interventions for chronic symptoms of mild traumatic brain injury: A systematic review and meta-analysis. *Applied Psychology: Health and Well-Being,* 13(1), 34-62.

Akamatsu, Y., & Hanafy, K. A. (2020). Cell death and recovery in traumatic brain injury. *Neurotherapeutics,* 17, 446-456.

Albert-Weissenberger, C., & Sirén, A. L. (2010). Experimental traumatic brain injury. *Experimental & translational stroke medicine*, 2(1), 1-8.

Ansari, M. A., Roberts, K. N., & Scheff, S. W. (2008). Oxidative stress and modification of synaptic proteins in hippocampus after traumatic brain injury. *Free Radical Biology and Medicine,* 45(4), 443-452.

Artuch, R., Salviati, L., Jackson, S., Hirano, M., & Navas, P. (2009). Coenzyme q 10 deficiencies in neuromuscular diseases. *Inherited Neuromuscular Diseases: Translation from Pathomechanisms to Therapies,* 117-128.

Badjatia, N., Carney, N., Crocco, T. J., Fallat, M. E., Hennes, H. M., Jagoda, A. S., Moriarty, T. M. (2008). Guidelines for prehospital management of traumatic brain injury 2nd edition. *Prehospital emergency care*, 12(sup1), S1-S52.

Berlot, G., La Fata, C., Bacer, B., Biancardi, B., Viviani, M., Lucangelo, U., Trillò, G. (2009). Influence of prehospital treatment on the outcome of patients with severe blunt traumatic brain injury: A single-centre study. *European Journal of Emergency Medicine,* 16(6), 312-317.

Bukur, M., Kurtovic, S., Berry, C., Tanios, M., Ley, E. J., & Salim, A. (2012). Pre-hospital hypothermia is not associated with increased survival after traumatic brain injury. *Journal of Surgical Research,* 175(1), 24-29.

Bulger, E. M., Guffey, D., Guyette, F. X., MacDonald, R. D., Brasel, K., Kerby, J. D., Morrison, L. J. (2012). Impact of prehospital mode of transport after severe injury: A multicenter evaluation from the resuscitation outcomes consortium. *Journal of Trauma and Acute Care Surgery,* 72(3), 567-575.

Busto, R., Dietrich, W. D., Globus, M., & Ginsberg, M. D. (1989). The importance of brain temperature in cerebral ischemic injury. *Stroke,* 20(8), 1113-1114.

Carney, N., Totten, A. M., O'Reilly, C., Ullman, J. S., Hawryluk, G. W., Bell, M. J., Kissoon, N. (2017). Guidelines for the management of severe traumatic brain injury. *Neurosurgery,* 80(1), 6-15.

Cernak, I. (2005). Animal models of head trauma. *NeuroRx,* 2(3), 410-422.

Chi, J. H., Knudson, M. M., Vassar, M. J., McCarthy, M. C., Shapiro, M. B., Mallet, S., Wisner, D. (2006). Prehospital hypoxia affects outcome in patients with traumatic brain injury: A prospective multicenter study. *Journal of Trauma and Acute Care Surgery,* 61(5), 1134-1141.

Cho, K. S., Shin, M., Kim, S., & Lee, S. B. (2018). Recent advances in studies on the therapeutic potential of dietary carotenoids in neurodegenerative diseases. *Oxidative medicine and cellular longevity,* 2018.

Clifton, G. L., Miller, E. R., Choi, S. C., Levin, H. S., McCauley, S., Smith Jr, K. R., Luerssen, T. G. (2001). Lack of effect of induction of hypothermia after acute brain injury. *New England Journal of Medicine,* 344(8), 556-563.

Comitato, R., Ambra, R., & Virgili, F. (2017). Tocotrienols: A family of molecules with specific biological activities. *Antioxidants,* 6(4), 93.

Cooper, D. J., Rosenfeld, J. V., Murray, L., Arabi, Y. M., Davies, A. R., D'Urso, P., Reilly, P. (2011). Decompressive craniectomy in diffuse traumatic brain injury. *New England Journal of Medicine,* 364(16), 1493-1502.

Das, M., Mohapatra, S., & Mohapatra, S. S. (2012). New perspectives on central and peripheral immune responses to acute traumatic brain injury. *Journal of neuroinflammation,* 9, 1-12.

DeMarchi, R., Bansal, V., Hung, A., Wroblewski, K., Dua, H., Sockalingam, S., & Bhalerao, S. (2005). Review of awakening agents. *Canadian journal of neurological sciences,* 32(1), 4-17.

Dietrich, W. D., Alonso, O., Busto, R., Globus, M. Y. T., & Ginsberg, M. D. (1994). Post-traumatic brain hypothermia reduces histopathological damage following concussive brain injury in the rat. *Acta neuropathologica,* 87, 250-258.

Failla, M. D., Conley, Y. P., & Wagner, A. K. (2016). Brain-derived neurotrophic factor (bdnf) in traumatic brain injury–related mortality: Interrelationships between genetics and acute systemic and central nervous system bdnf profiles. *Neurorehabilitation and neural repair, 30*(1), 83-93.

Ferraro, L., Antonelli, T., Tanganelli, S., O'Connor, W. T., de la Mora, M. P., Mendez-Franco, J., Fuxe, K. (1999). The vigilance promoting drug modafinil increases extracellular glutamate levels in the medial preoptic area and the posterior hypothalamus of the conscious rat: Prevention by local gabaa receptor blockade. *Neuropsychopharmacology,* 20(4), 346-356.

Fleminger, S., Greenwood, R. R., Oliver, D. L., & Group, C. I. (1996). Pharmacological management for agitation and aggression in people with acquired brain injury. *Cochrane database of systematic reviews*, 2008(3).

Forsyth, R., & Jayamoni, B. (2003). Noradrenergic agonists for acute traumatic brain injury. *The Cochrane Database of Systematic Reviews*(1), CD003984-CD003984.

Fox, J. L., Vu, E. N., Doyle-Waters, M., Brubacher, J. R., Abu-Laban, R., & Hu, Z. (2010). Prophylactic hypothermia for traumatic brain injury: A quantitative systematic review. *Canadian Journal of Emergency Medicine*, 12(4), 355-364.

Freire, M. A. M., Rocha, G. S., Bittencourt, L. O., Falcao, D., Lima, R. R., & Cavalcanti, J. R. L. P. (2023). Cellular and molecular pathophysiology of traumatic brain injury: What have we learned so far? *Biology*, 12(8), 1139.

Gallagher, C. N., Hutchinson, P. J., & Pickard, J. D. (2007). Neuroimaging in trauma. *Current opinion in neurology*, 20(4), 403-409.

Ganti, L., Stead, T., Daneshvar, Y., Bodhit, A. N., Pulvino, C., Ayala, S. W., & Peters, K. R. (2019). Gcs 15: When mild tbi isn't so mild. *Neurological Research and Practice*, 1(1), 1-8.

Goldstein, L. B. (1995). Common drugs may influence motor recovery after stroke. *Neurology*, 45(5), 865-871.

Graham, D., Adams, J. H., Nicoll, J., Maxwell, W., & Gennarelli, T. (1995). The nature, distribution and causes of traumatic brain injury. *Brain pathology*, 5(4), 397-406.

Gururaj, G. (2002). Epidemiology of traumatic brain injuries: Indian scenario. *Neurological Research*, 24(1), 24-28.

Haddad, S. H., & Arabi, Y. M. (2012). Critical care management of severe traumatic brain injury in adults. *Scandinavian journal of trauma, resuscitation and emergency medicine*, 20(1), 1-15.

Hall, K. M. (1997). Establishing a national traumatic brain injury information system based upon a unified data set. *Archives of physical medicine and rehabilitation*, 78(8), S5-S11.

Heegaard, W., & Biros, M. (2007). Traumatic brain injury. *Emergency medicine clinics of North America*, 25(3), 655-678.

Hoffe, B., & Holahan, M. R. (2022). Hyperacute excitotoxic mechanisms and synaptic dysfunction involved in traumatic brain injury. *Frontiers in Molecular Neuroscience*, 15, 831825.

Ingebrigtsen, T., Waterloo, K., Marup-Jensen, S., Attner, E., & Romner, B. (1998). Quantification of post-concussion symptoms 3 months after minor head injury in 100 consecutive patients. *Journal of neurology*, 245, 609-612.

Ismail, H., Shakkour, Z., Tabet, M., Abdelhady, S., Kobaisi, A., Abedi, R., Mondello, S. (2020). Traumatic brain injury: Oxidative stress and novel anti-oxidants such as mitoquinone and edaravone. *Antioxidants*, 9(10), 943.

Izzi, V., Masuelli, L., Tresoldi, I., Sacchetti, P., Modesti, A., Galvano, F., & Bei, R. (2012). The effects of dietary flavonoids on the regulation of redox inflammatory networks. *Frontiers in Bioscience-Landmark*, 17(7), 2396-2418.

Kim, E., & Humaran, T. J. (2002). Divalproex in the management of neuropsychiatric complications of remote acquired brain injury. *The Journal of neuropsychiatry and clinical neurosciences*, 14(2), 202-205.

Laurer, H. L., Lenzlinger, P. M., & McIntosh, T. K. (2000). Models of traumatic brain injury. *European Journal of Trauma,* 26, 95-110.

Lauritzen, L. a., Hansen, H., Jørgensen, M., & Michaelsen, K. (2001). The essentiality of long chain n-3 fatty acids in relation to development and function of the brain and retina. *Progress in lipid research,* 40(1-2), 1-94.

Len, T., & Neary, J. (2011). Cerebrovascular pathophysiology following mild traumatic brain injury. *Clinical physiology and functional imaging*, 31(2), 85-93.

Limongi, D., Baldelli, S., Checconi, P., Marcocci, M. E., De Chiara, G., Fraternale, A., Palamara, A. T. (2019). Gsh-c4 acts as anti-inflammatory drug in different models of canonical and cell autonomous inflammation through nfκb inhibition. *Frontiers in Immunology,* 10, 155.

Lin, J. S., Hou, Y., & Jouvet, M. (1996). Potential brain neuronal targets for amphetamine-, methylphenidate, and modafinil-induced wakefulness, evidenced by c-fos immunocytochemistry in the cat. *Proceedings of the National Academy of Sciences,* 93(24), 14128-14133.

Liu, Y. l., Xu, Z. M., Yang, G. Y., Yang, D. X., Ding, J., Chen, H., Tian, H. L. (2017). Sesamin alleviates blood-brain barrier disruption in mice with experimental traumatic brain injury. *Acta Pharmacologica Sinica*, 38(11), 1445-1455.

Maas, A. I., Menon, D. K., Adelson, P. D., Andelic, N., Bell, M. J., Belli, A., Chesnut, R. M. (2017). Traumatic brain injury: Integrated approaches to improve prevention, clinical care, and research. *The Lancet Neurology,* 16(12), 987-1048.

Maas, A. I., Stocchetti, N., & Bullock, R. (2008). Moderate and severe traumatic brain injury in adults. *The Lancet Neurology*, 7(8), 728-741.

Marklund, N., Lewander, T., Clausen, F., & Hillered, L. (2001). Effects of the nitrone radical scavengers pbn and s-pbn on *in vivo* trapping of reactive oxygen species after traumatic brain injury in rats. *Journal of Cerebral Blood Flow & Metabolism*, 21(11), 1259-1267.

Mascia, L., Zavala, E., Bosma, K., Pasero, D., Decaroli, D., Andrews, P., Berardino, M. (2007). High tidal volume is associated with the development of acute lung injury after severe brain injury: An international observational study. *Critical care medicine,* 35(8), 1815-1820.

McCrory, P. R. (2003). Brain injury and heading in soccer. In (Vol. 327): *British Medical Journal Publishing Group.*

McMahon, P. J., Hricik, A., Yue, J. K., Puccio, A. M., Inoue, T., Lingsma, H. F., Manley, G. T. (2014). Symptomatology and functional outcome in mild traumatic brain injury: Results from the prospective track-tbi study. *Journal of neurotrauma,* 31(1), 26-33.

Meythaler, J. M., Depalma, L., Devivo, M. J., Guin-Renfroe, S., & Novack, T. A. (2001). Sertraline to improve arousal and alertness in severe traumatic brain injury secondary to motor vehicle crashes. *Brain Injury,* 15(4), 321-331.

Mirończuk-Chodakowska, I., Witkowska, A. M., & Zujko, M. E. (2018). Endogenous non-enzymatic antioxidants in the human body. *Advances in medical sciences,* 63(1), 68-78.

Pearson, W. S., Ovalle Jr, F., Faul, M., & Sasser, S. M. (2012). A review of traumatic brain injury trauma center visits meeting physiologic criteria from the american college of surgeons committee on trauma/centers for disease control and prevention field triage guidelines. *Prehospital emergency care,* 16(3), 323-328.

Raghupathi, R. (2004). Cell death mechanisms following traumatic brain injury. *Brain pathology*, 14(2), 215-222.

Rockswold, S. B., Burton, P. C., Chang, A., McNally, N., Grant, A., Rockswold, G. L., Lenglet, C. (2019). Functional magnetic resonance imaging and oculomotor dysfunction in mild traumatic brain injury. *Journal of neurotrauma,* 36(7), 1099-1105.

Roof, R. L., Hoffman, S. W., & Stein, D. G. (1997). Progesterone protects against lipid peroxidation following traumatic brain injury in rats. *Molecular and chemical neuropathology*, 31, 1-11.

Saatman, K. E., Duhaime, A. C., Bullock, R., Maas, A. I., Valadka, A., & Manley, G. T. (2008). Classification of traumatic brain injury for targeted therapies. *Journal of neurotrauma,* 25(7), 719-738.

Saniova, B., Drobny, M., Kneslova, L., & Minarik, M. (2004). The outcome of patients with severe head injuries treated with amantadine sulphate. *Journal of neural transmission,* 111, 511-514.

Santos-Buelga, C., & Feliciano, A. S. (2017). Flavonoids: From structure to health issues. In (Vol. 22, pp. 477): *MDPI.*

Schneider, J. D. C., Tony M. Wong, Mary L. Dombovy, William N. (1999). Cognitive and behavioural efficacy of amantadine in acute traumatic brain injury: An initial double-blind placebo-controlled study. *Brain Injury*, 13(11), 863-872.

Siddall, O. R. M. (2005). Use of methylphenidate in traumatic brain injury. *Annals of Pharmacotherapy,* 39(7-8), 1309-1313.

Simpson, J. R. (2014). Dsm-5 and neurocognitive disorders. *Journal of the American Academy of Psychiatry and the Law Online*, 42(2), 159-164.

Steullet, P., Neijt, H., Cuénod, M., & Do, K. (2006). Synaptic plasticity impairment and hypofunction of nmda receptors induced by glutathione deficit: Relevance to schizophrenia. *Neuroscience,* 137(3), 807-819.

Tan, D., Yu, X., Chen, M., Chen, J., & Xu, J. (2017). Lutein protects against severe traumatic brain injury through anti-inflammation and antioxidative effects via icam-1/nrf-2. *Molecular Medicine Reports*, 16(4), 4235-4240.

Tavazzi, B., Signoretti, S., Lazzarino, G., Amorini, A. M., Delfini, R., Cimatti, M., Vagnozzi, R. (2005). Cerebral oxidative stress and depression of energy metabolism correlate with severity of diffuse brain injury in rats. *Neurosurgery,* 56(3), 582-589.

Temkin, N., Machamer, J., Dikmen, S., Nelson, L. D., Barber, J., Hwang, P. H., Giacino, J. (2022). Risk factors for high symptom burden three months after traumatic brain injury and implications for clinical trial design: A transforming research and clinical knowledge in traumatic brain injury study. *Journal of neurotrauma*, 39(21-22), 1524-1532.

Teng, C. J., Bhalerao, S., Lee, Z., Farber, J., Morris, H., Foran, T., & Tucker, W. (2001). The use of bupropion in the treatment of restlessness after a traumatic brain injury. *Brain Injury,* 15(5), 463-467.

Theadom, A., Mahon, S., Barker-Collo, S., McPherson, K., Rush, E., Vandal, A., & Feigin, V. (2013). Enzogenol for cognitive functioning in traumatic brain injury: A pilot placebo-controlled rct. *European Journal of Neurology*, 20(8), 1135-1144.

Tsai, H. Y., Ho, C. T., & Chen, Y. K. (2017). Biological actions and molecular effects of resveratrol, pterostilbene, and 3′-hydroxypterostilbene. *Journal of food and drug analysis,* 25(1), 134-147.

Tyurin, V. A., Tyurina, Y. Y., Borisenko, G. G., Sokolova, T. V., Ritov, V. B., Quinn, P. J., Kagan, V. E. (2000). Oxidative stress following traumatic brain injury in rats: Quantitation of biomarkers and detection of free radical intermediates. *Journal of neurochemistry*, 75(5), 2178-2189.

Valadka, A. B., Andrews, B. T., & Bullock, M. R. (2001). How well do neurosurgeons care for trauma patients? A survey of the membership of the american association for the surgery of trauma. *Neurosurgery,* 48(1), 17-25.

Vitarbo, E. A., Chatzipanteli, K., Kinoshita, K., Truettner, J. S., Alonso, O. F., & Dietrich, W. D. (2004). Tumor necrosis factor α expression and protein levels after fluid percussion injury in rats: The effect of injury severity and brain temperature. *Neurosurgery,* 55(2), 416-425.

Wang, K., Zhang, L., Rao, W., Su, N., Hui, H., Wang, L., ... Fei, Z. (2015). Neuroprotective effects of crocin against traumatic brain injury in mice: Involvement of notch signaling pathway. *Neuroscience letters,* 591, 53-58.

Wortzel, H. S., & Arciniegas, D. B. (2014). The dsm-5 approach to the evaluation of traumatic brain injury and its neuropsychiatric sequelae. *NeuroRehabilitation*, 34(4), 613-623.

Writer, B. W., & Schillerstrom, J. E. (2009). Psychopharmacological treatment for cognitive impairment in survivors of traumatic brain injury: A critical review. *The Journal of neuropsychiatry and clinical neurosciences,* 21(4), 362-370.

Wroblewski, B., Joseph, A., Kupfer, J., & Kalliel, K. (1997). Effectiveness of valproic acid on destructive and aggressive behaviours in patients with acquired brain injury. *Brain Injury,* 11(1), 37-48.

Xiao, G., Wei, J., Yan, W., Wang, W., & Lu, Z. (2008). Improved outcomes from the administration of progesterone for patients with acute severe traumatic brain injury: A randomized controlled trial. *Critical care,* 12, 1-10.

Zhang, M., Cui, Z., Cui, H., Wang, Y., & Zhong, C. (2017). Astaxanthin protects astrocytes against trauma-induced apoptosis through inhibition of nkcc1 expression via the nf-κb signaling pathway. *BMC neuroscience,* 18, 1-12.

Zhi, D., Zhang, S., & Lin, X. (2003). Study on therapeutic mechanism and clinical effect of mild hypothermia in patients with severe head injury. *Surgical neurology,* 59(5), 381-385.

Zhong, J., Cheng, C., Liu, H., Huang, Z., Wu, Y., Teng, Z., Cao, F. (2017). Bexarotene protects against traumatic brain injury in mice partially through apolipoprotein e. *Neuroscience,* 343, 434-448.

Zink, B. J. (2001). Traumatic brain injury outcome: Concepts for emergency care. *Annals of emergency medicine,* 37(3), 318-332.

Zwienenberg, M., & Muizelaar, J. P. (2001). Cerebral perfusion and blood flow in neurotrauma. *Neurological Research,* 23(2-3), 167-174.

Chapter 13

Oxidative Stress and Neuroinflammation in Neurodegenerative Disorders

Deepshi Arora[1]**, PhD,**
Yugam Taneja[2]**, M.Pharm,**
Diksha Gulati[1]**, M. Pharm,**
Manish Kumar[3,*]**, PhD,**
and Mohit Agrawal[4]

[1]Guru Gobind Singh College of Pharmacy, Yamunanagar, Haryana, India
[2]Nutrascience, Sidcul, Haridwar, India
3Department of Pharmaceutics, ISF College of Pharmacy, Moga, Punjab, India
[4]School of Medical & Allied Sciences, K. R. Mangalam University, Gurugram, Haryana, India

Abstract

Alzheimer's disease (AD) is a prevalent neurodegenerative condition marked by gradual memory loss and deterioration in cognitive function caused by amyloid-beta peptide (A) oligomer build-up, which results in amyloid deposits and neuronal degradation. Although the role of microglia and astrocytes in AD progression is becoming more widely recognized, their interaction with neurons in response to A, particularly in the early stages, is still poorly understood. Neuroinflammation and oxidative stress are crucial in the aetiology of Alzheimer's disease, with glial cells releasing pro-inflammatory cytokines, chemokines, and reactive oxygen and nitrogen species, resulting in synaptic dysfunction and memory impairment before late-stage neuronal death. Furthermore,

[*] Corresponding Author's Email: manish_singh17@rediffmail.com.

In: Neurogenerative Disorders
Editors: Mohit Agrawal, Manmohan Singhal, Amit Kumar Nayak et al.
ISBN: 979-8-89530-143-2

oxidative stress damages brain tissues, which are rich in easily oxidizable lipids and have a high oxygen demand, contributing to neurodegeneration. Understanding the complex interactions between neuro-inflammation and oxidative stress may be useful for creating therapeutic methods to control AD neurodegeneration by targeting microglial and astrocytic activation and reducing the production of pro-inflammatory and pro-oxidant factors, potentially opening up new avenues for effective AD treatment and management. This chapter looks at the part oxidative stress plays in Alzheimer's illness and emphasizes its significance in the disease's aetiology. Understanding the complicated relationships between neuro-inflammation and oxidative stress may provide useful insights into prospective treatment strategies for Alzheimer's disease.

Keywords: Alzheimer, clinical trials, artificial intelligence

Introduction

Overview of Alzheimer's Disease

Alzheimer's disease (AD) is a complicated neurological condition marked by memory loss and increasing cognitive deterioration. It affects Millions of people worldwide, making it the most typical cause of dementia. Dr. Alois Alzheimer made the first official diagnosis of AD in the early 20th century, and it has since grown to be a significant public health issue (Delay, 2022).

The pathological hallmarks of AD include the development of tau protein tangles and beta-amyloid plaques in the brain. The aberrant protein clumps cause neuronal disruption in function and communication, ultimately resulting in neurodegeneration and cognitive deficits (Delay, 2022).

The clinical course of AD typically progresses through stages, from mild cognitive impairment to severe dementia. The disease has a profound impact on individuals and places a significant burden on caregivers and healthcare systems (Delay, 2022).

The Significance of Investigating Oxidative Stress and Neuroinflammation

Role in Disease Progression

Oxidative stress and neuroinflammationplay a vital part in the pathogenesis and progression of Alzheimer's disease. Oxidative stress results from an unbalanced relationship between the body's antioxidant defences and reactive oxygen species (ROS) generationdefense mechanisms. This oxidative damage can assist with the accumulation of beta-amyloid and tau pathology and promote neurodegeneration (Butterfied et al., 2012).

Potential Therapeutic Targets

Investigating oxidative stress and neuroinflammation offers potential therapeutic targets. Antioxidants and anti-inflammatory agents are being explored as potential interventions to mitigate these processes and slow down the progression of AD (Pratico & Domenico, 2008).

Biomarker Discovery

Markers of oxidative stress and neuroinflammation have been studied as potential biomarkers for Alzheimer's disease. For example, increased levels of oxidative stress markers like 8-hydroxy-2'-deoxyguanosine (8-OHdG) are present in AD patients (Nunomura et al., 1999). Similarly, neuroinflammation markers, such as elevated levels of pro-inflammatory cytokines, have been observed in the brains and cerebrospinal fluid of AD patients (Tarkowski et al., 1999).

Lifestyle and Preventive Strategies

Understanding oxidative stress's function and neuroinflammation in AD can inform lifestyle modifications and preventive strategies. For instance, adopting antioxidant-rich diets, engaging in regular physical activity, and managing chronic inflammation may help reduce the risk or slow the progression of AD (Pritam et al., 2002).

Definition and Pathophysiology of AD

Alzheimer's disease (AD) is a chronic neurodegenerative disorder characterised by progressive cognitive decline, memory loss, and alterations in behaviour. It is the most prevalent type of dementia and often affects elderly people. AD is marked by the accumulation of abnormal protein deposits in the brain, primarily beta-amyloid plaques and tau protein tangles, which lead to neuronal damage and cell death (Bushman, Barbara & Madison, 2021).

The key pathological features of AD include:

Beta-Amyloid Plaques

These are clumps of beta-amyloid protein that accumulate between nerve cells. They disrupt cell-to-cell communication and trigger inflammation, leading to neuronal dysfunction and death.

Tau Protein Tangles

Abnormal tau protein forms tangles inside neurons. These tangles disrupt the cell's transport system, impairing the delivery of essential nutrients and molecules (Feter, 2021).

Neuroinflammation

The brain's immune cells, microglia, and astrocytes become activated, resulting in chronic inflammation. While inflammation is a protective response, chronic neuroinflammation can exacerbate neuronal damage.

Oxidative Stress

Oxidative stress results from an imbalance between the body's capacity to eliminate reactive oxygen species (ROS) and its ability to produce them. This damages neurons and contributes to AD progression (Jack et al., 2018).

Clinical Symptoms and Diagnostic Criteria

The clinical presentation of Alzheimer's disease typically includes the following symptoms:

Memory Loss

Initially, individuals may experience mild memory lapses, but as the disease progresses, significant memory impairment becomes evident.

Cognitive Decline

Patients often have difficulty with problem-solving, reasoning, and language. They may struggle with familiar tasks and experience disorientation.

Behavioural and Personality Changes

AD can lead to mood swings, agitation, and changes in personality and behaviour. Individuals may become anxious, depressed, or socially withdrawn.

Loss of Independence

As the disease advances, patients may lose the ability to perform daily tasks independently, such as dressing, grooming, and managing finances.

The diagnosis of Alzheimer's disease relies on clinical evaluation and may include neuroimaging and cognitive assessments. The most commonly used criteria for AD diagnosis are those established by the National Institute on Aging and the Alzheimer's Association (NIA-AA) (Jack et al., 2018).

These criteria emphasize:

Evidence of Cognitive Impairment

The presence of objective cognitive deficits, such as impaired memory and thinking skills.

Exclusion of Other Causes

Physicians should rule out other potential causes of cognitive decline, such as vitamin deficiencies or thyroid disorders.

Biomarker Evidence

The use of biomarkers, such as cerebrospinal fluid analysis or positron emission tomography (PET) scans, can provide evidence of beta-amyloid or tau pathology.

Prevalence and Impact on Society

Alzheimer's disease is a serious global health issue that has a significant effect on people, families, and society at large. Its prevalence continues to rise as the global population ages. Some key points regarding its prevalence and societal impact include:

Global Prevalence

As of my last knowledge update in September 2021, according to estimates from Alzheimer's disease International (2019), more than 50 million people worldwide suffer from Alzheimer's disease or an associated dementia.

Economic Burden

The economic burden of AD is immense. It encompasses healthcare costs, long-term care, and lost productivity. In the United States alone, the cost of caring for individuals with Alzheimer's was projected to reach trillions of dollars by the mid-21st century (Delay, 2022).

Caregiver Stress

AD places significant stress on caregivers, who often provide unpaid care to affected individuals. The emotional, physical, and financial toll on caregivers is substantial.

Oxidative Stress in Alzheimer's Disease

Overview of Oxidative Stress and Reactive Oxygen Species (ROS)

Oxidative Stress: A situation known as oxidative stress is characterised by an imbalance between the body's ability to neutralise reactive oxygen species (ROS) through antioxidants and the generation of ROS. Highly reactive chemicals known as ROS, which also include free radicals like superoxide anion (O2•) and hydroxyl radical (•OH), can harm biological components like lipids, proteins, and DNA.

Sources of ROS Generation in the Brain

Mitochondrial Dysfunction

The majority of ROS in the brain are generated within mitochondria during oxidative phosphorylation. Dysfunctional mitochondria produce excessive ROS (Tolar et al., 2021).

Inflammation

Activation of microglia and astrocytes during neuroinflammation leads to the release of ROS as part of the immune response.

Metal Ions

Transition metal ions like iron and copper, when dysregulated, can catalyze ROS production via Fenton chemistry.

Excitotoxicity

Overstimulation of glutamate receptors can lead to calcium influx and subsequent ROS production (Tolar et al., 2021).

Cellular and Molecular Mechanisms of Oxidative Damage

Lipid Peroxidation

ROS can attack lipids in cell membranes, leading to lipid peroxidation, which disrupts membrane integrity and function (Bloom and George, 2014).

Protein Oxidation

Oxidation of proteins can impair their structure and function, potentially leading to misfolding and aggregation.

DNA Damage

ROS-induced DNA damage can cause mutations and genomic instability (Bloom and George, 2014).

Link Between Oxidative Stress and AD Pathology

Beta-Amyloid Aggregation

ROS can promote the aggregation of beta-amyloid, a hallmark of AD pathology, and increase its neurotoxicity (de Paula et al., 2016).

Tau Hyper Phosphorylation

The hyper phosphorylation of tau protein, which results in the development of neurofibrillary tangles, has been linked to oxidative stress.

Neuronal Dysfunction and Death

ROS-induced damage to neurons can result in synaptic dysfunction and ultimately neuronal death, contributing to cognitive decline in AD (de Paula et al., 2016).

Neuroinflammation in Alzheimer's Disease

The central nervous system (CNS), which includes the brain and spinal cord, is subject to a complicated immune response known as neuroinflammation. It denotes the production of pro-inflammatory mediators together with the activation of the brain's resident immune cells, such as microglia and astrocytes (Heneka et al., 2015).

Causes of Neuroinflammation: Several factors can trigger neuroinflammation as shown in Table 1, including:

Pathogens

Infections by viruses, bacteria, or other pathogens can infiltrate the CNS, leading to an inflammatory response as the immune system attempts to eradicate the invaders.

Misfolded Proteins

The aggregation of mis-folded proteins, notably beta-amyloid and Hyperphosphorylated tau, can act as endogenous danger signals, inciting an immune response in the CNS (Heneka et al., 2015).

Oxidative Stress

Oxidative stress, characterised by an excess of reactive oxygen species (ROS), can result in cellular damage and inflammation within the brain.

Neurodegeneration

The progressive loss of neurons and associated cellular debris can activate immune cells, initiating an inflammatory cascade (Colonna, Marco and Oleg Butovsky, 2017).

The Role of Microglia and Astrocytes in Neuroinflammation

Microglia

The CNS's primary immune cells and initial line of defence are known as microglia. The phenotypes they can adopt are pro-inflammatory (M1) or anti-inflammatory (M2). In neuroinflammation, microglia can transition to an activated state, releasing pro-inflammatory cytokines, phagocytosing cellular debris, and contributing to inflammation (Colonna, Marco and Oleg Butovsky, 2017).

Table 1. Trigger factors for Alzheimer's disease

Triggering Factors	Description	Mechanisms and Consequences	Associated Conditions	Preventative Measures
Infections	CNS infections (viral, bacterial, fungal)	Microglial and astrocytic activation, cytokine release, immune cell recruitment, potential neuronal damage	Meningitis, encephalitis	Vaccination, hygiene measures
Trauma and Injury	TBI, stroke, spinal cord injury, trauma	Immediate tissue damage, DAMP release, secondary inflammation, potential neurodegeneration	Post-traumatic disorders	Injury prevention, rehabilitation
Autoimmune Diseases	MS, NMO, GBS	Dysregulated immune response, autoantibodies, demyelination, progressive neurological deficits	Autoimmune disorders	Immune-modulating therapies
Neurodegenerative Diseases	Alzheimer's, Parkinson's, ALS	Protein aggregation, microglial activation, chronic inflammation, neurotoxicity, cell death	Neurodegenerative disorders	Therapies targeting protein aggregates
Environmental Toxins	Heavy metals, pesticides, pollutants	Neurotoxic exposure, microglial and astrocytic activation, oxidative stress, neural damage	Environmental toxin-related disorders	Reduce exposure, detoxification
Chronic Stress	Psychological stress, isolation, trauma	HPA axis activation, stress hormone release, altered CNS immune responses, chronic neuroinflammation	Anxiety, depression, PTSD	Stress management, social support
Metabolic Disorders	Diabetes, obesity, metabolic syndrome	Systemic inflammation, blood-brain barrier dysfunction, neuro-inflammatory response, cognitive impairment	Type 2 diabetes, cognitive decline	Lifestyle changes, glucose control
Ageing	Normal ageing process	Microglial priming, chronic low-grade inflammation, increased susceptibility to neurodegenerative diseases	Age-related cognitive decline	Healthy lifestyle, cognitive training
Autoinflammatory Syndromes	Familial Mediterranean fever, CAPS	Genetic mutations leading to overactive inflammatory responses, including neuroinflammation	Auto-inflammatory disorders	Targeted anti-inflammatory therapies

Table 2. Signalling Pathways for Alzheimer's disease

Signalling Pathway	Activation Trigger	Key Components and Functions	Downstream Effects and Regulation
NF-κB (Nuclear Factor-κB)	- PAMPs (e.g., bacterial lipopolysaccharides) - DAMPs (e.g., cellular stress, DNA damage) - Cytokines (e.g., TNF-α, IL-1β)	- NF-κB transcription factors (p65, p50) - Inhibitor of κB (IκB) proteins - IKK complex (IKKα, IKKβ, IKKγ) - Toll-like receptors (TLRs) - TNF receptor	- Induction of pro-inflammatory gene expression (e.g., IL-6, IL-1β, TNF-α) - Promotion of cell survival and proliferation - Immune cell recruitment and activation - Tightly regulated by negative feedback mechanisms to prevent excessive inflammation.
MAPK (Mitogen-Activated Protein Kinase)	- Growth factors (e.g., EGF, PDGF) - Cytokines (e.g., IL-6) - Stress signals (e.g., oxidative stress) - Environmental stimuli (e.g., UV radiation)	-ERK (Extracellular signal-regulated kinase) - JNK (c-Jun N-terminal kinase) - p38 MAPK	- ERK: Promotes cell growth and proliferation - JNK: Regulates apoptosis and stress responses - p38 MAPK: Mediates inflammation and cell differentiation - Feedback loops and phosphatases control MAPK activity.
MAPK (Mitogen-Activated Protein Kinase)	- Growth factors (e.g., EGF, PDGF) - Cytokines (e.g., IL-6) - Stress signals (e.g., oxidative stress) - Environmental stimuli (e.g., UV radiation)	-ERK (Extracellular signal-regulated kinase) - JNK (c-Jun N-terminal kinase) - p38 MAPK	- ERK: Promotes cell growth and proliferation - JNK: Regulates apoptosis and stress responses - p38 MAPK: Mediates inflammation and cell differentiation - Feedback loops and phosphatases control MAPK activity.
NLRP3 Inflammasome	- DAMPs (e.g., ATP, uric acid crystals) - PAMPs (e.g., bacterial toxins) - ROS (Reactive Oxygen Species)	- NLRP3 (NOD-like receptor protein 3) -ASC (Apoptosis-associated speck-like protein containing a CARD) - Caspase-1	- Activation of caspase-1 leads to the maturation and release of IL-1β and IL-18. - Induction of pyroptosis, a pro-inflammatory form of cell death. - Dysregulation can result in chronic inflammatory conditions. - Negative regulators, such as NLRP3 inhibitors and autophagy, help control Inflammasome activation.

Table 3. Imaging Techniques to Assess Oxidative Stress and Neuroinflammation

Imaging Technique	Description	Targets and Biomarkers Assessed	Advantages	Limitations
Positron Emission Tomography (PET)	Uses radiolabelled tracers that bind to specific molecular targets in the brain.	- Glucose metabolism (FDG-PET) - Microglial activation (e.g., [11C]PK11195) - Neuroinflammation (e.g., TSPO ligands)	- High sensitivity and specificity. - Quantitative assessment of target density. - Suitable for longitudinal studies.	- Exposure to ionizing radiation. - Limited spatial resolution. - Costly and requires radiotracers.
Single Photon Emission Computed Tomography (SPECT)	Similar to PET but uses gamma-emitting radiopharmaceuticals.	- Regional cerebral blood flow (rCBF) - Dopamine transporter (DAT) - Serotonin transporter (SERT)	- Non-invasive and quantitative. - Widely available radiopharmaceuticals.	- Lower spatial resolution compared to PET. - Radiation exposure.
Magnetic Resonance Imaging (MRI)	Provides structural and functional information without radiation.	- Blood-brain barrier integrity (Gadolinium-enhanced MRI) - Blood oxygenation level (BOLD fMRI) - Neuroinflammation (e.g., T2-weighted, FLAIR, DTI)	- Excellent soft tissue contrast. - Multi-modal imaging options. - No ionizing radiation.	- Limited specificity for molecular targets. - Requires expensive equipment.
Magnetic Resonance Spectroscopy (MRS)	Measures chemical concentrations in brain tissue.	-Neuro-inflammatory markers (e.g., glutamate, myo-inositol) - Antioxidants (e.g., glutathione)	- Provides quantitative biochemical information. - Non-invasive.	- Limited spatial resolution. - Challenging data interpretation.
Optical Imaging (e.g., Near-Infrared Spectroscopy)	Uses near-infrared light to measure changes in tissue properties.	- Cerebral oxygenation (HbO2, HbR) - Cerebral blood volume (CBV) - Cellular metabolic activity	- Non-invasive and portable. - Suitable for continuous monitoring.	- Limited depth penetration. - Restricted to surface measurements.
Molecular Imaging (e.g., FLAP)	Employs specific molecular probes or contrast agents.	- Oxidative stress markers (e.g., ROS-sensitive probes) - Inflammatory markers (e.g., fluorinated nanoparticles)	- Targeted assessment of specific processes. - Potential for molecular specificity.	- Limited to preclinical research. - May require probe development.

Astrocytes

Astrocytes are multifunctional glial cells that become activated in response to CNS injury or inflammation. They are essential in controlling the immunological response in the brain. Activated astrocytes can release pro-inflammatory molecules, such as interleukin-1 alpha (IL-1α) and chemokines, while also participating in the maintenance of the blood-brain barrier (Colonna, Marco and Oleg Butovsky, 2017).

Release of Pro-Inflammatory Cytokines and Chemokines

Pro-Inflammatory Cytokines

Pro-inflammatory cytokines such as interleukin-1 beta (IL-1), tumour necrosis factor-alpha (TNF-), and interleukin-6 (IL-6) are secreted during neuroinflammation. These cytokines exert pleiotropic effects, contributing to immune activation and inflammation within the CNS (Heneka et al., 2015).

Chemokines

Chemokines are chemoattractant chemicals that help immune cells be attracted to inflamed areas of the brain. Involved in the recruitment of microglia and peripheral immune cells, examples include chemokine (C-C motif) ligand 2 (CCL2) and chemokine (C-X-C motif) ligand 10 (CXCL10) (Lopez et al., 2019).

The Association of Neuroinflammation with AD Progression

Neuroinflammation and AD

Neuroinflammation is intimately intertwined with the pathogenesis of Alzheimer's disease (AD). An inflammatory response is brought on by beta-amyloid plaques and tau tangles in the AD brain. Microglia and astrocytes become activated, releasing pro-inflammatory cytokines and exacerbating neurodegeneration (Lopez et al., 2019).

Neuroinfammation's Impact on AD

While neuroinflammation initially serves as a protective response aimed at mitigating damage, chronic and dysregulated inflammation can worsen neuronal injury in AD. It can further promote the aggregation of mis-folded proteins, disrupt synaptic function, and ultimately contribute to the progressive cognitive decline characteristic of AD (Wyss-Coray and Tony, 2006).

Interplay Between Oxidative Stress and Neuroinflammation

Reciprocal Relationship Between Oxidative Stress and Inflammation

Reciprocal Relationship: Oxidative stress and inflammation in the context of Alzheimer's disease (AD) often exist in a reciprocal relationship. Oxidative stress can trigger neuroinflammation, and conversely, inflammation can exacerbate oxidative stress (Wimo et al., 2017).

Amplification of Neurotoxicity and Neuronal Damage

Amplification: The interplay between oxidative stress and neuroinflammation amplifies neurotoxicity and neuronal damage in AD. When immune cells like microglia are activated by oxidative stress, they release pro-inflammatory cytokines known as reactive nitrogen species (RNS) and ROS. These cytokines, in turn, lead to further oxidative stress and neurotoxicity, creating a self-perpetuating cycle (Halliwell, Barry and John MC, 2015).

Activation of Signalling Pathways: NF-κB, MAPK, and NLRP3 Inflammasome (Table 2)

NF-κB

In neuroinflammation, nuclear factor-kappa B (NF-κB) is a crucial signalling route. It is turned on in response to pro-inflammatory stimuli and oxidative stress, which causes the transcription of pro-inflammatory genes (Sies, Helmut and Dean P. Jones, 2020).

MAPK

Oxidative stress also activates the Mitogen-Activated Protein Kinase (MAPK) pathways, which help to produce pro-inflammatory cytokines in neuroinflammation (Zhang et al., 2019).

NLRP3 Inflammasome

Pro-inflammatory cytokines like IL-1 are generated and released by the NLRP3 inflammasome, a multiprotein complex. The NLRP3 inflammasome can be activated by oxidative stress and improperly folded proteins like beta-amyloid, which exacerbates neuroinflammation (Uttara et al., 2009).

The Role of Aβ and Tau in Oxidative Stress and Neuroinflammation

Aβ

Beta-amyloid (Aβ) and its aggregates are central players in the oxidative stress and neuroinflammation observed in AD. Aβ can induce ROS production, impair mitochondrial function, and activate microglia, leading to the release of pro-inflammatory cytokines (Stadtman and Earl, 2006).

Tau

Hyperphosphorylated tau protein, forming neurofibrillary tangles, is associated with oxidative stress and inflammation in AD. Tau pathology can trigger microglial activation and pro-inflammatory responses, contributing to neuroinflammation (Cooke et al., 2003).

Oxidative Stress and Inflammatory Biomarkers in Alzheimer's Disease

Blood-Based Biomarkers

Blood Markers

Blood-based indicators for Alzheimer's disease (AD)-related oxidative stress and neuroinflammation are of significant interest due to their non-invasive nature and potential for widespread use in clinical settings. Some notable blood-based markers include:

Oxidative Stress Biomarkers

These include indicators of lipid peroxidation (8-isoprostane, for instance), protein oxidation (protein carbonyls, for instance), and antioxidant status (glutathione levels, for instance) (Butterfield, D. Allan and Barry Hali well, 2019).

Inflammatory Biomarkers

Neuroinflammation in AD is correlated with cytokines such as interleukin-6 (IL-6), C-reactive protein (CRP), and tumour necrosis factor-alpha (TNF-α) (Nunomura et al., 2001).

Cerebrospinal Fluid (CSF) Biomarkers

CSF Biomarkers

Cerebrospinal fluid provides direct access to biochemical changes occurring in the brain. Biomarkers measured in CSF can provide valuable insights into oxidative stress and neuroinflammation in AD. Prominent CSF biomarkers include:

Oxidative Stress Markers

These may include markers of lipid peroxidation products (e.g., 4-hydroxynonenal) and antioxidants (e.g., reduced glutathione) (Angelova, Plamena and Andrey Y., 2018).

Inflammatory Markers

Elevated levels of cytokines (e.g., IL-1β, IL-6), chemokines (e.g., CCl_2), and soluble receptors (e.g., TNF) have been observed in the CSF of AD patients, indicating neuroinflammation (Sultana, Rukhsanaand D. Allan, 2010).

Imaging Techniques to Assess Oxidative Stress and Neuroinflammation (Table 3)

Imaging Modalities

Advanced imaging techniques have been developed to visualize and quantify oxidative stress and neuroinflammation in AD brains. Key methods include:

Positron Emission Tomography (PET)

PET imaging using radiotracers like [^18F]-fluorodeoxyglucose (FDG) or [11C]-Pittsburgh compound B (PiB) can indirectly assess neuroinflammation and oxidative stress by measuring changes in glucose metabolism or amyloid deposition, respectively.

Magnetic Resonance Imaging (MRI)

MRI methods, such as magnetic resonance spectroscopy (MRS) and diffusion-weighted imaging (DWI), can shed light on changes in brain microstructure and metabolite concentrations linked to oxidative stress and inflammation (Quintanilla et al., 2012).

Novel PET Tracers

Emerging PET tracers, like [^18F]-FDG or [^11C]-DPA-713, specifically target microglia activation or reactive oxygen species, offering more direct measures of neuroinflammation and oxidative stress (Migliore et al., 2005).

Therapeutic Strategies for Oxidative Stress and Neuroinflammation in Alzheimer's Disease (AD)

Antioxidant Therapies

Antioxidant Supplementation

Antioxidant therapies aim to reduce oxidative stress in AD by neutralizing reactive oxygen species (ROS) and preventing cellular damage. Some common antioxidants investigated in AD include:

Vitamins

Studies on the possible neuroprotective effects of vitamins, such as vitamin E (-tocopherol) and vitamin C (ascorbic acid), have been conducted (Di Domenico et al., 2017).

Selenium

Selenium, often administered as selenomethionine, is another antioxidant that has shown promise in reducing oxidative stress (Edison et al., 2008).

Natural Compounds

Numerous naturally occurring substances with antioxidant characteristics are being researched for their potential advantages in AD, including resveratrol from grapes and curcumin from turmeric (Turner et al., 2020).

Anti-Inflammatory Interventions

Anti-Inflammatory Agents

Targeting neuroinflammation in AD involves the application of anti-inflammatory measures. These may include:

Non-Steroidal Anti-Inflammatory Drugs (NSAIDs)

Some studies have suggested that NSAIDs like ibuprofen may have a protective effect against AD by reducing inflammation (Villemagne et al., 2021).

Cytokine Modulators

Biologic agents or small molecules that modulate pro-inflammatory cytokines, such as TNF-α inhibitors, are being explored as potential therapies (Grundman, Michael and Patrick Delaney, 2002).

Microglial Modulation

Therapies aimed at regulating microglial activation and function, such as minocycline, are under investigation for their anti-inflammatory properties (Grundman, Michael and Patrick Delaney, 2002).

Combination Therapies and Challenges

Combination Approaches

Given the multifaceted nature of AD, combination therapies targeting both oxidative stress and neuroinflammation are being explored. These approaches may involve a blend of anti-inflammatory and antioxidant substances to address multiple pathogenic pathways simultaneously.

Challenges in Developing Effective Therapies for AD

Drug Efficacy

Many clinical trials targeting oxidative stress and neuroinflammation have shown limited efficacy, highlighting the complexity of AD pathology (Zucchi et al., 2008).

Timing of Intervention

Identifying the optimal stage of disease for intervention remains a challenge, as AD likely involves a long preclinical phase.

Safety Concerns

Some interventions, especially long-term use of anti-inflammatory drugs, may carry safety concerns, such as gastrointestinal or cardiovascular side effects (Szekely, C. A. and Zandi, 2010).

Potential Future Directions

Precision Medicine

Tailoring therapeutic approaches to an individual's unique genetic and molecular profile is an emerging area of research. Personalized treatment strategies may lead to more effective interventions.

Neuroprotection

Future therapies may focus on neuroprotective strategies that not only target oxidative stress and neuroinflammation but also promote neuronal survival and repair.

Lifestyle Interventions

Lifestyle modifications, including diet, exercise, and cognitive stimulation, are being investigated for their potential to reduce oxidative stress and inflammation and mitigate AD risk (Villarejo et al., 2020; Ngandu et al., 2015) In summary, therapeutic strategies targeting oxidative stress and neuroinflammation in Alzheimer's disease are a promising avenue for intervention. Antioxidant therapies, anti-inflammatory agents, and combination approaches are under investigation. However, challenges remain, and future directions may involve precision medicine, neuro-protection, and lifestyle interventions.

Conclusion

Cognitive decline and memory loss are hallmarks of the severe neurodegenerative condition Alzheimer's disease (AD). Even though the precise origin of AD is still unknown, substantial research has demonstrated the crucial roles that oxidative stress and neuroinflammation play in the course of the disease.

The cellular damage and neural dysfunction in AD are a result of oxidative stress, which is fuelled by an imbalance between the generation of reactive oxygen species (ROS) and the body's antioxidant defence mechanisms. This oxidative damage can exacerbate the accumulation of Misfolded proteins, including beta-amyloid plaques and tau tangles, hallmark pathologies of AD.

Neuroinflammation, on the other hand, involves the activation of immune responses within the central nervous system, including microglia and astrocytes. While initially a protective response, chronic neuroinflammation can lead to neuronal injury, synaptic dysfunction, and cognitive decline in AD.

The interplay between oxidative stress and neuroinflammation further complicates AD pathophysiology. Oxidative stress can trigger inflammation and inflammation, in turn, can exacerbate oxidative stress, creating a self-reinforcing cycle of damage.

Understanding the intricate relationship between these processes has led to the exploration of various therapeutic approaches. Antioxidant therapies aim to counteract oxidative stress, while anti-inflammatory interventions target neuroinflammation. Combination therapies and personalized approaches are also being investigated to address the multifaceted nature of AD.

Despite ongoing challenges and the need for further research, advancements in biomarker development and imaging techniques offer hope for earlier diagnosis and more effective treatments. Lifestyle interventions, promoting a healthy diet, regular exercise, and cognitive engagement, may also play a crucial role in reducing AD risk.

In conclusion, oxidative stress and neuroinflammation are central players in the complex puzzle of Alzheimer's disease. Continued research, innovative therapies, and a holistic approach to AD management are essential in the pursuit of effective treatments and, ultimately, a brighter future for those affected by this devastating condition.

Disclaimer

None.

References

Angelova, P. R., & Abramov, A. Y. (2018). Role of mitochondrial ROS in the brain: from physiology to neurodegeneration. *FEBS letters*, 592(5), 692-702.

Bloom, G. S. (2014). Amyloid-β and tau: the trigger and bullet in Alzheimer disease pathogenesis. *JAMA neurology*, 71(4), 505-508.

Bushman, B. A., & Pullen, M. E. (2021). Alzheimer's disease and Physical Activity. *ACSM's Health & Fitness Journal,* 25(4), 5-10.

Butterfield, D. A., Perluigi, M., Reed, T., Muharib, T., Hughes, C. P., Robinson, R. A., & Sultana, R. (2012). Redox proteomics in selected neurodegenerative disorders: from its infancy to future applications. *Antioxidants & redox signaling,* 17(11), 1610-1655.

Butterfield, D. Allan, and Barry Halliwell. "Oxidative stress, dysfunctional glucose metabolism and Alzheimer's disease." *Nature Reviews Neuroscience* 20, no. 3 (2019): 148-160.

Colonna, M., & Butovsky, O. (2017). Microglia function in the central nervous system during health and neurodegeneration. *Annual review of immunology,* 35(1), 441-468.

Cooke, M. S., Evans, M. D., Dizdaroglu, M., &Lunec, J. (2003). Oxidative DNA damage: mechanisms, mutation, and disease. *The FASEB Journal*, 17(10), 1195-1214.

Delay, P. G., Test, N. I. P., Sequencing, W. E., & Kits, T. I. (2022). What are neurodegenerative diseases? *Neurodegenerative diseases.*

de Paula, Jonas J., Maicon R. Albuquerque, Guilherme M. Lage, Maria A. Bicalho, Marco A. Romano-Silva, and Leandro F. Malloy-Diniz. "Impairment of fine motor dexterity in mild cognitive impairment and Alzheimer's disease dementia: association with activities of daily living." *Revistabrasileira de psiquiatria* 38, no. 3 (2016): 235-238.

Di Domenico, F., Tramutola, A., & Butterfield, D. A. (2017). Role of 4-hydroxy-2-nonenal (HNE) in the pathogenesis of alzheimer disease and other selected age-related neurodegenerative disorders. *Free Radical Biology and Medicine,* 111, 253-261.

Edison, P., Archer, H. A., Gerhard, A., Hinz, R., Pavese, N., Turkheimer, F. E., ...& Brooks, D. J. (2008). Microglia, amyloid, and cognition in Alzheimer's disease: An [11C](R) PK11195-PET and [11C] PIB-PET study. *Neurobiology of disease,* 32(3), 412-419.

Feter, N., Jayne Santos Leite, Ricardo Alt, and Airton José Rombaldi. "Ethnoracial disparity among patients with dementia during COVID-19 pandemic." Cadernos de SaúdePública 37 (2021).

Grundman, M., & Delaney, P. (2002). Antioxidant strategies for Alzheimer's disease. *Proceedings of the Nutrition Society,* 61(2), 191-202.

Halliwell, B., &Gutteridge, J. M. (2015). Free radicals in biology and medicine. Oxford university press, USA.

Heneka, M. T., Carson, M. J., El Khoury, J., Landreth, G. E., Brosseron, F., Feinstein, D. L., ...&Kummer, M. P. (2015). Neuroinflammation in Alzheimer's disease. *The Lancet Neurology,* 14(4), 388-405.

Jack Jr, C. R., Bennett, D. A., Blennow, K., Carrillo, M. C., Dunn, B., Haeberlein, S. B., ...& Silverberg, N. (2018). NIA-AA research framework: toward a biological definition of Alzheimer's disease. *Alzheimer's & dementia*, 14(4), 535-562.

Lopez, J. A. S., González, H. M., & Léger, G. C. (2019). Alzheimer's disease. *Handbook of clinical neurology*, 167, 231-255.

Migliore, L., Fontana, I., Trippi, F., Colognato, R., Coppede, F., Tognoni, G., ...&Siciliano, G. (2005). Oxidative DNA damage in peripheral leukocytes of mild cognitive impairment and AD patients. *Neurobiology of aging*, 26(5), 567-573.

Ngandu, T., Lehtisalo, J., Solomon, A., Levälahti, E., Ahtiluoto, S., Antikainen, R., ...&Kivipelto, M. (2015). A 2 year multidomain intervention of diet, exercise, cognitive training, and vascular risk monitoring versus control to prevent cognitive decline in at-risk elderly people (Finger): a randomised controlled trial. *The Lancet,* 385(9984), 2255-2263.

Nunomura, A., Perry, G., Hirai, K., Aliev, G., Takeda, A., Chiba, S., & Smith, M. A. (1999). Neuronal RNA oxidation in Alzheimer's disease and Down's syndrome. *Annals of the New York Academy of Sciences, 893*(1), 362-364.

Nunomura, A., Perry, G., Aliev, G., Hirai, K., Takeda, A., Balraj, E. K., ...& Smith, M. A. (2001). Oxidative damage is the earliest event in Alzheimer disease. *Journal of Neuropathology & Experimental Neurology,* 60(8), 759-767.

Praticò, D. (2008). Oxidative stress hypothesis in Alzheimer's disease: a reappraisal. *Trends in pharmacological sciences,* 29(12), 609-615.

Pritam, P., Deka, R., Bhardwaj, A., Srivastava, R., Kumar, D., Jha, A. K., ...&Jha, S. K. (2022). Antioxidants in Alzheimer's disease: Current therapeutic significance and future prospects. *Biology,* 11(2), 212.

Quintanilla, R. A., Orellana, J. A., & von Bernhardi, R. (2012). Understanding risk factors for Alzheimer's disease: interplay of neuroinflammation, connexin-based communication and oxidative stress. *Archives of Medical Research,* 43(8), 632-644.

Sies, H., & Jones, D. P. (2020). Reactive oxygen species (ROS) as pleiotropic physiological signalling agents. *Nature reviews Molecular cell biology,* 21(7), 363-383.

Stadtman, E. R. (1992). Protein oxidation and aging. *Science*, 257(5074), 1220-1224.

Sultana, R., & Butterfield, D. A. (2010). Role of oxidative stress in the progression of Alzheimer's disease. *Journal of Alzheimer's Disease*, 19(1), 341-353.

Szekely, C. A., & Zandi, P. P. (2010). Non-steroidal anti-inflammatory drugs and Alzheimer's disease: the epidemiological evidence. *CNS & Neurological Disorders-Drug Targets (Formerly Current Drug Targets-CNS & Neurological Disorders),* 9(2), 132-139.

Tarkowski, E., Blennow, K., Wallin, A., & Tarkowski, A. (1999). Intracerebral production of tumor necrosis factor-α, a local neuroprotective agent, in Alzheimer disease and vascular dementia. *Journal of clinical immunology,* 19, 223-230.

Tolar, M., Hey, J., Power, A., &Abushakra, S. (2021). Neurotoxic soluble amyloid oligomers drive Alzheimer's pathogenesis and represent a clinically validated target for slowing disease progression. *International journal of molecular sciences,* 22(12), 6355.

Turner, R. S., Stubbs, T., Davies, D. A., &Albensi, B. C. (2020). Potential new approaches for diagnosis of Alzheimer's disease and related dementias. *Frontiers in neurology,* 11, 496.

Uttara, B., Singh, A. V., Zamboni, P., & Mahajan, R. (2009). Oxidative stress and neurodegenerative diseases: a review of upstream and downstream antioxidant therapeutic options. *Current neuropharmacology,* 7(1), 65-74.

Villarejo-Galende, A., González-Sánchez, M., Blanco-Palmero, V. A., Llamas-Velasco, S., & Benito-León, J. (2020). Non-steroidal anti-inflammatory drugs as candidates for the prevention or treatment of Alzheimer's disease: do they still have a role? *Current Alzheimer Research,* 17(11), 1013-1022.

Villemagne, V. L., Barkhof, F., Garibotto, V., Landau, S. M., Nordberg, A., & van Berckel, B. N. (2021). Molecular imaging approaches in dementia. *Radiology,* 298(3), 517-530.

Wimo, A., Guerchet, M., Ali, G. C., Wu, Y. T., Prina, A. M., Winblad, B., ...& Prince, M. (2017). The worldwide costs of dementia 2015 and comparisons with 2010. *Alzheimer's & Dementia, 13*(1), 1-7.

Wyss-Coray, T. (2006). Inflammation in Alzheimer disease: driving force, bystander or beneficial response? *Nature medicine*, 12(9), 1005-1015.

Zhang, Lixiao, Xianwei Wang, Ramón Cueto, Comfort Effi, Yuling Zhang, Hongmei Tan, Xuebin Qin, Yong Ji, Xiaofeng Yang, and Hong Wang. "Biochemical basis and metabolic interplay of redox regulation." *Redox Biology* 26 (2019): 101284.

Zucchi, O. L. A. D., Faccioli, L. H., Nomizo, A., Moreira, S., Sá-Nunes, A., Bolzoni, R. M. F., ... & Salvador, M. J. (2008). Srtxrf Analysis of Trace Element on Inflammatory Immune Response. *Micronutrients and Health Research*, 293.

Chapter 14

Oxidative Stress and Neuroinflammation in Alzheimer's Disease

Himanshu Sharma[1],
Phool Chandra[1],
Vaibhav Rastogi[1],
Subhajit Mandal[2],
Radheshyam Pal[3,4],
and Sumel Ashique[3,4,*]

[1]Teerthanker Mahaveer College of Pharmacy, Teerthanker Mahaveer University, Moradabad (UP), India
[2]Department of Pharmaceutical Sciences, Faculty of Science and Engineering, Dibrugarh University, Dibrugarh, Assam, India
[3]Department of Pharmaceutical Sciences, Bengal College of Pharmaceutical Sciences & Research, Durgapur, West Bengal, India
[4]School of Pharmaceutical Sciences, Lovely Professional University, Phagwara, Punjab, India

Abstract

Oxidative stress, brought on by redox state imbalances, results in an excess of ROS being created or the antioxidant system malfunctioning. The brain is particularly susceptible to the effects of ROS because it has a high oxygen need and a large number of lipid cells that are prone to peroxidation. The theory that oxidative stress impairs cellular function with aging and contributes to several age-related disorders, including atherosclerosis, arthritis, and neurodegenerative diseases, is becoming

[*] Corresponding Author's Email: ashiquesumel007@gmail.com.

In: Neurogenerative Disorders
Editors: Mohit Agrawal, Manmohan Singhal, Amit Kumar Nayak et al.
ISBN: 979-8-89530-143-2

more and more supported by data. Alzheimer's disease (AD) is a well-researched neurodegenerative disorder that has generated a lot of attention. It is identified by a progressive deterioration in cognitive abilities. Pathological characteristics of AD include senile plaques, neurofibrillary tangles, and loss of synapses. Amyloid β-peptide (Aβ)-induced oxidative stress is one of the primary factors thought to play a part in the etiology and pathophysiology of AD. Oxidation of brain lipids, carbohydrates, proteins, and DNA has been demonstrated to be caused by AD. The primary histological alterations of the illness contain some byproducts of this oxidation. An increasing amount of evidence connects the pathophysiology of AD with oxidative stress caused by Aβ. Oxidative alterations in the context of AD are strongly linked to a moderate inflammatory response in the brain. There is strong evidence from several studies that oxidative stress has a role in the development of AD.

Keywords: Alzheimer's disease, amyloid plaque, inflammation, oxidative stress

Introduction

Alzheimer's disease is the most common neurological disease. Today, more than 60% of dementia patients have AD as their major cause, which presents a higher threat to society. In this condition, cognitive decline which mostly affects long-term memory progresses normally to severe dementia. Since AD affects older persons 60 to 64 years of age at a rate of around 1-2% and rises to about 30% in those 85 years of age and above, advanced age is a key risk factor for getting the condition (Sharma et al., 2023). There are about 20 to 30 million people with AD on the globe. The loss of brain cells has not been demonstrated to be slowed down by any of the treatments for AD now in use, and the illness is still not fully diagnosed. New aspects of the disease's diagnosis have been found by researchers, thanks in part to sample collecting and brain postmortems. Two neuropathological hallmarks are linked to AD (Asamu et al., 2023). These extracellular deposits of amyloid beta peptide are what give rise to diffuse plaques and NFTs. AD has a complex etiology that most likely involves several cellular and molecular mechanisms. However, the activation of AD requires amyloid β peptide. The evidence for the trigger action of AD has been described as the participation of amyloid β peptide and its precursor, amyloid precursor protein, which may raise the risk of AD (Song et al., 2021). The "Amyloid β cascade hypothesis," validated by new research, postulates that the essential metabolic process of amyloid β buildup causes neurodegeneration in both familial and sporadic AD. The current theory of the amyloid cascade states that these proteins build up chronologically and that this accumulation sets off a series of events that include the formation of NFT, mitochondrial malfunction, and neuroinflammation caused by abnormal activation of microglia and astrocytes (Ly et al., 2023). Neuroinflammation usually differs from exterior inflammation since it carries normal peripheral inflammation signals. The inflammatory processes that harm and eventually kill neurons are associated with neuroinflammation. It has also been connected to certain neurologic disorders, such as multiple sclerosis, and neurodegenerative disorders like AD. Nonetheless, the inflammatory response of the immune system may be a part of the neuropathological behavior of AD (Nayak et al., 2023). Despite causing neuronal dysfunction, some pathological research suggests that brain immune cells in AD induce neuroinflammation, which is important for Aβ accumulation. The high concentrations of inflammatory mediators surrounding Aβ plaques and neurofibrillary tangles demonstrated the connection between AD and neuroinflammation. Only a tiny portion of cases are in the early stages of AD (Yamini et al., 2022). The neuroprotective system, which also involves the antioxidant process, provides an efficient defense against the generation of reactive oxygen species. Conversely, the advancement of oxidative stress in AD may result in an excess of inflammation inside the brain. Microglia, astrocytes, and neurons are just a few of the cells in the CNS that have been shown to act as a precursor for neuroinflammation. According to the free-radical hypothesis of aging, an increase in ROS damages mitochondrial DNA and reduces mitochondrial function, which leads to senescence. It is well-accepted that ROS and intermediate free radicals are the main causes of oxidative damage (Mohammadi et al., 2021). However, a wealth of data also suggests that ROS are essential signaling molecules that facilitate physiological processes including cell division, proliferation, and survival. Redox signaling and oxidative stress appear to be the primary causes of illnesses ranging from neurological to cardiovascular diseases, despite studies over the past few decades tying oxidative stress to the etiology of various diseases. τ protein and the neurotoxic Aβ peptide are among the main contributors to decreased synaptic plasticity, neuroinflammation, part-vascular reactivity impairment, cholinergic denervation, neurotransmitter imbalance, neuronal loss, dendritic alterations, and significant synaptic loss due to oxidative stress (Lian et al., 2024).

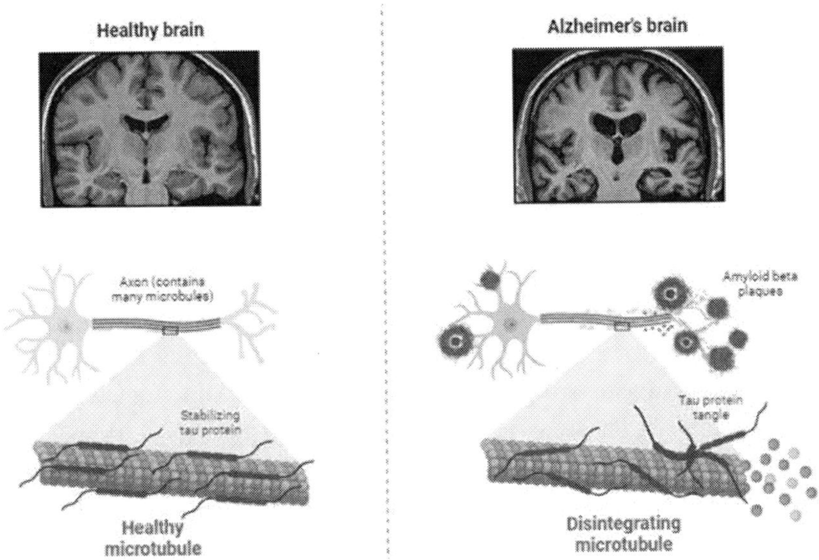

Figure 1. Pathogenesis of Alzheimer's disease.

Pathogenesis of Alzheimer's Disease

The main feature of the neurodegenerative illness known as Alzheimer's disease, which develops gradually, is the accumulation of abnormal protein deposits in the brain (Y. Wang et al., 2023). Amyloid-beta plaques and tau tangles impede brain transmission and ultimately result in neuronal death. Genetic factors, such as mutations in the APP, PSEN1, and PSEN2 genes, are involved even though rare instances are common. Memory loss and cognitive decline are caused by oxidative stress and inflammatory processes that further damage neurons. The accumulation of Aβ exacerbates the illness by initiating a cascade of events that includes synaptic impairment and neuroinflammation (Fonseca-Santos et al., 2023). Though the precise routes are still being investigated, these pathogenic changes are crucial to the genesis of Alzheimer's disease (see Figure 1).

β-Amyloid Peptide

The pathogenesis of AD-like is influenced by several factors, including age, sex, family history, lifestyle, depression, food, hypertension, medication, and cognitive activity. There is evidence that the new AD hallmark includes neurofibrillary tangles and amyloid plaque. A sequence of amino acids with more than 40-42 amino acids makes up the amyloid plaque. One of the main players in the synthesis of amyloid peptides is the APP (Nakanishi et al., 2021). Furthermore, there are two distinct kinds of enzymatic cleavage of the amyloid precursor protein (I) β & II) γ secretase; thus, these two enzymes aid in the production of amyloid β peptide in the central nervous system. Moreover, APP has several fantastic functions that promote synaptic plasticity, a process that strengthens the brain and memory. The peptide is released by neuronal cells in the stomach and other parts of the body, and it is then carried to the brain via the CSF and blood. The mechanism of action of the β-amyloid peptide is supported by the amyloid β cascade hypothesis (C. Wang et al., 2023). The amyloidogenic pathogenic route (I) and the nonamyloidogenic pathological pathway (II) are depicted in the cascade. The amyloidogenic pathway is important first. The β secretase enzyme binds the amyloid protein precursor to CTF-β using this mechanism (Erickson et al., 2023). As a result, different lengths of Aβ peptide are produced, some of which are longer than Aβ 40 and have a higher propensity to aggregate and lead to the formation of plaque. The second pathway produces certain substances that are neurotropic and neuroprotective for nerve cells and involves segments that are implicated in the synthesis of α & γ secretase. APP is sequentially cleaved by α & γ secretases to provide full-length Peptides Aβ (Liu et al., 2023). However, γ secretase is located in the transmembrane region. Extracellular Aβ peptides are mostly produced via the regulated secretory pathway. The APP enables proteolytic processing by β-γ secretase. While many BACE inhibitors have demonstrated target engagement in clinical studies, as seen by a decrease in patients' CSF, and no discernible adverse effects have been reported, the first phase 2 clinical research of a -secretase inhibitor was discontinued due to hepatotoxicity. The possibility that APP's amyloidogenic processing increased is another reason (Uddin et al., 2021).

Pathogenesis of Mitochondrial Alteration

Mitochondrial changes associated with oxidative stress are substantial in AD patients. Changes in the mitochondria cause several neurodegenerative diseases in the aged (Ghosh et al., 2021). The patient shows signs of age-related accumulation of mitochondrial DNA, which is especially common in AD, as well as changes in the mitochondrial DNA linked to the disease. The accumulation of mitochondrial DNA with age causes the brain to produce ROS, especially in neurons. It is commonly known that mitochondria are high oxygen consumers just by their function in ATP production. On the other hand, excessive ROS generation might result in cell death (Y. Zhang et al., 2022). Some studies suggest a link between mitochondrial alterations and the synthesis of amyloid β peptides. Therefore, excessive production of amyloid β peptide by the cell can alter the mitochondrial structure of the hippocampus and cortex. Because of structural abnormalities in their mitochondria, patients with AD have weaker memories (X. Zhang et al., 2023). Conversely, a limited amount of research suggests that the precursor protein and the accumulation of amyloid β contribute significantly to mitochondrial toxicity. AβPP695 is one of the protein molecules that targets the mitochondrial transmembrane to affect human cortical neurons. Furthermore, the accumulation of AβPP diminishes complex IV activity and mitochondrial ATP synthesis, hence decreasing the total quantity of ATP within the cell. Direct interactions between APP 450 and Tim23 (OMM 23 translocase) and Tom40 (OMM 40 translocase) 452. Nuclear-encoded protein cannot enter mitochondria due to APP 454's accumulation across the import channel, which 455 modifies the function of the organelles by generating a stable, high-molecular-weight complex. As a result, these proteins directly affect the cognitive impairment experienced by AD patients (Rehman et al., 2023).

ROS in Alzheimer's Disease

Oxidative Stress and Connexin-Based Channels in Brain Cells

Oxidative stress and connexin-based channels in brain cells are two important topics in cellular biology and neuroscience. Oxidative stress is the result of an imbalance between the body's ability to detoxify or neutralize ROS and the harmful effects they cause. ROS are naturally occurring byproducts of cellular metabolism, such as hydroxyl radicals, superoxide radicals, and hydrogen peroxide (M. Zhang et al., 2022). Numerous factors, including as inflammation, exposure to chemicals in the environment, and metabolic processes, can result in oxidative stress in the brain. Neurons are particularly vulnerable to oxidative damage due to their high concentration of polyunsaturated fatty acids, quick oxygen consumption, and restricted capacity for regeneration. Parkinson's and AD are among the neurological conditions that have been connected to oxidative stress. It can damage DNA, lipids, and proteins, among other components of cells (Lee and Kim, 2023). To combat oxidative stress, the neurons have developed several defense mechanisms. These consist of the presence of antioxidant molecules and enzymes such as glutathione, superoxide dismutase, and catalase. Gap junctions are intercellular channels that allow for direct cell-to-cell communication. They are produced by a class of transmembrane proteins called connexins. These channels are composed of connexin hexamers. Connexin-based channels are found in many different cell types in the brain, such as neurons, astrocytes, and oligodendrocytes (Song et al., 2021). These channels play a major role in the movement of ions, metabolites, and signaling molecules between neighboring cells. Gap junctions made by connexin-based channels allow neural networks to synchronize electrical activity and coordinate activities (Nayak et al., 2023). They play a particularly important role in spreading depolarization and controlling neural circuits. Connexins can also perform non-junctional tasks as hemichannels or unopposed connexons, allowing some cells to release ions and signaling molecules. Oxidative stress has the potential to impact brain connexin-based channels. Oxidative damage to connexins or the proteins that connect them can cause changes in the regulation of gap junctions or their dysfunction. Oxidative stress can also activate connexin hemichannels, allowing substances to be released that can either aggravate or avoid oxidative damage. For example, the release of glutathione by connexin hemichannels can help to reduce oxidative damage (M. Wang et al., 2023). On the other hand, excessive oxidative stress can lead to connexin-based channel dysfunction, which may interfere with intercellular communication and perhaps cause damage to brain cells. Research into the relationship between oxidative stress and connexin-based channels in brain cells is still ongoing to gain insight into the causes and mechanisms of various neurological conditions and to develop possible therapeutic interventions aimed at maintaining or restoring normal cellular communication and reducing oxidative damage in the brain (Mohammadi et al., 2021).

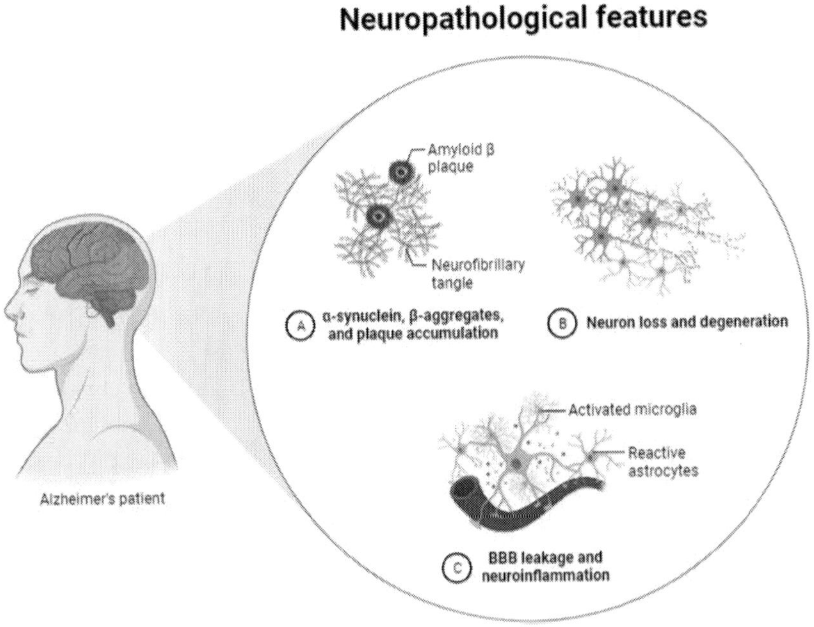

Figure 2. Alzheimer's disease-related neuropathology and neuroinflammation.

Alzheimer's Disease, Oxidative Stress, and NOX

In the context of AD pathophysiology, oxidative stress, AD, and NOX (NADPH oxidase) are related. Alzheimer's disease is a neurodegenerative condition marked by aberrant protein aggregation formation in the brain and a gradual decline in cognitive function. The onset and course of AD are influenced by oxidative stress and NOX involvement. Oxidative stress arises when the body's ability to eliminate ROS is out of balance with its creation (Lian et al., 2024). Some of the factors that contribute to oxidative stress in AD include the accumulation of beta-amyloid plaques and hyperphosphorylated tau tangles in the brain. NADPH oxidase (NOX) is an enzyme complex found in many different types of cells, including the immune cells known as microglia in the brain. NOX is one of the primary ways the brain generates ROS. Activated microglia in AD emit excessive ROS, mostly through NOX. Because they induce oxidative stress in the brain, these ROS have the potential to damage neurons and other brain cells. Oxidative stress and NOX activation are closely linked with AD (Ni et al., 2023). Microglia are activated in the brain by an immune response brought on by beta-amyloid plaque and tau tangle accumulation. Activated microglia emit ROS through

NOX, which can damage nearby neurons and exacerbate the neuroinflammatory response. Oxidative stress and NOX activation speed up AD neurodegeneration and cognitive decline (Fonseca-Santos et al., 2023). Prolonged oxidative stress and inflammation can also promote the aggregation of beta-amyloid and tau proteins, creating a vicious loop that accelerates the progression of disease. Researchers are examining potential therapies for AD that center on oxidative stress and NOX activity. This entails the development of antioxidant therapies to reduce ROS concentrations and the regulation of NOX to stop excessive ROS production (Liu et al., 2023). The use of antioxidants, such as vitamin E and other compounds, to lessen oxidative stress in AD has shown mixed results in the past; therefore, further research is needed. Understanding the complex link between oxidative stress, NOX, and AD is critical to developing medicines that can successfully halt or even reverse the progression of this terrible neurodegenerative condition. More research is being done to better understand the processes behind AD and discover new treatment options (Uddin et al., 2021).

NADPH Oxidase and Alzheimer's Disease

NADPH oxidase (NOX) and AD are related because NOX enzymes are involved in pathogenic processes associated with AD. The group of enzymes in cells that produce ROS is called NADPH oxidase. These ROS, which include superoxide radicals, can harm many cell components and induce oxidative stress and inflammation (Y. Zhang et al., 2022). In AD, there is a chronic inflammatory response in the brain. The microglia, which are the brain's native immune cells, become active. The NOX enzymes found in microglia are necessary for the production of ROS throughout the inflammatory response. NOX enzymes are a significant source of ROS production in the brain. An overabundance of ROS can lead to oxidative stress, a characteristic of AD pathogenesis (X. Zhang et al., 2023). Oxidative stress may damage the DNA, proteins, and lipids in brain cells, which can result in neurodegeneration. During AD, abnormal protein aggregates such as beta-amyloid plaques and hyperphosphorylated tau tangles accumulate in the brain. These aggregates can activate microglia, which via NOX-mediated ROS production raises oxidative stress and neuroinflammation. The ROS generated by NOX enzymes can be neurotoxic, impairing and damaging neuronal function. This neuronal loss causes cognitive decline in AD patients (Xiang et al., 2022). The significant roles that NOX enzymes play in the oxidative stress and inflammation associated with AD have made them attractive targets for treatment. Researchers are investigating drugs that inhibit NOX activity to reduce ROS production and neuroinflammation in AD (Gao et al., 2023). Chronic inflammation is a common feature of AD, and NOX-induced ROS production plays a crucial role in this inflammatory response. Strategies centered on NOX enzymes aim to reduce the ongoing inflammation linked to AD and may even prevent the illness from progressing. Even though targeting NOX enzymes as a therapeutic strategy for AD is becoming more popular, more research is required to develop effective treatments and get a better knowledge of the unique roles that different NOX isoforms play in the pathophysiology of AD. The complex interplay between NOX, inflammation, oxidative stress, and AD is a multidisciplinary area of study, and more research might provide fresh insights into potential treatment modalities for this crippling neurodegenerative condition (Rehman et al., 2023).

Neuroinflammation and Neuropathological in Alzheimer's Disease

Neuroinflammation in AD is closely linked to neuropathological changes in the brain. An inflammatory response is initiated by the activation of microglia and astrocytes brought on by the accumulation of abnormal proteins like tau and amyloid-beta. These immune cells release pro-inflammatory substances that lead to brain damage and the formation of tau tangles and amyloid plaques (M. Zhang et al., 2022). This chronic neuroinflammation impairs the blood-brain barrier, interferes with synapse function, and speeds up the process of neurodegeneration (Thu Thuy Nguyen and Endres, 2022). The connection between neuropathological changes and neuroinflammation is a key characteristic of Alzheimer's disease. To develop future treatment regimens that would address the underlying mechanisms of the illness, it is critical to understand these complex relationships. look at Figure 2.

Cell Mediators of Neuroinflammation

Many neurological and neurodegenerative illnesses, including Parkinson's disease, multiple sclerosis, and Alzheimer's disease, are mostly caused by neuroinflammation (Yan et al., 2021). It involves complex interactions in the central nervous system between various cell types and mediators. Microglia, which are immune cells that reside inside the central nervous system, are crucial for the onset and progression of neuroinflammation. When activated, microglia can release pro-inflammatory cytokines, chemokines, and reactive oxygen species. They also phagocytose debris from cells and pathogens (Y. Zhang et al., 2023). Astrocytes are a different type of glial cell found in the brain. It is possible to react reactively to neuroinflammatory signals. Activated astrocytes release pro-inflammatory cytokines and chemokines that help maintain the blood-brain barrier. Reactive astrocytes can either promote neuroinflammation or offer neuroprotection, depending on the circumstances (Quintanilla et al., 2012). Peripheral immune cells, such as T lymphocytes and monocytes, can penetrate the CNS in some neurological disorders (Wang et al., 2021). These cells may play a crucial role in the development of neuroinflammation because they generate more inflammatory mediators and support the immune response in the brain. These signaling molecules are essential mediators of neuroinflammation. Pro-inflammatory cytokines, such as TNF-α and IL-1β, are released by activated immune cells and can lead to inflammation and tissue damage. The inflammatory location attracts immune cells due to chemokines, which are chemotactic chemicals. The complement system, an element of the innate immune response, may be triggered in neuroinflammatory conditions (Azargoonjahromi, 2023). Complement proteins can promote phagocytosis, opsonize pathogens and cell debris, and cause inflammation. In response to inflammation, several cell types can produce eicosanoids, which are lipid mediators that include prostaglandins and leukotrienes. They affect pain perception, inflammation, and vasodilation in the CNS. The remodeling of the extracellular matrix is carried out by enzymes known as MMPs. In neuroinflammation, several MMPs may be overexpressed, resulting in tissue damage and a breach in the BBB. The generation of ROS and RNS during neuroinflammation can lead to oxidative stress (Goyal et al., 2021). These compounds can cause damage to cells and accelerate the aging process of the nervous system. Glutamate and Excitotoxicity: Inflammatory processes can lead to a dysregulation of the neurotransmitter glutamate. Overindulgence in glutamate can lead to excitotoxicity, which worsens neuroinflammation and destroys neurons. Certain mediators, such as BDNF, can function both pro- and anti-inflammatory in the central nervous system. Their role might vary depending on the neuroinflammatory context. Understanding the complex connections between different cell mediators in neuroinflammation is crucial to modifying the inflammatory response and protecting against neurological disorders and neurodegenerative diseases. If specific mediators or pathways are targeted, treatment and intervention may be possible (Al-Quraish et al., 2023).

Cytokine Production and Neuroinflammation

Cytokine production has a major role in mediating the inflammatory response known as neuroinflammation, which occurs in the CNS and is associated with certain neurological disorders and neurodegenerative diseases (Alqahtani et al., 2023). The immune response is coordinated by signaling molecules known as cytokines, which are produced by immune cells and other cell types. Depending on the specific cytokine and the conditions surrounding its synthesis, cytokines may be advantageous or detrimental in the context of neuroinflammation. These cytokines increase inflammation and the immune system of the central nervous system. IL-1β is a potent pro-inflammatory cytokine that is frequently implicated in neuroinflammation and is released by activated microglia and other immune cells (Bello-Corral et al., 2023). It might set off a series of inflammatory responses. TNF-α is secreted by microglia and astrocytes, causing inflammation and cell death, which in turn causes neuroinflammation. IL-6 is released by a variety of cell types, including microglia and astrocytes, and it plays a role in the acute phase response in neuroinflammation. Unlike pro-inflammatory cytokines, anti-inflammatory cytokines are produced to promote tissue repair and lessen inflammation. Among other immune cells, regulatory T cells can produce IL-10, an essential anti-inflammatory cytokine. It reduces inflammatory responses and decreases tissue damage. TGF-β lowers inflammation and aids in tissue repair (Jayaram and Krishnamurthy, 2021). These cytokines are among the subset that serve as chemoattractants, attracting immune cells to the site of inflammation in the central nervous system. Among them is monocyte chemoattractant protein-1 (MCP-1), which is produced and expressed by normal T cells and is activated by RANTES. The type I interferons, IFN-α and IFN-β, are produced in response to different inflammatory stimuli or during viral infections. Beyond their role in antiviral responses, they can intensify neuroinflammation. Certain cytokines may be pro- or anti-inflammatory, depending on the circumstance (Simões et al., 2023). For example, IL-4 and IL-13 may promote microglia's neuroprotective alternative activation. These are intracellular multiprotein complexes that induce the production of pro-inflammatory cytokines like IL-1β. Immune cell activation of inflammatory enzymes in microglia and other tissues may worsen neuroinflammation. In the CNS, pro- and anti-inflammatory cytokines must coexist. While pro-inflammatory cytokine production in excess can lead to tissue damage and neurodegeneration, an adequate anti-inflammatory response is required to reduce inflammation and facilitate recovery. The goal of this field's research is to develop strategies for altering the immune response in neurological conditions like multiple sclerosis, stroke, and Alzheimer's disease. It also aims to better understand the mechanisms underlying the production of cytokines in neuroinflammation and identify potential targets for treatment (Vaiserman et al., 2020).

Neuroinflammation and Connexin-Based Channels in Alzheimer's Disease

Neuroinflammation and connexin-based channels are associated in the AD context (Więckowska-Gacek et al., 2021). Connexin-based channels, which are important in facilitating cell-to-cell communication in the central nervous system, may be impacted by neuroinflammation in AD. Neuroinflammation is one of the typical features of AD. It entails the generation of cytokines that promote inflammation, the existence of immune cells within the brain, and the stimulation of microglia and astrocytes. Patients with AD may have inflammation as a result of the accumulation of tau tangles and beta-amyloid plaques, two of the disease's hallmark pathologies. Neurodegeneration and cognitive decline progress together with neuroinflammation in AD (Yang et al., 2023). Direct communication between nearby cells, including astrocytes, neurons, and other glial cells, is made possible by gap junctions called connexin-based channels. By creating channels that let ions, metabolites, and signaling molecules pass across cells, connexin proteins create gap junctions (Nayak et al., 2023). These channels are involved in the brain's electrical activity synchronization, neural circuit coordination, and homeostasis maintenance. During neuroinflammation, the release of inflammatory mediators has the power to modify connexin-based channel activity. Pro-inflammatory cytokines and oxidative stress modulate gap junction permeability and connexin protein expression (M. Wang et al., 2023). Activated microglia and astrocytes in neuroinflammation may release signaling molecules that alter connexin-based channels in neighboring cells. Changes in the way connexin-based channels work may affect the way glial cells and neurons communicate and signal. Dysregulation of connexin-based channels may influence the course of Alzheimer's disease. Modifications in intercellular communication may impede the functionality of neural networks and impact the dissemination of neuroinflammatory signals (Yamini et al., 2022). Modifying connexin-based channels may provide therapeutic benefits for AD, according to some studies. For example, promoting the opening or closing of certain channels may help stop the transmission of disease-causing proteins or restore normal network function. Further research is needed to completely understand the specific mechanisms by which neuroinflammation influences connexin-based channels in AD. Current investigations focus on how harmful proteins, such as tau and beta-amyloid, are transmitted through connexin-based channels since they can damage cells and induce neuroinflammation in AD. Currently, studies are being done to elucidate the precise mechanisms underlying the intricate relationship between connexin-based channels and neuroinflammation in AD, as well as to explore the potential for therapeutic strategies that specifically target these channels in the context of AD and other neurodegenerative diseases (Mohammadi et al., 2021).

Therapeutic Strategies for Inhibiting ROS in Alzheimer's Disease

Treatment strategies that reduce oxidative stress and inhibit ROS may be essential for possibly postponing the progression of AD (Ni et al., 2023). Chemicals known as ROS have been connected to AD neurodegeneration and can harm cells. Composite anti-oxidants help to stop oxidative damage and neutralize ROS. Common antioxidant supplements include vitamin C, vitamin E, and alpha-lipoic acid. These supplements can be used orally and have been evaluated for their potential to reduce oxidative stress in AD (Fonseca-Santos et al., 2023). Lowering oxidative stress may be achieved by eating a diet high in fruits, vegetables, and foods high in omega-3 fatty acids, which are abundant in natural antioxidants. Certain studies suggest that eating a diet high in antioxidants may help prevent AD. Since certain drugs have antioxidant properties, they may be utilized to treat AD. As one example, memantine, an NMDA receptor antagonist used to treat AD, may have antioxidant qualities. Additional drugs with antioxidant properties, such as creatine and idebenone, have been studied in clinical trials for AD. Berries, dark chocolate, and green tea are examples of foods rich in polyphenols and flavonoids that have anti-inflammatory and antioxidant properties (Nakanishi et al., 2021). There has been interest in these organic compounds because of their potential to reduce oxidative stress and neuroinflammation in AD (Liu et al., 2023). Exercise regularly has been shown to reduce oxidative stress and increase antioxidant defenses. Exercise can enhance general brain health and cognitive function in AD patients. Dysfunction of the cell's powerhouses, the mitochondria, may worsen oxidative stress. Researchers have looked at the possible benefits of substances that improve mitochondrial function in AD, such as coenzyme Q10 (CoQ10) and acetyl-L-carnitine. Chronic inflammation and oxidative stress are closely associated. Research has looked into the potential of NSAIDs and other anti-inflammatory medications to reduce inflammation and oxidative stress in AD (Erickson et al., 2023). A few studies have investigated the potential use of hormone replacement treatment, with an emphasis on estrogen, to reduce AD risk and oxidative stress in postmenopausal women. However, hormone therapy should be taken cautiously because there are certain risks involved. Lowering oxidative stress in AD patients may be achieved by lifestyle modifications that include reducing stress, obtaining adequate sleep, and avoiding environmental toxins. Given the complexity of both oxidative stress and AD, combination therapies that target many pathways simultaneously (e.g., antioxidants, anti-inflammatory medications, and lifestyle modifications) may be more effective in lowering ROS and slowing the progression of AD (Ghosh et al., 2021). It is important to keep in mind that AD cannot be cured and that individual outcomes may differ, even with the optimistic nature of many therapeutic approaches. To determine the best course of action for an individual with AD and to monitor for any potential drug interactions or bad effects, it is important to consult with a healthcare expert. Moreover, more research is required to refine and strengthen these strategies (Xiang et al., 2022).

Discussion

It is becoming evident that oxidative stress and neuroinflammation are important factors in the development of AD (Kopp et al., 2022). Excess reactive oxygen species lead to oxidative stress, which damages cellular components and exacerbates the AD-related protein misfolding. Furthermore, continuous neuroinflammation which is typified by the production of cytokines and the activation of microglia maintains neuronal injury (d'Avila, 2020). Because this dual interaction may both promote and aggravate neurodegeneration, it is the main focus of research on AD. By understanding these pathways, it may be possible to develop novel treatment options, delay the progression of AD, and enhance the quality of life for those who experience this debilitating condition (Mominur Rahman et al., 2022).

Prospects

The role of oxidative stress and neuroinflammation in AD is becoming more and more significant in the field of neurodegenerative research (Farooqui, 2022). Oxidative stress is caused by an imbalance between antioxidants and free radicals, which damages neuronal structures and intensifies the pathophysiology of AD. Concurrently, neuroinflammation characterized by the production of cytokines and the activation of microglia allows AD neurodegeneration. Prospects need an understanding of the intricate relationships between these systems and the potential use of these systems as therapeutic targets. There is hope for patients suffering from AD since new medicines aimed at lowering oxidative stress and neuroinflammation may be able to halt or slow the progression of the disease (Taylor et al., 2013).

Conclusion

Neuroinflammation and oxidative stress are key components of the intricate pathophysiology of AD. Reactive oxygen species imbalances cause oxidative stress, which damages cellular components and promotes the growth of diseases like tau tangles and beta-amyloid plaques that are characteristic of AD. Simultaneously, pro-inflammatory cytokines and activated microglia cause neuroinflammation, which accelerates cognitive decline and wipes out neurodegeneration. The interaction of these mechanisms creates a self-sustaining loop and accelerates the progression of AD. Comprehending their functions is essential for formulating remedial measures intended to curtail oxidative harm, alter inflammatory reactions, and maybe mitigate the incapacitating progression of this terrible neurodegenerative illness.

Acknowledgments

The authors are thankful to the Principal, Department of Pharmacy, Teerthanker Mahaveer University, Moradabad, and Pandaveswar School of Pharmacy, West Bengal for providing the necessary facilities.

Competing Interest Statement

The authors declare no conflict of interest.

Disclaimer

None.

Funding

NA.

References

Al-Kuraishy, H. M., Jabir, M. S., Albuhadily, A. K., Al-Gareeb, A. I., & Rafeeq, M. F. (2023). The link between Alzheimer disease and metabolic syndrome: a mutual relationship and long rigorous investigation. Ageing Research Reviews, 102084.

Asamu, M. O., Oladipo, O. O., Abayomi, O. A., & Adebayo, A. A. (2023). Alzheimer's disease: The role of T lymphocytes in neuroinflammation and neurodegeneration. Brain Research, 148589.

Bello-Corral, L., Alves-Gomes, L., Fernandez-Fernandez, J. A., Fernandez-Garcia, D., Casado-Verdejo, I., & Sanchez-Valdeon, L. (2023). Implications of gut and oral microbiota in neuroinflammatory responses in Alzheimer's disease. Life Sciences, 122132.

d'Avila, J. C. (2020). Neuroinflammation and oxidative stress in the aging brain: Linking in metabolism, stem cells, proteostasis, and stress adaptation. In Oxidative Stress and Dietary Antioxidants in Neurological Diseases (pp. 49-65). Academic Press.

Erickson, M. A., Logsdon, A. F., Rhea, E. M., Hansen, K. M., Holden, S. J., Banks, W. A., ... & Raber, J. (2023). Blood-brain barrier penetration of non-replicating SARS-CoV-2 and S1 variants of concern induce neuroinflammation which is accentuated in a mouse model of Alzheimer's disease. Brain, behavior, and immunity, 109, 251-268.

Farooqui, A. A. (2022). Contribution of neuroinflammation, resolution, and neuroprotection in neurotraumatic diseases. Neuroinflammation, Resolution, and Neuroprotection in the Brain; Farooqui, AA, Ed, 83-119.

Fonseca-Santos, B., Cazarin, C. A., da Silva, P. B., Dos Santos, K. P., da Rocha, M. C. O., Báo, S. N., ... & Chorilli, M. (2023). Intranasal in situ gelling liquid crystal for delivery of resveratrol ameliorates memory and neuroinflammation in Alzheimer's disease. Nanomedicine: Nanotechnology, Biology and Medicine, 51, 102689.

Gao, Q., Zhao, Y., Luo, R., Su, M., Zhang, C., Li, C., ... & Zhou, X. (2023). Intrathecal umbilical cord mesenchymal stem cells injection alleviates neuroinflammation and oxidative stress in the cyclophosphamide-induced interstitial cystitis rats through the Sirt1/Nrf2/HO-1 pathway. Life Sciences, 331, 122045.

Ghosh, P., Singh, R., Ganeshpurkar, A., Pokle, A. V., bhushan Singh, R., Singh, S. K., & Kumar, A. (2021). Cellular and molecular influencers of neuroinflammation in Alzheimer's disease: recent concepts & roles. Neurochemistry International, 151, 105212.

Goyal, D., Ali, S. A., & Singh, R. K. (2021). Emerging role of gut microbiota in modulation of neuroinflammation and neurodegeneration with emphasis on Alzheimer's disease. Progress in Neuro-Psychopharmacology and Biological Psychiatry, 106, 110112.

Jayaram, S., & Krishnamurthy, P. T. (2021). Role of microgliosis, oxidative stress and associated neuroinflammation in the pathogenesis of Parkinson's disease: The therapeutic role of Nrf2 activators. Neurochemistry international, 145, 105014.

Kopp, K. O., Glotfelty, E. J., Li, Y., & Greig, N. H. (2022). Glucagon-like peptide-1 (GLP-1) receptor agonists and neuroinflammation: Implications for neurodegenerative disease treatment. Pharmacological research, 186, 106550.

Lee, M. Y., & Kim, M. (2023). Effects of Red ginseng on neuroinflammation in neurodegenerative diseases. Journal of Ginseng Research.

Lian, X., Zhang, X., Chen, W., Xue, F., & Wang, G. (2024). Dexmedetomidine mitigates neuroinflammation in an Alzheimer's disease mouse model via the miR-204-3p/FBXL7 signaling axis. Brain Research, 1822, 148612.

Liu, P., Chen, W., Kang, Y., Wang, C., Wang, X., Liu, W., ... & Ikejima, T. (2023). Silibinin ameliorates STING-mediated neuroinflammation via downregulation of ferroptotic damage in a sporadic Alzheimer's disease model. Archives of Biochemistry and Biophysics, 744, 109691.

Ly, M., Gary, Z. Y., Mian, A., Cramer, A., Meysami, S., Merrill, D. A., ... & Raji, C. A. (2023). Neuroinflammation: a modifiable pathway linking obesity, alzheimer's disease, and depression. The American Journal of Geriatric Psychiatry, 31(10), 853-866.

Mohammadi, N., Asle-Rousta, M., Rahnema, M., & Amini, R. (2021). Morin attenuates memory deficits in a rat model of Alzheimer's disease by ameliorating oxidative stress and neuroinflammation. European Journal of Pharmacology, 910, 174506.

Rahman, M. M., Mim, S. A., Tumpa, M. A. A., Sarker, M. T., Ahmed, M., Alghamdi, B. S., ... & Ashraf, G. M. (2022). Exploring the management approaches of cytokines including viral infection and neuroinflammation for neurological disorders. Cytokine, 157, 155962.

Nakanishi, K., Sakakima, H., Norimatsu, K., Otsuka, S., Takada, S., Tani, A., & Kikuchi, K. (2021). Effect of low-intensity motor balance and coordination exercise on cognitive functions, hippocampal Aβ deposition, neuronal loss, neuroinflammation, and oxidative stress in a mouse model of Alzheimer's disease. Experimental neurology, 337, 113590.

Nayak, V., Patra, S., Rout, S., Jena, A. B., Sharma, R., Pattanaik, K. P., ... & Kerry, R. G. (2024). Regulation of neuroinflammation in Alzheimer's disease via nanoparticle-loaded phytocompounds with anti-inflammatory and autophagy-inducing properties. Phytomedicine, 122, 155150.

Ni, H., Liao, Y., Zhang, Y., Lu, H., Huang, Z., Huang, F., ... & Huang, Y. (2023). Levistilide A ameliorates neuroinflammation via inhibiting JAK2/STAT3 signaling for neuroprotection and cognitive improvement in scopolamine-induced Alzheimer's disease mouse model. International immunopharmacology, 124, 110783.

Quintanilla, R. A., Orellana, J. A., & von Bernhardi, R. (2012). Understanding risk factors for Alzheimer's disease: interplay of neuroinflammation, connexin-based communication and oxidative stress. Archives of Medical Research, 43(8), 632-644.

Rehman, M. U., Sehar, N., Dar, N. J., Khan, A., Arafah, A., Rashid, S., ... & Ganaie, M. A. (2023). Mitochondrial dysfunctions, oxidative stress and neuroinflammation as therapeutic targets for neurodegenerative diseases: an update on current advances and impediments. Neuroscience & Biobehavioral Reviews, 144, 104961.

Sharma, H., Chandra, P., Verma, A., Pandey, S. N., Kumar, P., & Sigh, A. (2023). Therapeutic approaches of nutraceuticals in the prevention of neurological disorders. Eur Chem Bull, 12(5), 1575-1596.

Simões, J. L., Sobierai, L. D., Leal, I. F., Dos Santos, M. V., Coiado, J. V., & Bagatini, M. D. (2023). Action of the Purinergic and Cholinergic Anti-inflammatory Pathways on Oxidative Stress in Patients with Alzheimer's Disease in the Context of the COVID-19 Pandemic. Neuroscience, 512, 110-132.

Song, T., Song, X., Zhu, C., Patrick, R., Skurla, M., Santangelo, I., ... & Du, F. (2021). Mitochondrial dysfunction, oxidative stress, neuroinflammation, and metabolic alterations in the progression of Alzheimer's disease: A meta-analysis of in vivo magnetic resonance spectroscopy studies. Ageing research reviews, 72, 101503.

Taylor, J. M., Main, B. S., & Crack, P. J. (2013). Neuroinflammation and oxidative stress: co-conspirators in the pathology of Parkinson's disease. Neurochemistry international, 62(5), 803-819.

Nguyen, V. T. T., & Endres, K. (2022). Targeting gut microbiota to alleviate neuroinflammation in Alzheimer's disease. Advanced drug delivery reviews, 188, 114418.

Uddin, M. S., Yu, W. S., & Lim, L. W. (2021). Exploring ER stress response in cellular aging and neuroinflammation in Alzheimer's disease. Ageing Research Reviews, 70, 101417.

Vaiserman, A., Koliada, A., & Lushchak, O. (2020). Neuroinflammation in pathogenesis of Alzheimer's disease: Phytochemicals as potential therapeutics. Mechanisms of Ageing and Development, 189, 111259.

Wang, C., Jiang, H., Liu, H., Chen, S., Guo, H., Ma, S., ... & Wang, D. (2023). Isoforsythiaside confers neuroprotection against Alzheimer's disease by attenuating ferroptosis and neuroinflammation in vivo and in vitro. Food Science and Human Wellness, 12(5), 1730-1742.

Wang, M., Tang, G., Zhou, C., Guo, H., Hu, Z., Hu, Q., & Li, G. (2023). Revisiting the intersection of microglial activation and neuroinflammation in Alzheimer's disease from the perspective of ferroptosis. Chemico-Biological Interactions, 375, 110387.

Wang, P., Li, X. L., & Cao, Z. H. (2021). STC1 ameliorates cognitive impairment and neuroinflammation of Alzheimer's disease mice via inhibition of ERK1/2 pathway. Immunobiology, 226(3), 152092.

Wang, Y., Zou, J., Wang, Y., Wang, J., Ji, X., Zhang, T., ... & Kang, Y. (2023). Hydralazine inhibits neuroinflammation and oxidative stress in APP/PS1 mice via TLR4/NF-κB and Nrf2 pathways. Neuropharmacology, 240, 109706.

Więckowska-Gacek, A., Mietelska-Porowska, A., Wydrych, M., & Wojda, U. (2021). Western diet as a trigger of Alzheimer's disease: From metabolic syndrome and systemic inflammation to neuroinflammation and neurodegeneration. Ageing research reviews, 70, 10139.

Xiang, X., Wang, X., Wu, Y., Hu, J., Li, Y., Jin, S., & Wu, X. (2022). Activation of GPR55 attenuates cognitive impairment, oxidative stress, neuroinflammation, and synaptic dysfunction in a streptozotocin-induced Alzheimer's mouse model. Pharmacology Biochemistry and Behavior, 214, 173340.

Yamini, P., Ray, R. S., Yadav, S., Dhaliwal, J., Yadav, M., Kondepudi, K. K., & Chopra, K. (2022). α7nAChR activation protects against oxidative stress, neuroinflammation and central insulin resistance in ICV-STZ induced sporadic Alzheimer's disease. Pharmacology Biochemistry and Behavior, 217, 173402.

Yan, T., Liu, B., Wang, N., Liao, Z., Wu, B., He, B., & Jia, Y. (2021). The flavonoids of okra insulates against oxidative stress, neuroinflammation and restores BDNF levels in Aβ1–42 induced mouse model of Alzheimer's disease. Experimental Gerontology, 147, 111263.

Yang, Y., Hao, T., Yao, X., Che, Y., Liu, Y., Fang, M., ... & Hou, Y. (2023). Crebanine ameliorates ischemia-reperfusion brain damage by inhibiting oxidative stress and neuroinflammation mediated by NADPH oxidase 2 in microglia. Phytomedicine, 120, 155044.

Zhang, M., Wu, Y., Gao, R., Chen, X., Chen, R., & Chen, Z. (2022). Glucagon-like peptide-1 analogs mitigate neuroinflammation in Alzheimer's disease by suppressing NLRP2 activation in astrocytes. Molecular and cellular endocrinology, 542, 111529.

Zhang, X., Guo, Y., Zhang, Z., Wu, X., Li, L., Yang, Z., & Li, Z. (2023). Neuroprotective effects of bavachin against neuroinflammation and oxidative stress-induced neuronal damage via activation of Sirt1/Nrf2 pathway and inhibition of NF-κB pathway. Journal of Functional Foods, 107, 105655.

Zhang, Y., Ma, R., Wang, W., Deng, Q., Cao, C., Yu, C., ... & Tian, J. (2023). Activation of α7nAChR by PNU282987 improves cognitive impairment through inhibiting oxidative stress and neuroinflammation in D-galactose induced aging via regulating α7nAChR/Nrf2/HO-1 signaling pathway. Experimental Gerontology, 175, 112139.

Zhang, Y., Liu, D., Yao, X., Wen, J., Wang, Y., & Zhang, Y. (2022). DMTHB ameliorates memory impairment in Alzheimer's disease mice through regulation of neuroinflammation. Neuroscience Letters, 785, 136770.

Chapter 15

Inflammation, Mitochondrial Dysfunction and Oxidative Stress Mechanisms in the Pathogenesis of Parkinson's Disease: Emerging Therapeutic and Clinical Approaches

Shahbaz Khan[1,*],
Alka Lohani[2],
Naina[3],
Amit Kumar[4],
Sunaina[3],
Ankita Singh[1],
and Mohit Agrawal[5]

[1]Pharmacy Academy, IFTM University, Moradabad, Uttar Pradesh, India
[2]Amity Institute of Pharmacy, Amity University Uttar Pradesh, Noida Campus, India
[3]ANA Institute of Pharmaceutical Sciences and Research, Bareilly, Uttar Pradesh, India
[4]School of Pharmaceutical Sciences IFTM University, Moradabad, Uttar Pradesh, India
[5]School of Medical & Allied Sciences, K. R. Mangalam University, Gurugram, Haryana, India

[*] Corresponding Author's Email: shahbazkhanmaju123@gmail.com.

In: Neurogenerative Disorders
Editors: Mohit Agrawal, Manmohan Singhal, Amit Kumar Nayak et al.
ISBN: 979-8-89530-143-2

Abstract

Parkinson's disease (PD) is a degenerative disorder of the nervous system that affects human mobility owing to the loss of brain cells. PD is regarded as the second most common disease to impact humans after Alzheimer's disease. Although the exact etiology of PD is unknown, some genetic risk factors and several genes that produce unusual family variants of the disease have recently been identified. The clinical pathology and diagnosis of PD are characterized by the continuous premature death of dopaminergic neurons in the substantia nigra pars compacta and the post-mortem detection of aberrant protein aggregates known as Lewy bodies, which contain α-synuclein. Numerous motor and non-motor processes are hampered by the dopaminergic neuron deficiency, which includes manifests as rigidity, tremor, bradykinesia and postural instability. The development of PD is significantly influenced by inflammation, oxidative stress, and mitochondrial dysfunction. Mitochondria are essential organelles with numerous roles. Dysfunctional mitochondria can result in decreased energy production, the generation of reactive oxygen species, and the activation of stress-induced apoptosis. A thorough history is taken as the first stage in the diagnosis of PD. Therapies for PD have mostly included compensatory methods that relieve clinical symptoms. Clinical methods to treat PD include symptomatic treatments, which help to offset the consequences of dopaminergic neuronal deficiencies, as well as more recently, a shift toward disease alteration, which aims to delay or halt the progression of the disease. This chapter focuses on the role of inflammatory, mitochondrial dysfunction & oxidative stress mechanisms in the pathogenesis of PD and the emerging therapeutic clinical approaches for PD.

Keywords: neurodegenerative disorder, Parkinson's disease, reactive oxygen species, mitochondrial dysfunction, oxidative stress

Introduction

Parkinson's disease (PD) is a progressive neurological disorder characterized by a combination of motor and non-motor symptoms. Named after James Parkinson, who first described its symptoms in 1817, the disease affects millions of people worldwide. PD primarily targets the brain's dopamine-producing neurons in a region called the substantia nigra, leading to a shortage of dopamine, a neurotransmitter crucial for coordinating movement. Symptoms typically manifest subtly and worsen over time, although the progression varies widely among individuals. The hallmark motor symptoms include tremors, rigidity, bradykinesia (slowness of movement), and postural instability. Non-motor symptoms may include cognitive impairment, mood changes, sleep disturbances, and autonomic dysfunction. While the exact cause of PD remains unclear, a combination of genetic and environmental factors likely contributes to its development. Approximately 3-5% of cases are attributed to monogenic forms linked to specific genetic mutations, while the majority of cases, classified as non-monogenic PD, involve complex interactions between multiple genetic variants and environmental triggers (Dickson and Dennis, 2012).

Hence, it is believed that Parkinson's disease begins to manifest long before any noticeable motor symptoms emerge. The progression of PD is typically gradual and continuous, unfolding through four distinct phases before diagnosis, as illustrated in Figure 1 (Poewe et al., 2017): (1) the phase of risk, during which many genetic, environmental, and other risk factors influence the onset of the illness; (2) the preclinical stage, in which neurodegeneration begins but there are no clinical signs at all; (3) the prodromal phase, during which mild to moderate motor symptoms may be present (Berg et al., 2014), whereas other non-motor symptoms are already noticeable and significant. These non-motor symptoms include (not necessarily in this chronological order) altered REM (rapid eye movement) sleep cycle and circadian disruption, olfactory dysfunction (hyposmia), autonomic dysfunction affecting the cardiovascular and gastrointestinal (GI) systems, among others, and depression (with or without anxiety; and (4) the clinical motor phase, which results in the diagnosis of PD when the characteristic motor symptoms are present (Zacharias et al., 2022).

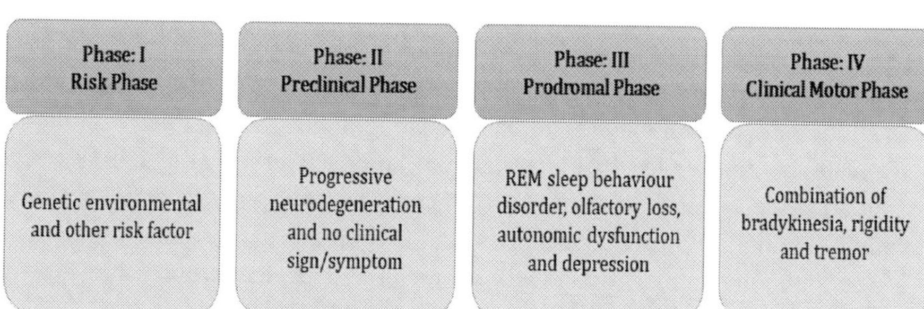

Figure 1. Development of Parkinson's Disease.

While the exact cause of PD remains elusive, emerging evidence suggests a complex interplay of inflammatory, mitochondrial dysfunction, and oxidative stress mechanisms in its pathogenesis. In recent years, research has increasingly focused on understanding how these mechanisms contribute to the degeneration of dopaminergic neurons and the progression of PD. Chronic inflammation within the brain, accompanied by the activation of microglia and the release of pro-inflammatory cytokines, has been implicated in neuronal damage and disease progression. Additionally, dysfunction in mitochondrial processes, including impaired energy production, oxidative phosphorylation, and mitochondrial dynamics, has emerged as a key factor in PD pathophysiology. Moreover, oxidative stress, resulting from an imbalance between the production of reactive oxygen species (ROS) and antioxidant defenses, contributes to cellular damage and exacerbates neurodegeneration in PD. These interconnected pathways form a complex network of cellular dysfunction, ultimately leading to neuronal demise and the clinical manifestations of PD. Understanding the underlying mechanisms driving PD pathogenesis has paved the way for the development of novel therapeutic approaches aimed at targeting these pathways. From anti-inflammatory agents to mitochondrial enhancers and antioxidants, a variety of emerging clinical interventions hold promise for slowing disease progression, alleviating symptoms, and improving the quality of life for individuals living with PD. In this chapter, we will explore the latest insights into the roles of inflammatory, mitochondrial dysfunction, and oxidative stress mechanisms in PD pathogenesis.

Epidemiology and Pathophysiology of Parkinson's Disease

PD is a prevalent neurodegenerative disorder, affecting approximately 1% of individuals over the age of 60, with its incidence rising with age (Ascherio & Schwarzschild, 2016). Although primarily diagnosed in older adults, a minority experience early-onset PD (Schapira et al., 2017). The disease shows a slight male predominance and exhibits geographical variability, with higher prevalence rates noted in industrialized nations (Dorsey et al., 2018). Age remains the most significant risk factor, though genetic predisposition, environmental toxins like pesticides, and certain occupations may also play a role. Pathophysiologically, PD is characterized by the progressive loss of dopaminergic neurons in the substantia nigra and the presence of Lewy bodies, abnormal protein aggregates primarily composed of alpha-synuclein

(Surmeier et al., 2017). Neuroinflammation, mitochondrial dysfunction, and genetic factors such as mutations in genes like SNCA and LRRK2 further contribute to neuronal degeneration (Poewe et al., 2017). Environmental factors, including exposure to toxins, also play a role in disease development. Understanding these epidemiological and pathophysiological aspects of PD is essential for the development of effective diagnostic and therapeutic strategies aimed at mitigating its impact on affected individuals.

Pathogenesis of Parkinson's Disease

The pathogenesis of PD is multifaceted, involving a complex interplay of genetic, environmental, and cellular factors. One of the key pathological hallmarks of PD is the accumulation of abnormal protein aggregates, predominantly composed of misfolded alpha-synuclein, known as Lewy bodies, within neurons. These aggregates are believed to contribute to neuronal dysfunction and death by disrupting cellular processes, impairing protein clearance mechanisms, and inducing oxidative stress (Spillantini et al., 1997).

Mitochondrial dysfunction is also implicated in PD pathogenesis, with evidence suggesting that impaired mitochondrial bioenergetics and increased oxidative stress contribute to dopaminergic neuronal degeneration (Schapira et al., 1990). Mutations in genes associated with mitochondrial quality control mechanisms, such as PINK1 and PARKIN, disrupt mitochondrial homeostasis and render neurons vulnerable to oxidative damage and cell death (Kitada et al., 1998).

Oxidative stress, arising from an imbalance between the production of reactive oxygen species (ROS) and antioxidant defences, plays a prominent role in PD pathogenesis. Excessive ROS production leads to oxidative damage to lipids, proteins, and DNA, exacerbating neuronal dysfunction and death (Dias et al., 2013). Neuroinflammation, characterized by the activation of microglia and astrocytes and the release of pro-inflammatory cytokines, further contributes to neurodegeneration in PD (Hirsch et al., 2012).

Furthermore, emerging evidence suggests a potential role for dysregulated protein homeostasis, excitotoxicity, and dysfunction of the gut-brain axis in PD pathogenesis (Anglade et al., 1997). Understanding the underlying mechanisms driving neuronal degeneration in PD is critical for the development of targeted therapeutic strategies aimed at slowing or halting disease progression.

Role of Inflammation in Parkinson's Disease

In PD, inflammation, particularly neuroinflammation, emerges as a pivotal contributor to disease pathogenesis and progression. Neuroinflammation, a type of brain inflammation. It is essential for the onset and development of PD. Overactive microglia and astrocytes have been found to release a number of pro-inflammatory cytokines in the brain of patients with PD, which helps to promote neuroinflammation. It's interesting to note that numerous research has examined how long-term NSAID medication regimens can reduce the occurrence and progression of neuroinflammation in PD (Frank-Cannon et al., 2008).

Biomarkers for Inflammation in Parkinson's Disease

Understanding and identifying biomarkers of inflammation are crucial for diagnosis, prognosis, and the development of targeted therapies. A myriad of studies have focused on elucidating various biomarkers associated with inflammatory processes in PD. Several biomarkers have been investigated in PD to assess the inflammatory state, providing valuable insights into the disease process.

Among the biomarkers studied, cytokines and chemokines have garnered significant attention. Tumor necrosis factor-alpha (TNF-α), interleukin-6 (IL-6), and C-reactive protein (CRP) are among the most extensively studied inflammatory markers in PD. Elevated levels of these markers have been consistently observed in the serum, cerebrospinal fluid (CSF), and post-mortem brain tissue of PD patients, indicating a systemic and central nervous system-specific inflammatory response (Qu et al., 2023).

Markers of oxidative stress and neuroinflammation have also been implicated in PD pathology. Reactive oxygen species (ROS), nitric oxide (NO), and microglial activation markers like CD68 are among the biomarkers associated with neuroinflammation in PD. These markers reflect the oxidative damage and immune response characteristic of PD pathophysiology. Understanding these biomarkers offers potential avenues for therapeutic intervention. Targeting inflammatory pathways may help mitigate neuroinflammation and slow disease progression in PD. By modulating specific biomarkers such as TNF-α or IL-6, novel therapeutic strategies could potentially preserve dopaminergic neurons and alleviate motor and non-motor symptoms associated with PD (Hirsch et al., 2009). However, further research is needed to validate the utility of these biomarkers in clinical practice.

Inflammatory Pathways in Parkinson's Disease

Inflammatory pathways play a significant role in the pathogenesis and progression of PD, contributing to neurodegeneration and disease pathology. Here are some key inflammatory pathways implicated in PD.

Microglial Activation

Microglia, the resident immune cells of the central nervous system, become activated in response to neuronal injury and inflammation in PD. Activated microglia release pro-inflammatory cytokines, such as tumor necrosis factor-alpha (TNF-α), interleukin-1β (IL-1β), and interleukin-6 (IL-6), exacerbating neuroinflammation and neuronal damage (Hirsch et al., 2009).

Astrocyte Activation

Astrocytes, another type of glial cell, also contribute to neuroinflammation in PD. Activated astrocytes release pro-inflammatory cytokines and chemokines, amplify neuroinflammatory responses, and impair neuronal function and survival (Liddelow et al., 2017).

Peripheral Immune Activation

Emerging evidence suggests that peripheral immune activation, characterized by increased levels of circulating pro-inflammatory cytokines and activated immune cells, may contribute to neuroinflammation and neuronal damage in PD. Peripheral inflammation can exacerbate central nervous system inflammation and influence disease progression (Williams-Gray et al., 2016).

Mitochondrial Dysfunction in Parkinson's Disease

Mitochondria

The majority of eukaryotic cells contain mitochondria, which provide cellular energy in the form of adenosine triphosphate (ATP) by oxidative phosphorylation. It is hypothesized that mitochondria evolved from the union of prokaryotic and eukaryotic organisms. Additionally, they have a role in the regulation of cell division and growth as well as processes like iron-sulfur (Fe-S) cluster formation and export, calcium homeostasis, haem production and apoptosis. Contrary to other cellular organelles, mitochondria have their own circular, double-stranded DNA (mtDNA). This DNA codes for 37 mitochondrial genes, 13 of which produce oxidative phosphorylation-related proteins.

Mitochondrial dysfunction refers to abnormalities in the structure or function of mitochondria, the cellular organelles responsible for producing energy in the form of adenosine triphosphate (ATP) through oxidative phosphorylation. Mitochondria play a crucial role in various cellular processes, including energy metabolism, calcium homeostasis, reactive oxygen species (ROS) generation, and apoptosis. Dysfunction in mitochondria can have profound effects on cellular function and has been implicated in a wide range of diseases, including neurodegenerative disorders,

Mitochondrial Dysfunction in Parkinson's Disease

Mitochondrial dysfunction refers to abnormalities in the structure or function of mitochondria, the cellular organelles responsible for producing energy in the form of adenosine triphosphate (ATP) through oxidative phosphorylation. Mitochondria play a crucial role in various cellular processes, including energy metabolism, calcium homeostasis, reactive oxygen species (ROS) generation, and apoptosis. Dysfunction in mitochondria can have profound effects on cellular function and has been implicated in a wide range of neurodegenerative disorders including PD. Here are the key aspects of intricate relationship between mitochondrial dysfunction and PD-

Energy Production Deficits

Mitochondria play a critical role in cellular energy production through oxidative phosphorylation, generating adenosine triphosphate (ATP) to meet the high energy demands of neurons, particularly dopaminergic neurons affected in PD. Dysfunction in mitochondrial complex I, a key component of the electron transport chain, leads to impaired ATP synthesis and energy deficits in PD-affected neurons (Schapira & Jenner, 2011).

Reactive Oxygen Species (ROS) Generation

Mitochondria are a primary source of ROS, which are natural byproducts of oxidative phosphorylation. Excessive ROS production overwhelms cellular antioxidant defences, leading to oxidative stress and damage to cellular components, including proteins, lipids, and DNA. Oxidative stress is implicated in neuronal damage and death observed in PD pathology (Jenner, 2003).

Mitochondrial DNA (mtDNA) Damage

Mitochondria possess their own genome (mtDNA), which is particularly susceptible to oxidative damage and mutations due to its proximity to ROS production sites. Accumulation of mtDNA mutations impairs mitochondrial function, further exacerbating oxidative stress and contributing to neurodegeneration in PD. Studies have identified mtDNA mutations and deletions in PD patients, suggesting a role in disease pathogenesis (Reeve & Turnbull, 2008).

Alpha-Synuclein Interactions

Alpha-synuclein, a protein associated with PD pathology, interacts with mitochondria and disrupts mitochondrial function. Alpha-synuclein aggregates localize to mitochondria, impairing mitochondrial dynamics, membrane potential, and calcium homeostasis. Mitochondrial dysfunction induced by alpha-synuclein contributes to neuronal toxicity and degeneration in PD.

Toxin-Induced Mitochondrial Damage

Environmental toxins such as rotenone and 1-methyl-4-phenyl-1,2,3,6-tetrahydropyridine (MPTP) selectively target mitochondrial complex I, inhibiting electron transport chain activity and inducing dopaminergic neurodegeneration. These toxins are commonly used to model PD in experimental studies and provide insights into the role of mitochondrial dysfunction in disease pathogenesis (Sherer & Betarbet, 2002).

Oxidative Stress in Parkinson's Disease

Oxidative Stress

An imbalance between a biological system's ability to detoxify these reactive by-products and the production and accumulation of Reactive Oxygen Species (ROS) in cells and tissues results in the phenomenon known as oxidative stress. Numerous vital bodily metabolic activities lead to oxidative stress. On the other side, it can have a harmful and poisonous effect on the body. The residues of oxygen consumption called ROS are typically created and have a wide range of physiological functions, involving cell signaling. Although this, xenobiotics like antiblastic medications and outside factors like UV, ionizing radiation, pollution, and heavy metals all dramatically enhance the production of ROS, which in turn causes an equilibrium that leads to cell and tissue damage (oxidative stress). Oxidative stress has been linked to PD and there is overwhelming mark that altered mitochondrial function that play an important role in the disease. Increased iron, protein oxidation, and lipid peroxidation appear to be particularly frequent in the SN. Glutathione (GSH) levels that are lower in the midbrain may indicate higher levels of free radicals (Sian et al., 1991). Figure 2 shows the connection between oxidative stress and PD.

The intricate relationship between oxidative stress and PD, highlighting the underlying mechanisms and implications for disease progression and therapeutic interventions are-

Mitochondrial Dysfunction and ROS Production

Mitochondria are the primary cellular organelles responsible for energy production through oxidative phosphorylation. However, they are also a major source of ROS generation, particularly during electron transport chain activity. In PD, mitochondrial dysfunction is a central pathological feature, characterized by impaired mitochondrial respiration, decreased ATP production, and increased ROS production. Dysfunctional mitochondria accumulate mutations in their DNA, leading to further impairment of respiratory chain complexes and ROS overproduction. The resulting oxidative stress damages cellular components, including lipids, proteins, and DNA, contributing to neuronal degeneration in PD (Bose et al., 2016).

Dopaminergic Neuron Vulnerability

Dopaminergic neurons are particularly vulnerable to oxidative stress due to their high metabolic activity, elevated levels of iron and dopamine, and limited antioxidant defenses. Dopamine metabolism generates ROS as byproducts, leading to oxidative damage to cellular components. Moreover, iron ions released from damaged mitochondria can participate in Fenton reactions, generating highly reactive hydroxyl radicals. Oxidative stress-induced damage to proteins, lipids, and DNA in dopaminergic neurons disrupts cellular homeostasis and impairs neuronal function, ultimately contributing to their degeneration in PD (Dias et al., 2013).

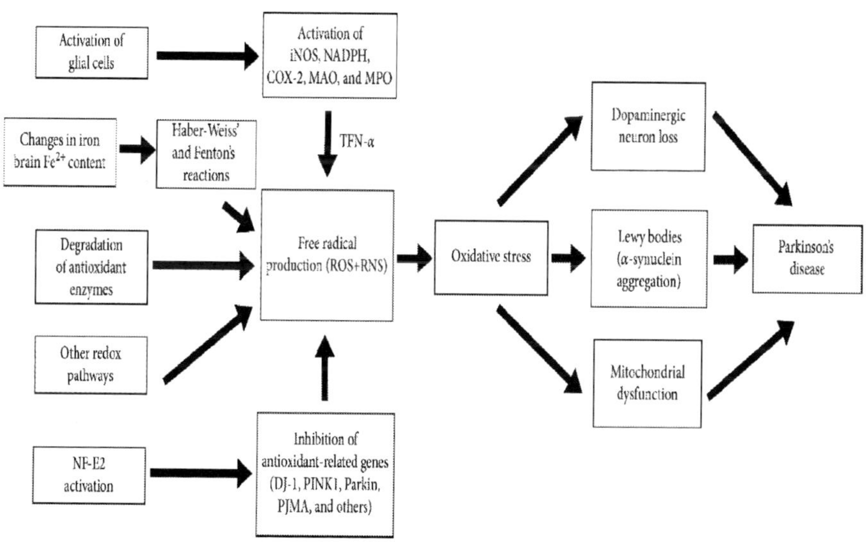

Figure 2. Oxidative Stress in Parkinson's disease.

Protein Aggregation and Oxidative Stress

Abnormal protein aggregation, including the aggregation of alpha-synuclein into Lewy bodies, is a pathological hallmark of PD. Oxidative stress plays a critical role in promoting the misfolding, aggregation, and accumulation of alpha-synuclein and other proteins involved in PD pathogenesis. ROS can modify proteins, leading to their misfolding and aggregation. Additionally, oxidative stress-induced damage to cellular chaperones and proteolytic systems impairs protein quality control mechanisms, facilitating the accumulation of toxic protein aggregates. These protein aggregates further exacerbate oxidative stress, mitochondrial dysfunction, and neuroinflammation, contributing to neuronal dysfunction and death in PD (Cookson 2009).

Emerging Clinical Approaches for Parkinson's Disease

Emerging clinical approaches for PD are continuously evolving, aiming to address the complex pathophysiology of the condition and provide more effective treatments to improve patients' quality of life. Several promising approaches have emerged, ranging from novel pharmacotherapies to advanced surgical interventions and innovative non-pharmacological strategies.

Gene Therapy

Gene therapy holds promise as a potential disease-modifying treatment for PD. Experimental studies and clinical trials have explored the use of viral vectors to deliver therapeutic genes into specific regions of the brain affected by PD. For example, one approach involves delivering genes encoding for neurotrophic factors, such as glial cell line-derived neurotrophic factor (GDNF) or brain-derived neurotrophic factor (BDNF), to promote neuronal survival and function. Other strategies target alpha-synuclein or other proteins implicated in PD pathology to mitigate their toxic effects. While gene therapy for PD is still in the early stages of development, preliminary results from clinical trials show encouraging signs of efficacy and safety (Olanow et al., 2019).

Deep Brain Stimulation (DBS)

Deep brain stimulation has emerged as a valuable therapeutic option for managing motor symptoms in advanced PD patients who are refractory to medication. DBS involves the surgical implantation of electrodes into specific brain regions, such as the subthalamic nucleus (STN) or globus pallidus interna (GPi), followed by the delivery of electrical impulses to modulate abnormal neural activity. Recent advancements in DBS technology, including the development of directional leads and closed-loop stimulation systems, aim to optimize treatment outcomes and minimize side effects. Moreover, ongoing research is exploring the potential benefits of adaptive DBS strategies, where stimulation parameters are dynamically adjusted based on real-time feedback from neural signals or biomarkers (Okun et al., 2012).

Immunotherapy

Immunotherapy approaches targeting alpha-synuclein aggregation represent a promising avenue for slowing disease progression in PD. Antibodies, vaccines, and small molecules designed to stimulate the immune system to recognize and clear abnormal alpha-synuclein aggregates are currently under investigation in preclinical and early clinical trials. These immunotherapeutic strategies aim to halt the spread of alpha-synuclein pathology and preserve neuronal function in PD patients (Chu et al., 2012).

Personalized Medicine

Advances in precision medicine and biomarker discovery are paving the way for personalized approaches to PD management. By identifying genetic, molecular, and clinical biomarkers associated with disease progression and treatment response, clinicians can tailor therapies to individual patients' specific needs. Personalized medicine strategies may involve optimizing medication regimens, selecting the most suitable candidates for surgical interventions like DBS, or identifying individuals at higher risk of developing PD for early intervention and risk mitigation (Espay et al.,2019).

Conclusion

In conclusion, the convergence of inflammatory processes, mitochondrial dysfunction, and oxidative stress mechanisms underscores their pivotal roles in Parkinson's disease (PD) pathogenesis. These interconnected pathways contribute synergistically to neuronal degeneration, protein aggregation, and neuroinflammation, hallmark features of PD pathology. However, the emergence of therapeutic clinical approaches offers promising avenues for disease management and potential disease modification. Immunotherapy targeting aberrant protein aggregates, interventions addressing mitochondrial dysfunction, and antioxidant therapies aimed at restoring redox balance represent key strategies in this endeavor. Additionally, lifestyle modifications and personalized medicine approaches hold promise in optimizing treatment outcomes for PD patients. By targeting these fundamental pathways, therapeutic interventions seek to slow disease progression, alleviate symptoms, and ultimately improve the quality of life for individuals living with PD. Continued research efforts are crucial for deepening our understanding of PD pathophysiology and translating these insights into effective clinical therapies, with the ultimate goal of finding a cure for this debilitating neurodegenerative disorder.

Disclaimer

None.

References

Anglade, P., Vyas, S., Javoy-Agid, F., Herrero Ezquerro, M. T., Michel, P. P., Marquez, J., & Agid, Y. (1997). Apoptosis and autophagy in nigral neurons of patients with Parkinson's disease. *Histology and histopathology*.

Ascherio, A., & Schwarzschild, M. A. (2016). The epidemiology of Parkinson's disease: risk factors and prevention. *The Lancet Neurology*, 15(12), 1257-1272.

Berg, D., Postuma, R. B., Bloem, B., Chan, P., Dubois, B., Gasser, T., & Deuschl, G. (2014). Time to redefine PD? Introductory statement of the MDS Task Force on the definition of Parkinson's disease. *Movement Disorders*, 29(4), 454-462.

Bose, A., & Beal, M. F. (2016). Mitochondrial dysfunction in Parkinson's disease. *Journal of neurochemistry*, 139, 216-231.

Breen, D. P., Nombela, C., Vuono, R., Jones, P. S., Fisher, K., Burn, D. J., & Barker, R. A. (2016). Hypothalamic volume loss is associated with reduced melatonin output in Parkinson's disease. *Movement Disorders,* 31(7), 1062-1066.

Cannon, J. R., Tapias, V., Na, H. M., Honick, A. S., Drolet, R. E., & Greenamyre, J. T. (2009). A highly reproducible rotenone model of Parkinson's disease. *Neurobiology of disease*, 34(2), 279-290.

Chu, Y., & Kordower, J. H. (2018). Immunotherapy strategies for Parkinson's disease. Parkinsonism & related disorders, 46, S20-S24.

Cookson, M. R. (2009). α-Synuclein and neuronal cell death. *Molecular neurodegeneration*, 4, 1-14.

Dickson, D. W. (2012). Parkinson's disease and parkinsonism: neuropathology. *Cold Spring Harbor perspectives in medicine,* 2(8), a009258.

Dorsey, E., Sherer, T., Okun, M. S., & Bloem, B. R. (2018). The emerging evidence of the Parkinson pandemic. *Journal of Parkinson's disease*, 8(s1), S3-S8.

Frank-Cannon, T. C., Tran, T., Ruhn, K. A., Martinez, T. N., Hong, J., Marvin, M., & Tansey, M. G. (2008). Parkin deficiency increases vulnerability to inflammation-related nigral degeneration. *Journal of Neuroscience,* 28(43), 10825-10834.

Hirsch, E. C., & Hunot, S. (2009). Neuroinflammation in Parkinson's disease: a target for neuroprotection? *The Lancet Neurology*, 8(4), 382-397.

Hirsch, E. C., Hunot, S., & Hartmann, A. (2005). Neuroinflammatory processes in Parkinson's disease. *Parkinsonism & related disorders,* 11, S9-S15.

Jenner, P. (2003). Oxidative stress in Parkinson's disease. Annals of Neurology: Official *Journal of the American Neurological Association and the Child Neurology Society,* 53(S3), S26-S38.

Kitada, T., Asakawa, S., Hattori, N., Matsumine, H., Yamamura, Y., Minoshima, S., & Shimizu, N. (1998). Mutations in the parkin gene cause autosomal recessive juvenile parkinsonism. *Nature,* 392(6676), 605-608.

Liddelow, S. A., & Barres, B. A. (2017). Reactive astrocytes: production, function, and therapeutic potential. *Immunity,* 46(6), 957-967.

Okun, M. S. (2012). Deep-brain stimulation for Parkinson's disease. *New England Journal of Medicine,* 367(16), 1529-1538.

Olanow, C. W., Savolainen, M., Chu, Y., Halliday, G. M., & Kordower, J. H. (2019). Temporal evolution of microglia and α-synuclein accumulation following foetal grafting in Parkinson's disease. *Brain,* 142(6), 1690-1700.

Poewe, W., Seppi, K., Tanner, C. M., Halliday, G. M., Brundin, P., Volkmann, J., & Lang, A. E. (2017). Parkinson disease. *Nature reviews Disease primers,* 3(1), 1-21.

Reeve, A. & Turnbull, D. (2008). Mitochondrial DNA mutations in disease: A review. *Clinical Science,* 115(3-4), 147-158.

Schapira, A. H. V., Cooper, J. M., Dexter, D., Jenner, P., Clark, J. B., & Marsden, C. D. (1989). Mitochondrial complex I defi ciency in Parkinson's disease.

Schapira, A. H. V., Mann, V. M., Cooper, J. M., Dexter, D., Daniel, S. E., Jenner, P., & Marsden, C. D. (1990). Anatomic and disease specificity of NADH CoQ1 reductase (complex I) deficiency in Parkinson's disease. *Journal of neurochemistry,* 55(6), 2142-2145.

Schapira, A. H., & Jenner, P. (2011). Etiology and pathogenesis of Parkinson's disease. *Movement disorders,* 26(6), 1049-1055.

Schapira, A. H., Chaudhuri, K. R., & Jenner, P. (2017). Non-motor features of Parkinson disease. *Nature Reviews Neuroscience*, 18(7), 435-450.

Sherer, T. B., Betarbet, R., Testa, C. M., Seo, B. B., Richardson, J. R., Kim, J. H., & Greenamyre, J. T. (2003). Mechanism of toxicity in rotenone models of Parkinson's disease. *Journal of Neuroscience,* 23(34), 10756-10764.

Sian, J., Dexter, D. T., Jenner, P., & Marsden, C. D. (1991). Decrease in nigral reduced glutathione in Parkinson's Disease. In *Brit J Pharmacol* (Dec., London meeting).

Spillantini, M. G., Schmidt, M. L., Lee, V. M. Y., Trojanowski, J. Q., Jakes, R., & Goedert, M. (1997). α-Synuclein in Lewy bodies. *Nature,* 388(6645), 839-840.

Surmeier, D. J., Obeso, J. A., & Halliday, G. M. (2017). Selective neuronal vulnerability in Parkinson disease. *Nature Reviews Neuroscience*, 18(2), 101-113.

Zacharias, H. U., Kaleta, C., Cossais, F., Schaeffer, E., Berndt, H., Best, L., & Berg, D. (2022). Microbiome and metabolome insights into the role of the gastrointestinal–brain axis in Parkinson's and Alzheimer's disease: Unveiling potential therapeutic targets. *Metabolites,* 12(12), 1222.

Chapter 16

Pharmacological and Physical Therapy Intervention in the Clinical Management for Neurodegenerative Disorders

Charu Chhabra[1], MPT,
Harsirjan Kaur[2,*], MPT,
Sohrab Ahmed Khan[1], PhD,
Rabia Aziz[1], MPT,
Habiba Sundus[1], MPT,
and Kusum Yadav[3], MPT

[1]Department of Physiotherapy, Jamia Hamdard, New Delhi, India
[2]Faculty of Physiotherapy, S.G.T. University, Haryana, India
[3]Department of Physiotherapy, Jagannath University, India

Abstract

Since they cause a gradual decline in an individual's cognitive and functional abilities, neurodegenerative disorders are a class of neurological pathologies that cause the structure and function of the nervous system to gradually deteriorate. These disorders pose a significant challenge to modern healthcare. Pharmaceutical treatments are essential for symptom relief, delaying the onset of the illness, and enhancing enhancing the quality of life for those with neurodegenerative diseases. The chapter will cover the state of pharmacotherapy at the moment, including new and existing medications that target important pathways connected to these illnesses. It will provide an understanding

* Corresponding Author's Email: sirjan4242@gmail.com.

In: Neurogenerative Disorders
Editors: Mohit Agrawal, Manmohan Singhal, Amit Kumar Nayak et al.
ISBN: 979-8-89530-143-2

of the efficaciousness, possible adverse effects, and current research about medications such as dopamine agonists, acetylcholinesterase inhibitors, N-methyl-D-aspartate (NMDA) receptor antagonists, and disease-modifying compounds. The chapter will also explore the limitations of pharmacotherapy and the difficulties of customized treatment in neurodegenerative illnesses, emphasizing the value of physical therapy and individualized pharmaceutical therapies. Exercise, gait training, exercise, and occupational therapy are some of the techniques used in physiotherapy, which is a crucial part of the treatment of neurodegenerative diseases. These techniques work together to preserve or improve motor function, movement, and the patient's quality of life. This section will highlight the value of interdisciplinary care by summarizing evidence-based physical therapy techniques that target certain symptoms linked to a range of neurodegenerative illnesses. The chapter will also look at how neuroplasticity and neurorehabilitation are becoming more and more important in improving treatment results. It investigates the possibility for novel techniques in the treatment of neurodegenerative disorders, including virtual reality, robotic-assisted therapy, and non-invasive brain stimulation. The combination of pharmaceutical and physical therapy treatments offers a comprehensive strategy for addressing the many problems associated with neurodegenerative diseases. Clinicians are able to provide patients with the best possible care by integrating physical therapy regimens with disease-modifying medications to address both the motor and cognitive elements of these diseases.

Keywords: patient-centered, pharmacological, neurodegenerative diseases, physiotherapy

Introduction

Neurodegenerative illnesses impact millions of individuals globally. The most prevalent neurodegenerative illnesses are Parkinson's and Alzheimer's diseases. According to Alzheimer's Disease Association forecast from 2022, there may be as many as 6.2 million Americans who have Alzheimer's disease. The Parkinson's Foundation estimates that around one million people in America have Parkinson's disease. Dementia, with the majority of cases being Alzheimer's disease-related, appears to be the most well studied and common neurodegenerative disorder in sub-Saharan Africa (Lamptey et al., 2022).

A class of pathological illnesses known as neurodegenerative disorders (NDDs) are defined by the gradual loss and malfunctioning of particular neuronal populations, which results in a variety of issues with mobility and mental function. While Huntington's disease and ALS frequently manifest earlier, both ailments have a significant age correlation and are far more common in those over 65. According to projections made by the World Health Organization (WHO), the population over 65 will at least double over the next 30 years, which means that the number of persons suffering from neurodegenerative diseases will rise at a comparable pace (Jellinger, 2010).

Neurodegenerative disorders present with a wide range of symptoms. Without particular medical testing, some may seem wholly unrelated, while others may show clear links to a degenerative brain illness. **Table 1** displays the symptoms of the most prevalent neurodegenerative disorders. Two known risk factors for neurological illness are advancing age and certain genetic variants. Additional factors that might contribute to this illness include gender, low educational attainment, hormonal disorders, oxidative stress, inflammation, stroke, high blood pressure, diabetes, tobacco use, brain injuries, depression, infections, tumors, vitamin deficiencies, immune system and metabolic disorders, and exposure to chemicals. As people age, their risk of acquiring a neurological illness increases significantly (Hou Y., 2019).

Table 1. Symptoms of common neurodegenerative conditions

S.NO.	Type of Disease	Symptoms
1	Dementia-type diseases	Confusion, memory loss, trouble thinking or concentrating, and behaviour changes.
2	Demyelinating diseases	Problems with movement, balance, and coordination
3	Motor neuron diseases	Muscle weakness, twitching, and wasting
4	Spinocerebellar ataxias	Problems with movement, balance, and coordination
5	Parkinson's disease	Tremors, stiffness, and problems with balance and coordination

Evaluating neurologic symptoms separately and early, prior to clinical diagnosis, might be one way to address the difficulties involved in identifying neurodegenerative illnesses. Formal neuropsychologic assessments can offer some impartial confirmation. With this aim, several lines of evidence have been presented. A population-based prevalence and incidence research involving both urban and rural populations is required and achievable in order to further our understanding of each neurodegenerative disorder (Errkeinnin, 2018).

Pharmacological Interventions for Neurodegenerative Conditions

Pharmacological treatments can help control symptoms and reduce the rate at which a disease develops. The following are a few pharmacological treatments for neurodegenerative diseases that are now available:

Amantadine

Amantadine exhibits modest antiparkinsonian action and is an antiviral drug. In the early 2000s, amantadine was used to treat influenza A. But recently, strong resistance has surfaced - first in Asia and now in North America. Due to significant levels of resistance, the CDC does not recommend treatment or prevention for influenza A as of 2011. Parkinson's disease is currently the primary indication for amantadine use. In the context of an interprofessional team administering the care of Parkinson disease patients, this activity provides an overview of the indications, contraindications, activity, adverse drug reactions, warning, precautions, toxicity, and limitations of amantadine in a clinical setting (Chang C., 2023)

Amantadine's exact mode of action is unknown. The main effect of antiviral action is to impede virus replication. Amantadine inhibits the entrance of infectious viral nucleic acids into the host cell by rupturing the transmembrane domain of the viral M2 protein. Additionally, during replication, it could prevent influenza A virus isolates from the H1N1, H2N2, and H3N2 subtypes from assembling. Amantadine is ineffective against influenza B due to the structural differences in the M2 protein (Okigbo A., 2019).

Investigations have demonstrated that amantadine operates on dopamine neurons in the treatment of Parkinson disease. Amantadine inhibits dopamine absorption and enhances dopamine release by acting as a weak, non-competitive antagonist of the NMDA receptor. Despite not having anticholinergic action, amantadine may have clinically significant anticholinergic side effects, such as dry mouth, urine retention, and constipation (Chang & Ramphul, 2023).

Apoptomine

This dopaminergic agonist may activate the regions of the brain responsible for motor control. It acts quickly and has a wide therapeutic index, although large doses are needed for severe toxicity. The possible adverse effects of hallucinations, hyperpyrexia during withdrawal, somnolence throughout the day, hypotension, irritation of the oral mucosa, falls, and lengthening of the QT interval should be explained to patients.

Apomorphine, a non-ergoline dopamine agonist, binds to the D2, D3, and D5 dopamine receptors with great affinity. Apomorphine is N-demethylated by CYP2B6, 2C8, 3A4, and 3A5. It can be glucuronidated by a range of UGTs or sulfated by SULTs 1A1, 1A2, 1A3, 1E1, and 1B1. Although it is difficult to find out the composition of these sulfate conjugates, around 60% of sublingual apomorphine is eliminated as one. Apomorphine glucuronide and norapomorphine glucuronide are the byproducts of an apomorphine dosage that is not entirely consumed. Just 0.3% of subcutaneous apomorphine is retrieved as the original parent material. How apomorphine's cellular actions might alleviate hypomobility brought on by Parkinson's disease is yet unknown, though.

This medication stimulates the brain's dopamine receptors to treat Parkinson's disease. Furthermore, apomorphine has antagonistic effects on serotonergic 5HT2A, 5HT2B, and 5HT2C receptors as well as agonistic effects on adrenergic α2A, α2B, and α2C receptors (Jenner P, 2016). Since the landmark study in the 1980s, apomorphine has shown successful in returning severe, sudden "off" episodes in advanced Parkinson's disease (PD) despite appropriate oral therapy, as shown by many open-label studies. A reduction in the amount of time spent "off" was usually the primary outcome of intermittent subcutaneous pen injections or continuous subcutaneous apomorphine infusion (CSAI). Prolonged subcutaneous infusions were also demonstrated to reduce dyskinesia, albeit the results differed between the trials that followed (Carbone et al., 2019).

Carbidopa

When used to treat Parkinson's disease (PD), carbidopa prevents levodopa from being converted to dopamine outside of the central nervous system (CNS), which reduces the medication's undesirable side effects on organs outside of the CNS. Increased numbers of activated/memory T cells, immune cell infiltration into the brain, and elevated expression of inflammatory genes in the peripheral and central nervous systems (CNS) are all linked to Parkinson's disease (PD). This medication is used to treat Parkinson's disease in addition to levodopa (Zhu et al., 2017).

It functions by blocking levodopa's breakdown before it reaches the brain, which increases dopamine production. It also prevents levodopa's undesirable side effects on organs outside of the central nervous system (CNS) (Huabin Zhu, 2017). The chemical designation of carbidepa is N-amino-alpha-methyl-3-hydroxy-L-tyrosine monohydrate. A powerful inhibitor of aromatic amino acid decarboxylase (DDC), it does not penetrate the blood-brain barrier because of its chemical makeup. Carbidopa and levodopa are always supplied together because of their action. A unique formulation made entirely of carbidopa was created to treat individuals who do not respond well to the combined therapy of levodopa and carbidopa in terms of nausea reduction.

Levodopa/Carbidopa

Carbidopa is a drug used to treat and manage Parkinson's disease (PD). The medication belongs to the class of decarboxylase inhibitors. Carbidopa is prescribed in combination with levodopa (L-dopa) to treat parkinsonism symptoms resulting from carbon monoxide or manganese intoxication, post-encephalitic parkinsonism, and motor symptoms associated with Parkinson disease (PD). This combination medication acts by raising dopamine levels in the brain to treat Parkinson's disease (Tadi & Leyden, 2023).

Carbidopa, sometimes referred to as 1-methyldopahydrazine, functions by obstructing the PLP-dependent enzyme l-aromatic amino acid decarboxylase (AADC) and irreversibly binding pyridoxal 5′-phosphate (PLP). L-dopa and 5-HTP are converted by AACD into serotonin and dopamine, respectively. Carbidopa has minimal effects on enzyme activity and cannot cross the blood-brain barrier, while levodopa is absorbed by the central nervous system. When peripheral levodopa metabolism is decreased, the central nervous system can absorb more L-dopa. This increased potency results in a reduction in the dosage of levodopa needed to successfully treat parkinsonian motor symptoms by up to 75%. Furthermore, as this keeps the GI system from absorbing too much dopamine, the absence of peripheral conversion of levodopa to dopamine lessens the likelihood of adverse effects from the drug, such as nausea, vomiting, and/or diarrhea (Tadi & Leyden, 2023).

Combinations of levodopa and carbidopa are available in a range of formulations and modes of administration. The dose of levodopa to carbidopa is determined by weight and is either 10:1 or 4:1. Motor fluctuations known as "off time" and "on time" are frequent when levodopa is delivered and also occur when coadministering carbidopa with levodopa. The phrase "off time" describes the periods of time during which a patient experiences parkinsonian motor symptoms, meaning that the medication is not working as planned. On the other hand, "on-time" describes the resolution of symptoms or the likely beginning of dyskinesias and unpredictable, erratic movements. The erratic symptoms are most likely caused by pulsatile, non-physiological activation of the dopamine receptors (Tadi & Leyden, 2023).

Dopamine levels can be affected by Parkinson disease severity, even with the same dosage of levodopa. The severity of the condition may need the use of different medication formulations.

Dantrolene

This medication is used to treat spinal cord injuries and multiple sclerosis-related muscular spasms and stiffness. In skeletal muscle, dantrolene functions intracellularly to decrease the actin-myosin excitation-contraction coupling interaction inside each individual sarcomere. By opposing ryanodine receptors, or RyR1 and RyR3, in the sarcoplasmic reticulum, this function is carried out by preventing the release of calcium ions that are essential to the contraction process (Dominic Ratto, 2023). As a result, DS has positive effects on a number of illnesses, including stroke, ischemia/reperfusion damage, and neurodegenerative disorders, that are brought on by the disruption of calcium homeostasis in addition to mental health disorders. By directly interacting with RYR1 and RYR3, DS lowers the Ca2+sensitivity of channel activation by reducing the amount of channel activation caused by CaM. DS is a therapy option for MH and other disorders like RyRs that are caused by anomalies in L-type calcium channel receptors (Pinder and others, 2017).

Fast twitch muscles are more impacted by dandrolene than slow twitch muscle fibers. Dizziness, sleepiness, weakness, rashes, facial, lip, tongue, and neck swelling, jaundice, breathing difficulties, chest discomfort, persistent vomiting, diarrhea, constipation, issues with speech or vision, headedness, and seizures are some of the side symptoms of DS. Oral usage over an extended period of time may cause liver damage. The following side effects are uncommon: rash, weakness, and exhaustion (Yang and others, 2023).

Donepezil

A piperidine derivative, donepezil hydrochloride is a fast-acting, reversible, centrally acting acetylcholinesterase inhibitor that is mostly used to treat Alzheimer's disease. The enzyme acetylcholinesterase breaks down acetylcholine after its release from the presynapse. Donepezil increases the quantity of acetylcholine available at synapses and enhances cholinergic transmission by inhibiting acetylcholine hydrolysis by binding reversibly to acetylcholinesterase. This medication is used to treat Alzheimer's disease by increasing acetylcholine levels, which are essential for memory and learning (Shin C. Y., 2018).

A piperidine derivative, donepezil hydrochloride is a fast, reversible, centrally acting acetylcholinesterase inhibitor. After acetylcholine is released from the presynapse, the enzyme acetylcholinesterase breaks it down. Donepezil's reversible binding to acetylcholinesterase inhibits acetylcholine hydrolysis, which increases acetylcholine availability at synapses and enhances cholinergic transmission. Donepezil's anticholinesterase action is mainly targeted towards the brain's acetylcholinesterase. In terms of structure, donepezil is distinct from other anticholinesterase medications like tacrine and physostigmine. According to recent research, neuroinflammation is a key player in the etiology of neurodegenerative illnesses. Interestingly, donepezil has been shown to significantly reduce neuroinflammatory responses, such as activation of astrocytic and microglial cells, which are linked to Alzheimer's disease (Kim J., 2021).

The gastrointestinal (GI) side effects of donepezil, which might include vomiting, diarrhea, and nausea, are the most frequent adverse effects. Moreover, additional typical side effects such anorexia, weariness, cramping in the muscles, and sleeplessness are more commonly associated with greater donepezil dosages. But in the majority of individuals, these side effects are usually modest and temporary, lasting up to three weeks, and they normally go away even if the medicine is prolonged (Kumar et al., 2023).

Entacapone

Entacapone only partially inhibits COMT activity. Since it requires frequent liver function monitoring and carries a risk of hepatotoxicity, tolcapone is the most effective COMT inhibitor currently available on the market in terms of shorter OFF times; nonetheless, its application is practically restricted to second-line therapy. This medication is used to treat Parkinson's disease in conjunction with levodopa and/or carbidopa. It is a particular inhibitor of the key enzyme in the levodopa metabolic pathway, cathechol-O-methyltransferase (COMT). Consequently, levodopa's metabolism is slowed by entacapone, increasing the drug's bioavailability and duration of effect (Najib, 2021).

Therefore, the two choices for first-line oral COMT inhibitors are entacapone and opicapone. Meta-analyses suggested that entacapone increased ON times more on average than opicapone did, but the BI-PARK-I trial, the only direct comparative research with data, could not demonstrate any superiority for either drug (Regensburger M. 2023).

Schacht (2016) conducted a critical assessment of the literature on the COMT Val158Met moderation of dopaminergic medication effects on cognitive performance. Several studies show that there is conflicting evidence for this pharmacogenetic impact for stimulants and COMT inhibitors, which are more likely to affect D1 receptors. Data clearly support the action of antipsychotics, which affect D2 receptors more than other medications. It has been demonstrated that the genotype COMT Val158Met is a viable target for identifying those who are more likely to benefit from dopaminergic drugs (Ma et al., 2021).

Memantine

In 1966, memantine was identified as a drug for the treatment of hyperglycemia. It has not been shown to have a substantial impact on blood glucose decrease. However, there was optimism that this drug might help cure Parkinson's disease, seizures, depression, migraines, and eventually Alzheimer's disease as soon as it went into clinical trials. Memantine and cholinergic inhibitors together cause less decline than a placebo, but in terms of cognitive performance, psychological and behavioral symptoms, and functioning, memantine is probably no better in people with moderate AD than a placebo (Willenborg B., 2011).

Memantine is an antagonist of the glutamatergic N-methyl-D-aspartate acid (NMDA) receptor that is non-competitive. These calcium channels are ultimately responsible for neuronal dysfunction and death because they regulate significant quantities of glutamate (Olivares D., 2012).

Memantine's primary mechanism of action is thought to be the inhibition of current flow through N-methyl-d-aspartate (NMDA) receptor channels, a glutamate receptor subfamily implicated in brain function to a great extent. Surprisingly, some medications that inhibit NMDA receptor channels, such as ketamine, have extremely harmful adverse effects. Along with shared inhibitory mechanisms with ketamine, memantine's exceptional therapeutic success is probably due to its unique actions. Two potentially important differences between memantine and ketamine are its effect on blocked channel gating and its binding to two NMDA receptor sites (Johnson et al., 2006).

Memantine has been shown to improve cognition, general clinical status, activities of daily living, and behavioral changes in both mild and severe AD cases. Although memantine has a mild overall impact, its interindividual response varies, much like that of cholinergic inhibitors. Tablets containing memantine can be taken with or without food. However, memantine dosages in patients with renal impairment must be adjusted, especially when creatinine clearance approaches 50 ml/min/1.73 m2. In this case, the recommended daily dosage of memantine is around 10 mg (Kavirajan H., 2007).

Rivastigmine

Rivastigmine inhibits both brain AChE and BuChE. This medication has therapeutic importance in treating dementia associated with Parkinson's disease in addition to its primary usage in treating Alzheimer's disease. This functions by blocking cholinesterase, an enzyme critical to memory and learning, raising acetylcholine levels in the brain. The medication's specific mode of action is unclear. (Kandiah N., 2017) Rivastigmine bonds to cholinesterase's esteratic and ionic locations, preventing acetylcholine (ACh) from being degraded by enzymes. The G1 form of AChE predominates in dementia patients due to the selective elimination of the membrane-bound globular tetrameric form of AChE, or G4, which is found in the cortical and hippocampal areas of the normal brain. The G1 form of AChE is selectively inhibited by rivastigmine. When both AChE and BuChE are suppressed, rivastigmine also lowers the activity of BuChE, which raises ACh levels in the brain; however, the advantage of inhibiting BuChE is more theoretical (Grossberg G. T., 2003).

When used orally, rivastigmine has a 36% bioavailability (at a dosage of 3 mg). It absorbs quickly and completely, reaching its maximal plasma concentration in around an hour. Rivastigmine appears to have linear pharmacokinetics up to 3 mg, but when the dose is raised, these properties become nonlinear. In general, rivastigmine treatment with meals delays absorption by delaying t max by 90 minutes, lowering C max by 30%, and raising AUC by 30% (t max is around 0.5-2.0 h). Rivastigmine is more accessible and tolerated when taken with meals since gastrointestinal undesirable effects are coupled with elevated plasma levels (Kandiah N., 2017).

Baclofen

Available from the FDA, Baclofen is used to treat reversible spasticity caused by muscular spasms. It is especially useful in treating flexor spasms, clonus, and associated discomfort, which are frequent side effects of spinal cord injuries and multiple sclerosis. There are several off-label applications for baclofen. This exercise describes how to use Baclofen in a therapeutic environment, including the indications, mechanism of action, safe administration, side effects, contraindications, toxicity, and monitoring of a wide range of physiological variables. The FDA has authorized Baclofen for the treatment of reversible spasticity, with specific benefits for clonus, concurrent pain, flexor spasms, multiple sclerosis, and common sequelae of spinal cord injuries (Ghanavatian et al., 2022).

Baclofen (beta-[4-chlorophenyl]-GABA) functions as an agonist at the beta subunit of gamma-aminobutyric acid on mono and polysynaptic neurons in the brain and spinal cord (Albright et al., 1996). It is hypothesized that baclofen alleviates spasticity by inhibiting the release of excitatory neurotransmitters in presynaptic neurons and stimulating inhibitory neuronal signals in postsynaptic neurons (Gracies et al., 1997). Additionally, it has been found that Baclofen attracts voltage-gated calcium channels. However, its therapeutic effectiveness in this regard is currently unknown. Orally administered baclofen has a bioavailability of 70% to 85% and is rapidly absorbed through the digestive tract. Typically, peak plasma concentrations occur two to three hours after consumption. A dose-dependent increase in absorption occurs when the dosage is increased. Due to the brief half-life of two to six hours, frequent administration is required for optimal results. 70% of unchanged baclofen is eliminated via renal excretion, while the remaining 30% is eliminated via faeces. Therefore, baclofen is an effective treatment for patients with liver disease or a high risk of cytochrome P450-mediated drug-drug interactions. The absorption and elimination processes of baclofen exhibit considerable inter-individual variability. Insufficient evidence supporting the use of baclofen in patients with Parkinson disease and stroke is another reason why the drug is not recommended. Additionally, skeletal muscular spasms linked to rheumatologic illnesses are not suggested for baclofen as shown in Figure 1 mechanisms of action of medications used to treat neurodegenerative disorders (Ghanavatian et al., 2022).

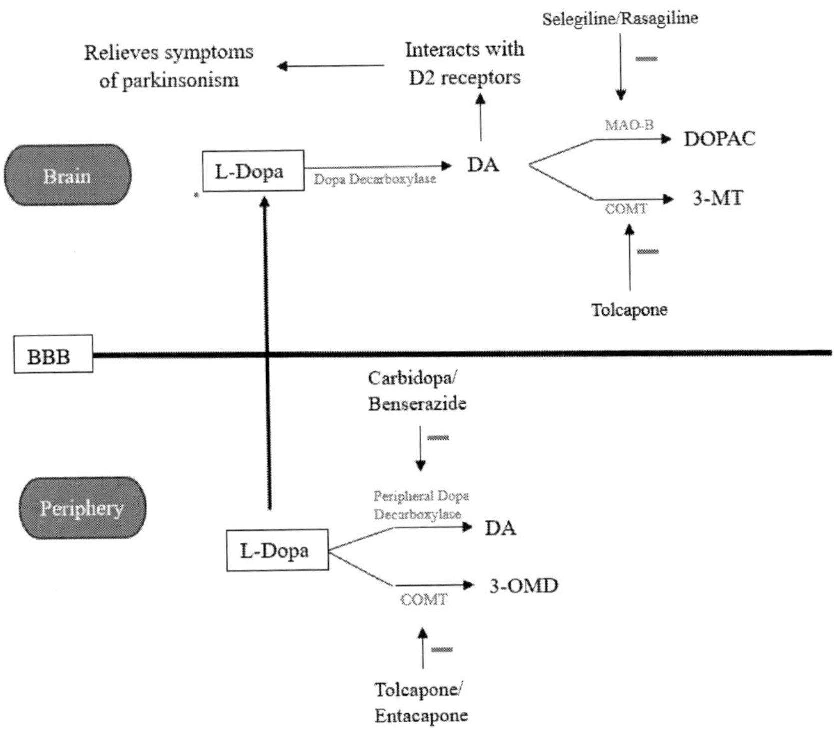

Figure 1. Mechanisms of action of medications used to treat neurodegenerative (Da- Dopamine; BBB- Blood Brain Barrier; MAO- Monoamine Deoxidase; COMT- Catechol-O- methyltransferase; 3 MT- 3-methoxytyramine; DOPAC- 3,4- dihydroxyphenylacetic acid; 3-O-MD- 3-O-methyldopa; L-Dopa- Levodopa).

Promising biological targets exist for pharmacological treatment of neurodegenerative illnesses in addition to these medications. HDAC inhibitors, for instance, have been demonstrated to lessen cognitive impairments in animal models of neurodegenerative diseases. Additional medications possessing antioxidative, antiapoptotic, steroid-like, and neuroprotective properties are being studied for the treatment of uncommon neurodegenerative illnesses (Shukla et al., 2021).

It is significant to highlight that there are few medication therapies available for neurodegenerative disorders, and that the varied and poorly known etiologies of these illnesses make it difficult to find effective treatments.

Pharmacological treatments can help control symptoms and reduce the rate at which a disease develops. A few medications can help Alzheimer's patients with their cognitive abilities. There are medications that can extend the time that levodopa works for Parkinson's disease patients. Many adverse effects, such as nausea, vomiting, diarrhoea, disorientation, and confusion, can be brought on by these medications. Certain medications can wear off in Parkinson's disease and induce dyskinesias when taken long-term. Drugs can sometimes result in liver issues. Patients should closely follow their doctor's instructions and report any negative effects see in Table 2 exhibits the list of specific drugs for Neurodegenerative disorders and their side effects The dosage and administration of these medications varies based on the medication and the patient's condition.

Table 2. List of specific drugs for neurodegenerative disorders and their side effects

S.No	Disease	Drug	Side Effects
1	Parkinson's Disease	• Amantadine • Apomorphine • Carbidopa/levodopa • Entacapone	Dizziness, confusion, and hallucinations. Nausea, vomiting, and low blood pressure. Long-term use can cause dyskinesias (involuntary movements) and wearing-off (loss of effectiveness) Diarrhea and liver problems
2	Alzheimer's Disease	• Donepezil • Memantine • Rivastigmine	Nausea, vomiting, and diarrhea Dizziness, headache, and confusion Nausea, vomiting, and diarrhea
3	Multiple Sclerosis	• Baclofen • Dantrolene	Drowsiness, dizziness, and weakness. Drowsiness, dizziness, and weakness

Challenges and Limitations of Current Pharmacological Treatments

The many and poorly understood etiologies of neurodegenerative disorders provide a major obstacle to the development of effective therapeutics for these ailments. It is challenging to create specialized therapies for these illnesses since their causes are complicated and frequently unknown. The development of tau protein tangles and beta-amyloid plaques, for instance, are hallmarks of Alzheimer's disease; nevertheless, the precise processes behind these abnormalities remain poorly known (Irvine G. B., 2008).

The limited ability of existing pharmacological therapies to change disease progression is another drawback of these treatments for neurodegenerative illnesses. Numerous medications already in use, such acetylcholinesterase inhibitors and NMDA-receptor antagonists, have only moderately controlled symptoms and have not shown any discernible benefits on the course of the disease. Cholinesterase inhibitors, for instance, do not slow down the underlying neurodegenerative process, even if they can help Alzheimer's patients with their cognitive function (Colović M. B., 2013).

Another issue impeding the development of neurodegenerative disease therapies is inadequate characterisation of the condition. The inability to fully comprehend these disorders makes it challenging to pinpoint possible pharmacological targets and create efficient treatment plans. For instance, inadequate understanding of Alzheimer's disease may be the reason for the failure of several clinical studies (Yiannopoulou K. G., 2019).

Another drawback of the pharmacological therapies for neurodegenerative illnesses that are now available is the absence of reliable animal and cell-culture models. It will be easier to develop and test drugs if there are better models available for investigating these disorders. To better understand the underlying processes of neurodegeneration and discover possible therapeutic targets, for instance, researchers may find it useful to utilize animal models that closely resemble the human disease process (Tello J. A., 2022).

The Necessity of Supplementary or Substitute Nonpharmacological Therapies

Because neurodegenerative illnesses are complicated and multidimensional, it is critical to have alternate or complementary nonpharmacological therapies in the therapeutic management of these problems. Neurodegenerative disorders, including Parkinson's disease, ALS, and Alzheimer's disease, are characterized by the progressive deterioration and loss of neurons in the central nervous system. Pharmaceutical therapies are necessary for managing symptoms and delaying the progression of disease, but they frequently have drawbacks, such as insufficient efficacy and potential side effects (Lamptey R. N. L., 2022).

A number of significant benefits are provided by non-pharmacological therapies when it comes to meeting the holistic requirements of people with neurodegenerative diseases. First off, by treating symptoms and functional restrictions that medicine might not be able to completely relieve, they can improve patients' overall quality of life. In addition, non-pharmacological interventions can be incorporated into a holistic care approach to support a patient's physical, mental, and emotional well-being. For example, cognitive rehabilitation and psychotherapy can help manage the emotional and cognitive challenges associated with neurodegenerative disorders. Secondly, these interventions are generally safer and less likely to produce adverse effects, making them suitable for individuals who may be sensitive to medications or have contraindications. In addition, these interventions are generally safer and less likely to produce adverse effects, making them suitable for people who may be sensitive to medications or have contraindications (Rodakowski J., 2015, Coleman J. J., 2016).

Nonpharmacological approaches are also used to treat the complex elements of neurodegenerative diseases. Exercise regimens, physical therapy, and occupational therapy, for instance, can help patients keep their independence and improve their general well-being by enhancing their mobility, coordination, and overall physical function. Dietary therapies and nutritional counseling can improve brain function and lessen the nutritional deficits that are frequently linked to these conditions. In the face of illnesses like ALS, speech therapy can help people retain their communicative abilities (Castellano-Tejedor C., 2022).

Nonpharmacological therapies also support a more individualized and patient-centered approach to care. Since every patient has a unique experience with neurodegenerative conditions, nonpharmacological therapies can be customized to meet their requirements and preferences. Patients' mental health can be greatly enhanced by therapeutic modalities that provide opportunities for emotional expression and stress reduction, such as music therapy, art therapy, and mindfulness-based activities (Herholz S. C., 2022).

Physical Therapy Interventions

The possibility of using exercise as a preventative measure or as a treatment to lessen the severity of neurodegenerative illnesses is becoming more widely acknowledged. These conditions, which include multiple sclerosis, Parkinson's disease, and Alzheimer's disease, frequently result in movement impairments, cognitive decline, and a general reduction in quality of life. Exercise programs customized to each patient's unique requirements and capabilities have become increasingly popular as effective treatments (Mahalakshmi et al., 2020 (Chhabra et al., 2023).

Aerobic Exercise

It has been demonstrated that aerobic exercise can be used as a therapeutic intervention for neurodegenerative diseases. Among the main advantages of aerobic exercise are:

Reducing the Risk of Neurodegenerative Diseases

According to studies, engaging in aerobic exercise can lower the chance of contracting neurodegenerative illnesses including Parkinson's and Alzheimer's. Increased blood flow from the brain to the hippocampus, as well as an increase in hippocampal size in humans and a decrease in neuro-inflammation, are all positive consequences of exercise (Cass, 2017).

Lack of sufficient physical activity may increase the risk of Parkinson's disease, Alzheimer's disease, and stroke. Cognitive function was enhanced in the elderly by aerobic exercise. To explain the underlying mechanism, Monteiro et al., (2015) proposed two hypotheses: (a) PE reduces chronic oxidative stress in PD by stimulating mitochondria biogenesis and upregulating autophagy; and (b) exercise stimulates the synthesis of trophic factors such as fibroblast growth factor 2 (FGF-2) and neuro-transmitters such as dopamine and glial-derived neurotrophic factor (GDNF), insulin-like growth factor-1 (IGF 1), brain (Mahalakshmi et al., 2020).

PE has an impact on several neurophysiological processes and features, including neurogenesis, autophagy, neuronal plasticity, antioxidant defense systems, and more. Additionally, it lessens neurodegeneration and neuronal apoptosis. Although the effects of PE on neuro-plastic alterations in the human brain vary greatly across individuals. Frequent PE enhances brain function and is a potent inducer of autophagy. Additionally, it increases mitochondrial biogenesis and lessens long-term oxidative stress. In addition, it decreases the expression of Bax and neuro-inflammatory cytokines in the hippocampal regions while increasing the production of neurotrophic factors such as GDNF and BDNF, neurotransmitters such as dopamine, and the hormone irisin. Since

BDNF is a multifunctional molecule involved in neuronal plasticity, synaptic transmission and plasticity, neuronal stress resistance, neuronal differentiation and maturation, activation of other supporting molecules such as NFB, and dopamine in neurons, it is essential to regulate BDNF through physical activity. Therefore, PE has multiple interconnected positive impacts on the brain (Farì G., 2021).

Improving Cognitive Function

The mechanisms of neuroprotection and neuroplasticity are responsible for maintaining cognitive function. Learning and the acquisition of abilities are the outcome of neuroplasticity, which is the brain's capacity to change its structural and functional characteristics in response to shifting demands. It is commonly recognized that PE enhances cognitive abilities by facilitating the neuroplasticity of specific brain areas. Farmer et al., showed that exercise causes hippocampus neurons to proliferate and differentiate from a single population of stem cells (Deng W., 2021). Because they may form connections more freely than mature neurons, young neurons support healthy learning, memory function, and mood control. Additionally, the hippocampus contributes to the proper functioning of many brain activities by secreting certain stimulating factors like insulin-like growth factor (IGF-1), glial-derived neurotrophic factor (GDNF), and brain-derived neurotrophic factor (BDNF). These factors, when combined with synapsins and synaptophysins, induce a downregulation of apoptotic and oxidative stress functions. In research involving both humans and animals, PE is linked to an increased release of protective neurotrophins. It has been shown that aerobic exercise helps patients with neurodegenerative illnesses think more clearly. In healthy individuals, it has also been demonstrated to enhance memory and learning. One non-pharmacological technique that may help prevent cognitive decline and lower the risk of AD is exercise. In addition to reducing and delaying the onset of severe neuro-psychiatric symptoms including apathy, confusion, and depression, PE helps maintain and enhance cognitive performance in AD patients. It has also been demonstrated that exercise produces neurotrophic factors and anti-inflammatory benefits. Despite considerable weight gain, exercise appears to protect against obesity-induced white matter damage by decreasing neuro-inflammation and vascular dysfunction, according to a mouse experiment research. The mRNA expression of ABCA1 is considerably increased by aerobic exercise, and this may enhance cognitive function by mitigating and perhaps avoiding the symptoms of AD. Treatment possibilities for age-related neurodegenerative illnesses, such as AD, are offered by all these results. BDNF is a member of the small-secreted protein family, which also includes neurotrophin 3 and 4, nerve growth factor, and neurotrophin 4. In addition to its antiapoptotic and antioxidant properties, it tends to inhibit every autophagy process that is brought on by proinflammatory cytokines and microglia. Among all the neurotrophins, BDNF is unique because of its strong actions at synapses and its high levels of expression in the brain. Additionally, BDNF neurotrophin has been linked to information storage mechanisms in long-term memory and learning, according to research done in 2002 by Churchill et al., (Molinari C., 2020).

Physiologically, following an ischemic insult, the microglia are activated and act with proinflammatory activity, leading to an increase in free oxidative radicals (ROS), to which neuronal cells try to respond by consuming ATP and ultimately dying. Increasing the levels of BDNF through PE could mitigate the effects of these events. PE actually upregulates the production of both BDNF and IGF-1, which, when combined with BDNF, mediates the cognitive benefits of exercise.

As there is currently no disease-modifying treatment for degenerative illnesses, individuals with AD, PD, and dementia are often treated with a combination of pharmaceutical medications, social care, and counseling in attempt to slow down the course of their conditions (Farì G., 2021).

Improving Physical Function

Many disease conditions, including sarcopenia, metabolic diseases, cardiovascular problems, and osteoporosis, are protected against by physical activity. By lowering the development of neurotoxic protein aggregates like β-amyloid protein plaques and lewy bodies, physical activity can also help prevent the onset and progression of neurodegenerative disorders including Parkinson's and Alzheimer's (Bonanni R., 2022). Consequently, physical exercise has a protective effect by enhancing cognitive and motor abilities and lowering neuroinflammation, mitochondrial malfunction, and cell death. For those suffering from neurodegenerative disorders, aerobic exercise can help with physical function, including balance and fall risk in Parkinson's disease patients. Numerous exercise regimens have been examined in people with Parkinson's disease (PD), and the phrases physical therapy and exercise are sometimes used interchangeably. Exercise is a subtype of physical activity that involves deliberate, systematic, and repetitive motions of the body that are carried out to enhance or maintain one or more aspects of physical activity, according to the American College of Sports Medicine (ACSM). Physical activity, on the other hand, is any movement of the body caused by the contraction of skeletal muscles that increases energy expenditure. This can include both home duties and activities like walking the dog. In order to promote more efficient movement, physical therapy makes use of a variety of techniques, including cognitive tactics, which are not usually associated with exercise (Caspersen C. J., 1985).

Over the past twenty years, there has been a significant surge in both clinical and scientific interest in the use of exercise as a remedy for mobility issues in Parkinson's disease patients. A growing body of excellent research is demonstrating specific features of improved mobility following exercise, owing to exciting developments in fundamental science research that point to neurochemical and neuroplastic changes following exercise. Exercise can aid with Parkinson's disease's nonmotor (fatigue, apathy, depression, constipation), motor (gait, balance, strength), and secondary consequences (cardiovascular, osteoporosis) of immobility. This viewpoint essay emphasizes the significance of focused exercise intervention for optimizing the benefits of exercise, especially focusing on current findings about the effects of exercise in increasing mobility (van der Kolk N. M., 2013).

Inducing Neuroplasticity

Aerobic exercise has been found to promote neuroplasticity in healthy individuals, or the brain's capacity for adaptation and change. For those suffering from neurodegenerative illnesses, this may assist to delay the disease's course (Stellmann J. P., 2020).

It is significant to remember that research is currently ongoing to determine the ideal frequency, length, and intensity of aerobic exercise for neurodegenerative illnesses. But moderate-to-intense aerobic activity that raises heart rate might potentially halt Parkinson's disease development. Overall, aerobic exercise has demonstrated promise as a non-pharmacological strategy to alleviate or lessen the symptoms of neurodegenerative disorders without incurring the additional costs or side effects of pharmaceutical therapy. Long-term aerobic exercise has been demonstrated to enhance life quality (Goodman et al., 2016; Mang et al., 2013). the paradigm of persistent aerobic exercise-induced neuroplasticity. The effects of exercise on the body may be quantified using a variety of methods, which can indicate modifications to the structure, function, molecular makeup, and behavior. The following lists the supporting data for each level of this model. Chronic aerobic exercise alters the concentrations of vascular endothelial growth factor (VEGF), insulin-like growth factor 1 (IGF-1) and peripheral brain-derived neurotrophic factor (BDNF) (Cotman and colleagues 2007). According to

Monteggia et al., (2004) and Poo (2001), BDNF stimulates neuroplasticity during development and maturity. The enzyme-ligand immunosuppressant assay (ELISA) can be used to measure it in blood serum or plasma.

Consistent exercise upregulates transcription and signaling cascades and increases the absorption efficiency of BDNF into the central nervous system (CNS) (Currie and others 2009). Cross-sectional studies or research examining the differences between fit and inactive individuals have yielded contradictory results regarding the relationship between fitness and BDNF levels. Certain studies show that individuals with higher Those with high cardiorespiratory fitness and who engage in regular physical activity had lower levels of serum and plasma BDNF (refer to Huang et al., 2014 review). According to Huang et al., (2014), the negative correlation between BDNF and fitness may indicate that increases in fitness are accompanied by improvements in the brain's capacity to absorb BDNF. On the other hand, long-term exercise programs show that after exercise training, serum and plasma BDNF levels rise.

Molecular and cellular alterations brought on by exercise are essential for bringing about structural changes in the brain. Long-term exercise alters cortical regions as revealed by neuroimaging-based differentiation of gray and white matter. In the hippocampus, cerebellum, basal ganglia, cingulate, frontal, parietal, occipital, temporal, and insular cortices, exercise is associated with an increase in gray matter volume. Prolonged activity also increases the volume of the frontal, parietal, and occipital lobes' white matter.

The duration of the intervention and the number of sessions within an intervention are crucial factors to take into account when using long-term fitness programs. It is feasible to recommend likely intervention durations that support modifications in brain architecture and neuronal activity based on the evaluated research. All studies that demonstrated improvements in gray matter volume and brain activity employed the same frequency of exercise sessions in the intervention (i.e., three per week), despite variations in the length of the intervention. Training in aerobic exercise appears to be an effective way to induce neuroplasticity at this frequency.

Balance Training

To enhance physical function and overall health, balance training is advised in addition to strength, cardio, and flexibility activities. The goal of balancing training programs is to improve balance control during daily activities, which will enhance walking speed, decrease fear of falling, and improve fall-related self-efficacy. Improving stability and reducing the risk of falls is one of the main goals of balance training in the treatment of neurodegenerative disorders (Halvarsson A., 2015). Due to diminished sensory input, muscular weakness, and poor proprioception, people with these diseases are more likely to fall. The muscles that govern posture and balance may be strengthened with the use of balancing exercises, which will increase general stability and lower the chance of injury. Programs for training in balance are usually customized to meet the unique requirements and skills of each participant. When creating these plans, physical therapists and rehabilitation experts are essential in considering the patient's present function level and the disease's development (Conradsson D., 2019). Combinations of static and dynamic balancing exercises are common in exercise programs. Examples of such exercises include walking on uneven terrain, standing on one leg, and using stability balls for controlled movements.

Enhancement of cognitive function can be achieved by balance training. Exercises for balance put the brain's capacity to coordinate motions and adjust to changing circumstances to the test. For those suffering from neurodegenerative diseases like Alzheimer's disease, this cognitive engagement can help reduce the rate at which their cognitive function declines. Furthermore, balance training helps lessen anxiety and elevate mood, both of which are prevalent in patients dealing with these difficult circumstances (Dunsky A., 2019).

Crucially, balancing training is included into an all-encompassing management plan rather than existing as a stand-alone treatment. The total plan may also include medication, physical therapy, occupational therapy, and lifestyle changes. In order to keep the exercises interesting and productive, balance training should also be gradual and constant, with frequent monitoring and changes.

Tai Chai

The ancient Chinese mind-body discipline of tai chi has acquired popularity recently due to its possible benefit in the treatment of neurological diseases such multiple sclerosis, Parkinson's disease, and Alzheimer's disease. In order to improve both physical and emotional well-being, this kind of exercise is soft and elegant and incorporates deep breathing, awareness, and slow, flowing movements (Klein P. J., 2008).

Regarding neurodegenerative conditions, tai chi has several advantages. First of all, it helps with balance and coordination, which are frequently hampered under these circumstances. The methodical, slow motions promote a more acute awareness of one's body and lower the danger of falls and associated injuries - which may be especially crippling for those suffering from Parkinson's disease (Wang R., 2022).

Second, studies have indicated that Tai Chi improves memory and cognitive performance. According to studies, practicing Tai Chi on a daily basis may help prevent cognitive loss and perhaps reduce the onset of conditions like Alzheimer's. Tai chi, which cultivates the mind-body link, can improve mental clarity and attention, which enhances overall wellbeing. Tai Chi also functions as a method for stress relief. As too much stress can worsen symptoms and hasten the course of the disease, stress management is crucial to the treatment of neurodegenerative illnesses. Tai Chi incorporates relaxation methods that assist lower the body's stress response, improving the mental and physical well-being of persons who are impacted by these disorders (Wang R., 2022).

Furthermore, Tai Chi is an exercise style that can be modified to accommodate different physical capacities and fitness levels, making it suitable for a broad spectrum of people with neurodegenerative diseases. Being inclusive is crucial because people who have these diseases frequently have limited opportunities for physical activity. According to Nocera J. R. (2013), Tai Chi offers a secure and pleasurable workout option for those who qualify.

Participating in Tai Chi courses or groups frequently fosters the development of a social network of like-minded people dealing with related health challenges. This sense of community helps fight against depressive and isolated thoughts that are frequently linked to neurodegenerative diseases. In a group setting, individuals may trade coping mechanisms, swap experiences, and develop a support network that extends beyond the exercise. In order to manage the emotional components of these diseases, it might be very helpful to establish a mind-body connection. Because of their illness, many people with neurodegenerative disorders feel helpless, anxious, and that they're losing something. The emphasis on mindfulness and relaxation methods in tai chi can improve people's mental health by fostering emotional resilience and a more upbeat attitude on life. In addition, Tai Chi is a gentle, low-impact exercise that is appropriate for individuals of all ages, including the elderly and those with restricted mobility. Because of its inclusivity, people with neurodegenerative disorders can continue to benefit from it and modify their practice to accommodate their evolving physical capabilities. Although tai chi has demonstrated potential in enhancing functionality and quality of life in those with neurodegenerative diseases, it shouldn't be seen as a stand-alone therapy. Included in a complete care plan should be medical supervision and suitable therapies. On the other hand, Tai Chi's holistic approach, which addresses both mental and physical elements, makes it a useful adjunct in the treatment of these difficult disorders. Tai Chi's significance in managing neurodegenerative disorders is likely to become even more established as research in this field develops and becomes more integrated into holistic healthcare approaches (Zhu M., 2020).

Strength Training

For the treatment of many clinical aspects that people with neurodegenerative illnesses exhibit, strength training has been demonstrated to be effective. The following information relates to the use of strength training in the treatment of neurodegenerative diseases:

Alzheimer's Disease

Studies have shown that strength training for six months can help shield brain regions that are particularly susceptible to Alzheimer's disease up to a year later. The long-term study discovered that strength training improved cognitive function generally and was associated with protection against hippocampal atrophy in certain subregions. One intricate brain structure that plays a key part in memory and learning is the hippocampus. Strength training was intended to target certain hippocampal subregions that were more susceptible to Alzheimer's disease (Ahlskog J. E., 2011).

Multiple Sclerosis

Increasing muscular strength in multiple sclerosis can be achieved by strength training. It is believed that central (spinal and supraspinal) and muscle deficiencies underlie the strength impairments associated with multiple sclerosis (Cruickshank T. M., 2015).

Parkinson's Disease

Increasing muscular strength during strength training is helpful for those with Parkinson's disease. Strength impairments in Parkinson's disease are believed to be solely the product of cerebral deficiencies. Strength training, when done against a resistance other than body weight, has been shown to be beneficial in reducing motor and nonmotor symptoms in people with Parkinson's disease, according to a systematic review and meta-analysis of the subject (Ramazzina I., 2017).

Resistance Training

Research has shown that resistance training is an easy and reasonably priced treatment for Alzheimer's sufferers. Resistance training for a brief period of time enhanced cognitive performance in 3xTg mice and had positive impacts on neuroinflammation, tau and amyloid pathology, and synaptic plasticity. Another workout regimen for slowing the course of Alzheimer's disease may be resistance training. In an animal model of Alzheimer's disease, resistance training also reverses the atrophy of skeletal muscle and increases the content of satellite cells.

In general, it has been discovered that strength training is an effective treatment for a number of the clinical symptoms that people with neurodegenerative diseases exhibit. It can improve muscular strength in multiple sclerosis and Parkinson's disease, protect brain regions susceptible to Alzheimer's disease, and slow the illness's progression in Alzheimer's disease (Liu Y., 2020).

The Effects of Exercise on Physical Function

Exercise has a significant effect on many facets of human health and wellbeing, including quality of life, mood, motor function, brain structure and function, physical skills, and even the likelihood of being institutionalized. The significance of consistent physical exercise as the foundation of a healthy lifestyle is highlighted by these benefits (Mandolesi L., 2018).

Firstly, improving motor function is greatly aided by exercise. Frequent exercise maintains and enhances fine motor abilities, balance, and coordination. It can promote independence and lower the risk of accidents and injuries by preventing or lessening the decrease in motor function that is frequently linked to aging.

Exercise has a major impact on the structure and function of the brain as well. Research indicates that it can promote the development of new neurons and enhance synaptic plasticity, which can enhance cognitive abilities including memory, attention, and executive functioning. Furthermore, exercise can help maintain a healthy brain structure throughout an individual's life and shield the brain against age-related illnesses like Alzheimer's (Gomez-Pinilla F., 2013).

Fitness, strength, and endurance are all aspects of physical function that are significantly impacted by exercise. higher muscular growth, better cardiovascular health, and higher stamina are the results of regular exercise. Higher levels of physical independence result from this, making it easier for people to carry out everyday duties and lowering their chance of developing physical disabilities. The impact of exercise on mood and mental health is well-established. Stress, anxiety, and sadness are lessened when physical exercise releases endorphins and other mood-enhancing neurotransmitters. Frequent exercise can have a strong antidepressant effect on the body and mind, enhancing mental clarity and overall wellbeing (Pinckard K., 2019).

Exercise also significantly improves quality of life. An individual's general sense of contentment and happiness is closely correlated with maintaining their physical and mental health. People who have improved physical and cognitive performance may participate in a greater variety of activities, which leads to a more satisfying and joyful existence. Finally, exercise has an impact on institutionalization risk, especially for older persons. Regular physical exercise can postpone or even eliminate the need for long-term care in assisted living facilities or nursing homes by maintaining cognitive and physical abilities. This protects human liberty and dignity while also lessening the financial burden on people and society (McPhee J. S., 2016).

Recommendations and Guidelines for an Exercise Prescription Based on Individual Characteristics

For people with neurodegenerative diseases, exercise can be a useful non-pharmacological method to improve cognitive performance, delay deterioration, and improve quality of life. A variety of illnesses are included in the category of neurodegenerative disorders, including multiple sclerosis (MS), Alzheimer's disease, Parkinson's disease, amyotrophic lateral sclerosis (ALS), and Huntington's disease. Every one of these ailments offers different difficulties and things to keep in mind while prescribing exercise. Exercise recommendations, however, must be customized for each patient's unique needs (Santiago J. A., 2023).

Type of Exercise

For individuals with neurodegenerative illnesses, aerobic, resistance, and balance training are advised. For instance, in individuals with Parkinson's disease (PD), aerobic exercise can significantly raise the evoked dopamine release in the caudate nucleus and the ventral striatum's responsiveness. Patients suffering from multiple sclerosis (MS) may find that their muscular strength and function improve with resistance training. For PD patients, balance training can lower their chance of falling.

Exercise Intensity

The degree of exercise should be adjusted based on the patient's fitness level and the severity of their illness. For instance, people with MS are advised to engage in low-to-moderate intensity exercise, but those with Parkinson's disease may benefit from high-intensity exercise (Sacheli M. A., 2019).

Exercise Duration

The length of time spent exercising should also be customized based on the fitness level and severity of the ailment in the individual. For instance, it is advised that MS patients engage in 30 minutes a day of moderate-intensity aerobic activity.

Exercise Frequency

The amount of exercise a person does should be based on their degree of fitness and the severity of their illness. For instance, it is advised that PD patients engage in aerobic activity three to five days a week (Kim Y., 2019).

Safety Concerns

When recommending exercise to people suffering from neurodegenerative diseases, safety concerns need to be taken into mind. Exercise should be done in a cool atmosphere since people with MS may be heat intolerant. Balance training should be carried out under the guidance of a healthcare provider since patients with Parkinson's disease (PD) may experience balance problems. Because neurodegenerative illnesses affect motor skills and balance, people may be more likely to fall and sustain injuries. Perhaps supervision is required. When exercising, think about using assistive technology to help with balance and movement, such walkers or canes.

Other Non-Pharmacological Interventions

In addition to physical therapy, there are a number of different non-pharmacological therapies that are intended to improve the general well-being of those living with these disorders, slow down the disease's course, and increase their quality of life (Berg Weger M., 2017). Several important non-pharmacological therapies for neurodegenerative diseases consist of:

Occupational Therapy

OTs assist patients in regaining or preserving their capacity to carry out routine tasks including eating, taking a shower, and getting dressed. In order to compensate for cognitive and motor deficits, they provide adaptive approaches and technologies that enhance independence and quality of life.

Speech and Language Therapy

Communication problems can arise in people suffering from illnesses such as frontotemporal dementia or Alzheimer's disease. In order to promote improved social interaction and nutrition, speech therapists focus on enhancing speech, language, and swallowing abilities (Dixon L., 2007).

Cognitive Rehabilitation

Neurodegenerative diseases frequently result in cognitive impairment. A variety of methods are used in cognitive rehabilitation to improve executive functioning, memory, attention, and problem-solving skills. People can efficiently handle daily chores with the use of cognitive exercises and methods (Barman A., 2016).

Psychological Counseling

Receiving a neurodegenerative diagnosis can have a significant emotional impact. Support, coping mechanisms, and psychotherapy are offered by psychologists and counselors to treat the sadness, anxiety, and stress that frequently accompany these diseases. Counseling aids in coping with the difficulties for families and carers as well (Barman A., 2016).

Social Support and Education

Individuals and their families can greatly benefit from social support groups and educational initiatives. These discussion boards assist patients and their caregivers in navigating the intricacies of their illness by providing emotional support, a feeling of community, and information exchange.

Diet and Nutrition

People with neurodegenerative diseases can benefit from a balanced diet that is customized to meet their unique needs, since it can improve their general health. Nutritionists offer advice on food selections that can help control symptoms and preserve ideal body weight and energy levels.

Music and Art Therapy

These forms of creative therapy offer a means of expressing emotions while also stimulating the mind. By involving patients in engaging activities, these therapies might enhance their mood and cognitive abilities.

Mindfulness and Relaxation Techniques

Stress can be reduced, and general well-being can be enhanced through practices like mindfulness and meditation. They could also aid in the management of symptoms including anxiety and sleep problems.

Conclusion

Interventions including medication and physical therapy play an important role in the treatment of neurodegenerative disorders. Despite the fact that there is now no treatment for these illnesses, medications can aid in the management of Parkinson's disease (PD) motor symptoms, however they may have unfavorable side effects. In adult neurologic populations, secondary prevention management strategies are required to prevent further decline in health and to promote health. Parkinson's disease, multiple sclerosis (MS), and Huntington's disease are examples of neurodegenerative disorders. Non-pharmacological treatments like physical activity and lifestyle changes have also been investigated as potential remedies. In order to cure neurodegenerative disorders, a combination of strategies may work best.

The chapter emphasizes the need for a comprehensive strategy that combines pharmaceutical treatments with physical therapy techniques for the clinical management of neurodegenerative illnesses. Healthcare professionals can work to provide comprehensive care that not only manages symptoms but also improves patients' overall well-being and functional capacity by addressing the complex and multifaceted nature of these disorders. In the end, this can give patients affected by these debilitating conditions hope and an improved quality of life.

Disclaimer

None.

References

Ahlskog, J. Eric, Yonas E. Geda, Neill R. Graff-Radford, and Ronald C. Petersen. 2011. "Physical Exercise as a Preventive or Disease-Modifying Treatment of Dementia and Brain Aging." *Mayo Clinic Proceedings* 86 (9): 876–84. https://doi.org/10.4065/mcp.2011.0252.

Albright, A. Leland. "Topical review: Baclofen in the treatment of cerebral palsy." *Journal of Child Neurology* 11, no. 2 (1996): 77-83.

Barman, A., Ahana Chatterjee, and Rohit Bhide. 2016. "Cognitive Impairment and Rehabilitation Strategies after Traumatic Brain Injury." *Indian Journal of Psychological Medicine* 38 (3): 172–81. https://doi.org/10.4103/0253-7176.183086.

Berg-Weger, M., and Daniel B. Stewart. "Non-pharmacologic interventions for persons with dementia." *Missouri medicine* 114, no. 2 (2017): 116.

Bonanni, R., Ida Cariati, Umberto Tarantino, Giovanna D'Arcangelo, and Virginia Tancredi. 2022. "Physical Exercise and Health: A Focus on Its Protective Role in Neurodegenerative Diseases." *Journal of Functional Morphology and Kinesiology* 7 (2): 38. https://doi.org/10.3390/jfmk7020038.

Carbone, F., AtbinDjamshidian, Klaus Seppi, and Werner Poewe. "Apomorphine for Parkinson's disease: efficacy and safety of current and new formulations." *CNS drugs* 33 (2019): 905-918.

Caspersen, C. J., Kenneth E. Powell, and Gregory M. Christenson. "Physical activity, exercise, and physical fitness: definitions and distinctions for health-related research." *Public health reports* 100, no. 2 (1985): 126.

Cass, S. P. 2017. "Alzheimer's Disease and Exercise." *Current Sports Medicine Reports* 16 (1): 19–22. https://doi.org/10.1249/jsr.0000000000000332.

Castellano-Tejedor, C. 2022. "Non-Pharmacological Interventions for the Management of Chronic Health Conditions and Non-Communicable Diseases." *International Journal of Environmental Research and Public Health* 19 (14): 8536. https://doi.org/10.3390/ijerph19148536.

Chang, C., and Kamleshun Ramphul. 2019. "Amantadine." *Nih.gov.* StatPearls Publishing. October 12, 2019. https://www.ncbi.nlm.nih.gov/books/NBK499953/.

Chhabra, C., Kaur, H., Bano, S., & Bhattacharjee, B. (2023). Recent Advancements In Physiotherapy for Parkinsons disease. In *Recent Advances in* Physiotherapy (Vol. 1, pp. 199–215). Kayva Publishers.

Coleman, J. J, and Sarah K Pontefract. 2016. "Adverse Drug Reactions." *Clinical Medicine* 16 (5): 481–85. https://doi.org/10.7861/clinmedicine.16-5-481.

Colovic, M. B., Danijela Z. Krstic, Tamara D. Lazarevic-Pasti, Aleksandra M. Bondzic, and Vesna M. Vasic. 2013. "Acetylcholinesterase Inhibitors: Pharmacology and Toxicology." *Current Neuropharmacology* 11 (3): 315–35. https://doi.org/10.2174/1570159x11311030006.

Conradsson, D., and Alexandra Halvarsson. 2019. "The Effects of Dual-Task Balance Training on Gait in Older Women with Osteoporosis: A Randomized Controlled Trial." *Gait & Posture* 68 (February): 562–68. https://doi.org/10.1016/j.gaitpost.2019.01.005.

Cruickshank, T.M., Alvaro R. Reyes, and Melanie R. Ziman. 2015. "A Systematic Review and Meta-Analysis of Strength Training in Individuals with Multiple Sclerosis or Parkinson Disease." *Medicine* 94 (4): e411. https://doi.org/10.1097/md.0000000000000411.

Deng, W., James B. Aimone, and Fred H. Gage. 2010. "New Neurons and New Memories: How Does Adult Hippocampal Neurogenesis Affect Learning and Memory?" *Nature Reviews Neuroscience* 11 (5): 339–50. https://doi.org/10.1038/nrn 2822.

Dixon, L., Dawn C Duncan, Paul Johnson, Liz Kirkby, Helen O'Connell, Hilary J Taylor, and Katherine Deane. 2007. "Occupational Therapy for Patients with Parkinson's Disease." *The Cochrane Database of Systematic Reviews* 2007 (3). https://doi.org/10.1002/14651858.CD002813.pub2.

Dunsky, A. 2019. "The Effect of Balance and Coordination Exercises on Quality of Life in Older Adults: A Mini-Review." *Frontiers in Aging Neuroscience* 11 (318). https://doi.org/10.3389/fnagi.2019.00318.

Erkkinen, M. G., Mee-Ohk Kim, and Michael D. Geschwind. 2018. "Clinical Neurology and Epidemiology of the Major Neurodegenerative Diseases." *Cold Spring Harbor Perspectives in Biology* 10 (4): a033118. https://doi.org/10.1101/cshperspect.a033118.

Farì, G., Paola Lunetti, Giovanni Pignatelli, Maria Vittoria Raele, Alessandra Cera, Giulia Mintrone, Maurizio Ranieri, Marisa Megna, and Loredana Capobianco. 2021. "The Effect of Physical Exercise on Cognitive Impairment in Neurodegenerative Disease: From Pathophysiology to Clinical and Rehabilitative Aspects." *International Journal of Molecular Sciences* 22 (21): 11632. https://doi.org/10.3390/ijms222111632.

Ghanavatian, S., and Armen Derian. 2019. "Baclofen." *Nih.gov.* StatPearls Publishing. October 2019. https://www.ncbi.nlm.nih.gov/books/NBK526037/.

Gomez-Pinilla, F., and Charles Hillman. 2013. "The Influence of Exercise on Cognitive Abilities." *Comprehensive Physiology* 3 (1). https://doi.org/10.1002/cphy.c110063.

Grossberg, G. T. 2003. "Cholinesterase Inhibitors for the Treatment of Alzheimer's Disease": *Current Therapeutic Research* 64 (4): 216–35. https://doi.org/10.1016/s0011-393x(03)00059-6.

Halvarsson, A., Ing-Mari Dohrn, and Agneta Ståhle. 2014. "Taking Balance Training for Older Adults One Step Further: The Rationale for and a Description of a Proven Balance Training Programme." *Clinical Rehabilitation* 29 (5): 417–25. https://doi.org/10.1177/0269215514546770.

Herholz, S. C, Regina S Herholz, and Karl Herholz. 2013. "Non-Pharmacological Interventions and Neuroplasticity in Early Stage Alzheimer's Disease." *Expert Review of Neurotherapeutics* 13 (11): 1235–45. https://doi.org/10.1586/14737175.2013.845086.

Hou, Y., Xiuli Dan, Mansi Babbar, Yong Wei, Steen G. Hasselbalch, Deborah L. Croteau, and Vilhelm A. Bohr. 2019. "Ageing as a Risk Factor for Neurodegenerative Disease." Nature Reviews. *Neurology* 15 (10): 565–81. https://doi.org/10.1038/s41582-019-0244-7.

Irvine, G. B., Omar M. El-Agnaf, Ganesh M. Shankar, and Dominic M. Walsh. 2008. "Protein Aggregation in the Brain: The Molecular Basis for Alzheimer's and

Parkinson's Diseases." *Molecular Medicine* 14 (7-8): 451–64. https://doi.org/10.2119/2007-00100.irvine.

Johnson, J. W., and Shawn E. Kotermanski. "Mechanism of action of memantine." *Current opinion in pharmacology* 6, no. 1 (2006): 61-67.

Kabir, Tanvir, Md. Sahab Uddin, Abdullah Al Mamun, Philippe Jeandet, Lotfi Aleya, Rasha A. Mansouri, Ghulam Md Ashraf, Bijo Mathew, May N. Bin-Jumah, and Mohamed M. Abdel-Daim. 2020. "Combination Drug Therapy for the Management of Alzheimer's Disease." *International Journal of Molecular Sciences* 21 (9). https://doi.org/10.3390/ijms21093272.

Kandiah, N., Ming-Chyi Pai, VorapunSenanarong, Irene Looi, Encarnita Ampil, Kyung Won Park, Ananda Krishna Karanam, and Stephen Christopher. 2017. "Rivastigmine: The Advantages of Dual Inhibition of Acetylcholinesterase and Butyrylcholinesterase and Its Role in Subcortical Vascular Dementia and Parkinson's Disease Dementia." *Clinical Interventions in Aging* Volume 12 (April): 697–707. https://doi.org/10.2147/cia.s129145.

Kavirajan, H., and Lon S Schneider. 2007. "Efficacy and Adverse Effects of Cholinesterase Inhibitors and Memantine in Vascular Dementia: A Meta-Analysis of Randomised Controlled Trials." *The Lancet Neurology* 6 (9): 782–92. https://doi.org/10.1016/s1474-4422(07)70195-3.

Kim, J., Hyun-ju Lee, Seon Kyeong Park, Jin-Hee Park, Ha-Ram Jeong, Soojung Lee, Heeyong Lee, Eunyoung Seol, and Hyang-Sook Hoe. 2021. "Donepezil Regulates LPS and Aβ-Stimulated Neuroinflammation through MAPK/NLRP3 Inflammasome/STAT3 Signaling." *International Journal of Molecular Sciences* 22 (19): 10637. https://doi.org/10.3390/ijms221910637.

Kim, Y., Byron Lai, Tapan Mehta, Mohanraj Thirumalai, Sangeetha Padalabalanarayanan, James H. Rimmer, and Robert W. Motl. 2019. "Exercise Training Guidelines for Multiple Sclerosis, Stroke, and Parkinson Disease." *American Journal of Physical Medicine & Rehabilitation* 98 (7): 613–21. https://doi.org/10.1097/phm.0000000000001174.

Klein, P. J. 2008. "Tai Chi Chuan in the Management of Parkinson's Disease and Alzheimer's Disease." *Medicine and Sport Science,* 173–81. https://doi.org/10.1159/000134298.

Kolk, N. M. van der, and Laurie A. King. 2013. "Effects of Exercise on Mobility in People with Parkinson's Disease." *Movement Disorders* 28 (11): 1587–96. https://doi.org/10.1002/mds.25658.

Kumar, A. and Sandeep Sharma. 2019. "Donepezil." *Nih.gov.* StatPearls Publishing. May 23, 2019. https://www.ncbi.nlm.nih.gov/books/NBK513257/.

Lamptey, R. Nii Lante, Bivek Chaulagain, Riddhi Trivedi, Avinash Gothwal, Buddhadev Layek, and Jagdish Singh. 2022. "A Review of the Common Neurodegenerative Disorders: Current Therapeutic Approaches and the Potential Role of Nanotherapeutics." *International Journal of Molecular Sciences* 23 (3): 1851. https://doi.org/10.3390/ijms23031851.

Leyden, E., and Prasanna Tadi. 2020. "Carbidopa." *PubMed.* Treasure Island (FL): StatPearls Publishing. 2020. https://www.ncbi.nlm.nih.gov/books/NBK554552/.

Liu, Y., John Man Tak Chu, Tim Yan, Yan Zhang, Ying Chen, Raymond Chuen Chung Chang, and Gordon Tin Chun Wong. 2020. "Short-Term Resistance Exercise Inhibits Neuroinflammation and Attenuates Neuropathological Changes in 3xTg Alzheimer's Disease Mice." *Journal of Neuroinflammation* 17 (1). https://doi.org/10.1186/s12974-019-1653-7.

Ma, J., Mingzhe Zhao, Wei Zhou, Mo Li, Cong Huai, Lu Shen, Ting Wang, et al., 2021. "Association between the COMT Val158Met Polymorphism and Antipsychotic Efficacy in Schizophrenia: An Updated Meta-Analysis." *Current Neuropharmacology* 19 (10): 1780–90. https://doi.org/10.2174/1570159x18666201023154049.

Mahalakshmi, B., Nancy Maurya, Shin-Da Lee, and V. Bharath Kumar. 2020. "Possible Neuroprotective Mechanisms of Physical Exercise in Neurodegeneration." *International Journal of Molecular Sciences* 21 (16): 5895. https://doi.org/10.3390/ijms21165895.

Mandolesi, L., Arianna Polverino, Simone Montuori, Francesca Foti, Giampaolo Ferraioli, Pierpaolo Sorrentino, and Giuseppe Sorrentino. 2018. "Effects of Physical Exercise on Cognitive Functioning and Wellbeing: Biological and Psychological Benefits." *Frontiers in Psychology* 9 (9). https://doi.org/10.3389/fpsyg.2018.00509.

McPhee, J. S., David P. French, Dean Jackson, James Nazroo, Neil Pendleton, and Hans Degens. 2016. "Physical Activity in Older Age: Perspectives for Healthy Ageing and Frailty." *Biogerontology* 17 (3): 567–80. https://doi.org/10.1007/s10522-016-9641-0.

Molinari, C., Vera Morsanuto, Sara Ruga, Felice Notte, MahitabFarghali, Rebecca Galla, and Francesca Uberti. 2020. "The Role of BDNF on Aging-Modulation Markers." *Brain Sciences* 10 (5): 285. https://doi.org/10.3390/brainsci10050285.

Najib, J. 2001. "Entacapone: A Catechol-O-Methyltransferase Inhibitor for the Adjunctive Treatment of Parkinson's Disease." *Clinical Therapeutics* 23 (6): 802–32. https://doi.org/10.1016/s0149-2918(01)80071-0.

Okigbo, A. A., Michael S. Helkowski, Brittany J. Royes, Isabel H. Bleimeister, Tracey R. Lam, Gina C. Bao, Jeffrey P. Cheng, Corina O. Bondi, and Anthony E. Kline. "Dose-Dependent Neurorestorative Effects of Amantadine after Cortical Impact Injury." *Neuroscience Letters* 694 (February 2019): 69–73. https://doi.org/10.1016/j.neulet.2018.11.030.

Olivares, D., Varun K Deshpande, Ying Shi, Debomoy K Lahiri, Nigel H Greig, Jack T Rogers, and Xudong Huang. 2012. "N-Methyl D-Aspartate (NMDA) Receptor Antagonists and Memantine Treatment for Alzheimer's Disease, Vascular Dementia and Parkinson's Disease." *Current Alzheimer Research* 9 (6): 746–58. https://doi.org/10.2174/156720512801322564.

Pinckard, K., Kedryn K. Baskin, and Kristin I. Stanford. 2019. "Effects of Exercise to Improve Cardiovascular Health." *Frontiers in Cardiovascular Medicine* 6 (69). https://doi.org/10.3389/fcvm.2019.00069.

Pinder, R. M., R. N. Brogden, T. M. Speight, and G. S. Avery. 1977. "Dantrolene Sodium." *Drugs* 13 (1): 3–23. https://doi.org/10.2165/00003495-197713010-00002.

Rabins, P. V., and Constantine G Lyketsos. 2006. "Cholinesterase Inhibitors and Memantine Have a Role in the Treatment of Alzheimer's Disease." *Nature Clinical Practice Neurology* 2 (11): 578–79. https://doi.org/10.1038/ncpneuro0269.

Ramazzina, I., Benedetta Bernazzoli, and Cosimo Costantino. 2017. "Systematic Review on Strength Training in Parkinson's Disease: An Unsolved Question." *Clinical Interventions in Aging* Volume 12 (March): 619–28. https://doi.org/10.2147/cia.s131903.

Regensburger, M., Chi Wang Ip, Zacharias Kohl, Christoph Schrader, Peter P Urban, Jan Kassubek, and Wolfgang H Jost. 2023. "Clinical Benefit of MAO-B and COMT Inhibition in Parkinson's Disease: Practical Considerations." *Journal of Neural Transmission* 130 (6): 847–61. https://doi.org/10.1007/s00702-023-02623-8.

Rodakowski, J., Ester Saghafi, Meryl A. Butters, and Elizabeth R. Skidmore. 2015. "Non-Pharmacological Interventions for Adults with Mild Cognitive Impairment and Early Stage Dementia: An Updated Scoping Review." *Molecular Aspects of Medicine* 43-44 (June): 38–53. https://doi.org/10.1016/j.mam.2015.06.003.

Sacheli, M. A., Jason L. Neva, Bimal Lakhani, Danielle K. Murray, Nasim Vafai, Elham Shahinfard, Carolyn English, et al., 2019. "Exercise Increases Caudate Dopamine Release and Ventral Striatal Activation in Parkinson's Disease." *Movement Disorders: Official Journal of the Movement Disorder Society* 34 (12): 1891–1900. https://doi.org/10.1002/mds.27865.

Santiago, J. A., and Judith A. Potashkin. 2023. "*Physical Activity and Lifestyle Modifications in the Treatment of Neurodegenerative Diseases*" 15 (May). https://doi.org/10.3389/fnagi.2023.1185671.

Shin, C. Y., Hae-Sun Kim, Kwang-Ho Cha, Dong Han Won, Ji-Yun Lee, Sun Woo Jang, and Uy Dong Sohn. 2018. "The Effects of Donepezil, an Acetylcholinesterase Inhibitor, on Impaired Learning and Memory in Rodents." *Biomolecules & Therapeutics* 26 (3): 274–81. https://doi.org/10.4062/biomolther.2017.189.

Shinichi A., Joe R Nocera, and Srikanth VVallabhajosula Chris J Hass. 2013. "Tai Chi Exercise to Improve Non-Motor Symptoms of Parkinson's Disease." *Journal of Yoga & Physical Therapy* 03 (03). https://doi.org/10.4172/2157-7595.1000137.

Shukla, S., and Babu L. Tekwani. 2020. "Histone Deacetylases Inhibitors in Neurodegenerative Diseases, Neuroprotection and Neuronal Differentiation." *Frontiers in Pharmacology* 11 (April). https://doi.org/10.3389/fphar.2020.00537.

Stellmann, J. P., Adil Maarouf, Karl-Heinz Schulz, Lisa Baquet, Jana Pöttgen, Stefan Patra, Iris-Katharina Penner, et al., 2020. "Aerobic Exercise Induces Functional and Structural Reorganization of CNS Networks in Multiple Sclerosis: A Randomized Controlled Trial." *Frontiers in Human Neuroscience* 14 (June). https://doi.org/10.3389/fnhum.2020.00255.

Tello, J. A., Haley E. Williams, Robert M. Eppler, Michelle L. Steinhilb, and May Khanna. 2022. "Animal Models of Neurodegenerative Disease: Recent Advances in Fly Highlight Innovative Approaches to Drug Discovery." *Frontiers in Molecular Neuroscience* 15 (April). https://doi.org/10.3389/fnmol.2022.883358.

U.S. Department of Health and Human Services. Neurodegenerative Diseases. *National Institute of Environmental Health Sciences.* https://www.niehs.nih.gov/research/supported/health/neurodegenerative/index.cfm

Wang, R., Hao Zhou, Yu-Chen Wang, Xiao-Long Chang, and Xue-Qiang Wang. 2022. "Benefits of Tai Chi Quan on Neurodegenerative Diseases: A Systematic Review."

Ageing Research Reviews 82 (December): 101741. https://doi.org/10.1016/j.arr.2022.101741.

Willenborg, B., André Schmoller, J Caspary, Uwe H Melchert, Harald G Scholand-Engler, Kamila Jauch-Chara, Fritz Hohagen, Ulrich Schweiger, and Kerstin M Oltmanns. 2011. "Memantine Prevents Hypoglycemia-Induced Decrements of the Cerebral Energy Status in Healthy Subjects." *The Journal of Clinical Endocrinology and Metabolism* 96 (2): E384–88. https://doi.org/10.1210/jc.2010-1348.

Yang, H. S., Jae Moon Choi, Junyong In, Tae-Yun Sung, Yong Beom Kim, and Shofina Sultana. 2023. "Current Clinical Application of Dantrolene Sodium." *Anesthesia and Pain Medicine* 18 (3): 220–32. https://doi.org/10.17085/apm.22260.

Yiannopoulou, K. G., Aikaterini I. Anastasiou, Venetia Zachariou, and Sygkliti-Henrietta Pelidou. 2019. "Reasons for Failed Trials of Disease-Modifying Treatments for Alzheimer Disease and Their Contribution in Recent Research." *Biomedicines* 7 (4): 97. https://doi.org/10.3390/biomedicines7040097.

Zhu, H., Henrique Lemos, Brinda Bhatt, Bianca N. Islam, Abhijit Singh, Ashish Gurav, Lei Huang, et al., 2017. "Carbidopa, a Drug in Use for Management of Parkinson Disease Inhibits T Cell Activation and Autoimmunity." *PloS One* 12 (9): e0183484. https://doi.org/10.1371/journal.pone.0183484.

Zhu, M., Yonghua Zhang, Jiafei Pan, Changyong Fu, and Yaqun Wang. 2020. "Effect of Simplified Tai Chi Exercise on Relieving Symptoms of Patients with Mild to Moderate Parkinson's Disease." *The Journal of Sports Medicine and Physical Fitness* 60 (2). https://doi.org/10.23736/s0022-4707.19.10104-1.

Chapter 17

Nanocarrier-Based Approaches for Alzheimer's Disease Treatment

Farheen[1],
Debashish Paramanick[1],
Deepika Modi[1],
Swati Arya[2,*]
and Subodh Kumar Dubey[3]

[1]School of Medical Allied Sciences, K. R Mangalam University Sohna Gurugram, Haryana, India
[2]SGT College of Pharmacy, Shree Guru Gobind Singh Tricentenary University, Badli Road Chandu, Budhera, Gurugram, Haryana, India
[3]School of Pharmacy, ITM University, Gwalior, M. P., India

Abstract

Alzheimer's disease (AD) is a progressive neurodegenerative disorder marked by cognitive decline, memory loss, and impaired daily functioning, making it the primary cause of dementia. Amyloid beta and tau proteins' accumulation, resulting in disrupted neuronal communication and dysfunction. Genetic mutations in APP, PSEN1, and PSEN2 genes are associated with familial AD cases, while sporadic cases stem from intricate interactions between genetics and the environment. Current treatments, although lacking a cure, manage symptoms and slow progression, such as Donepezil, Rivastigmine, Galantamine, which are cholinesterase inhibitors which are used to slow the propagation of disease. Whereas many drugs are reported potency to treat AD however

* Corresponding Author's Email: aryaswati2020@gmail.com.

In: Neurogenerative Disorders
Editors: Mohit Agrawal, Manmohan Singhal, Amit Kumar Nayak et al.
ISBN: 979-8-89530-143-2

enzymatic degradation, Slow bioavailability and poor BBB permeability are major obstacles in treatments of AD. Nanotechnology has emerged as a promising avenue for enhancing drug delivery to the brain, overcoming BBB limitations, enhancing drug delivery, and targeting key pathological features. The unique capabilities of nanocarriers offer a promising avenue to address the challenges associated with delivering therapeutic agents to the brain, ultimately enhancing the efficacy of interventions for this complex neurodegenerative disorder. Nanocarriers, such as nanoparticles and liposomes, nanotubes, Micelles, Dendrimers, Nanocrystals, Nanogels and Exosomes act as microscopic delivery vehicles, ferrying therapeutic payloads across this barrier and precisely releasing them at the intended site of action. These minuscule carriers are engineered to encapsulate various types of drugs, including small molecules and nucleic acids, providing protection and controlled release. Additionally, nanocarriers can be functionalized with specific ligands or antibodies, allowing them to selectively recognize and bind to pathological targets, such as amyloid-beta plaques or tau protein tangles. In this chapter we will cover challenges of brain drug delivery and modern impact of nanotechnology for treatment of AD.

Keywords: Alzheimer's, neurodegenerative disorder, nanocarrier, blood-brain barrier, drug delivery, amyloid-beta, tau protein, neuroinflammation, therapeutic targeting

Introduction

Alzheimer's disease (AD) is a neurodegenerative disorder that disturbs motor and cognitive function and may lead to complete disability and the death of neurons. It affects the function of the central nervous system (Bollen & Prickaerts, 2012). More than 6 million people are suffering from AD in America, and that number will increase to 6.5 million in 2022, whereas it will reach up to 12.7 million in 2050(Alzheimer's Association, 2021). According to recent findings, AD has become the 7th leading cause of death after other diseases in the United States (Tahami Monfared et al., 2022). Whereas it is estimated that the number of people with the disease in India will increase significantly in the coming years. Dementia is a neurological syndrome caused by AD that affects the brain. Memory impairment is one of the most common symptoms of dementia. There is a 3% prevalence of dementia in people aged 65 to 75 years of age, but it will rise to 19% at 75 to 85 years of age in AD, memory impairment is often one of the first symptoms to be noticed. As the disease progresses, people with AD may become confused and disoriented and may have difficulty remembering recent events, recognizing people, handling money, and other everyday tasks (Schönecker et al., 2018). It starts with the hippocampus, a brain region that plays a key role in learning and memory. Damage to the hippocampus can lead to memory loss and cognitive decline. AD is thought to originate in the hippocampus and then spread to other parts of the brain (Ju et al., 2023). The actual cause of the disease is still unknown. However, the most accepted hallmark of Alzheimer's disease is the presence of neurofibrillary tangles (NFTs) and senile plaques (SPs) in the brain. NFTs are made up of twisted, thread-like proteins called tau, and SPs are clusters of a protein called beta-amyloid (Sehar et al., 2022, Theerasri et al., n.d.). There is no drug to cure AD; however, there are drugs available to manage the symptoms, such as Cholinesterase inhibitors (Donepezil, Rivastigmine, and Galantamine) are a class of drugs that are used to treat Alzheimer's disease. They work by blocking the action of the enzyme cholinesterase, which breaks down acetylcholine. This results in an increase in the amount of acetylcholine in the brain, which is thought to be beneficial in treating Alzheimer's disease (Grossberg, 2003). Furthermore, NMDA receptor antagonists are being studied as potential treatments for Alzheimer's disease. The rationale for this approach is that over-activation of NMDA receptors may play a role in the development of the disease. Drugs that block NMDA receptors could help protect neurons from damage (Colović et al., 2013). These drugs are effective for mild to moderate Alzheimer disease, but they are not effective for severe Alzheimer disease. The cholinesterase inhibitors may also cause side effects such as nausea, vomiting, diarrhea, and muscle cramps. They also have low permeability, poor bioavailability.

Recently, nanotechnology has been playing an emerging approach for diagnosis and treatment of AD. Uses of nanotechnology improved drug permeability, pharmacokinetic profile such as bioavailability. Nanotechnology advancements have led to the development of various nano-drug delivery systems, enabling precise drug delivery to specific molecular targets and sites of action. The controlled and safe release of drugs through these systems reduces the required dosage. Such as Baysal et al., developed Donepezil loaded PLGA-b-PEG nanoparticles via double emulsion method. Their result suggested that developed nanoparticles easily cross the BBB and showed control release manner of Donepezil (Baysal et al., 2017). Furthermore, Fazil et al., prepared rivastigmine loaded chitosan nanoparticles by ionic gelation method for brain delivery. Their result suggested that rivastigmine loaded chitosan nanoparticles have easily crossed BBB as compared to free rivastigmine (Fazil et al., 2012). Despite the progress made in AD research, reliable treatments remain limited. Further investigation is needed to better understand the mechanisms involved in these disorders. However, due to the growing aging population worldwide, there is an urgent need to accelerate diagnostic and therapeutic approaches for neurodegenerative diseases. This chapter aims to provide an overview of AD, discuss current obstacles and available strategies for overcoming them, and explore the status of nanomaterials and their application in drug delivery systems for neurological disorders.

Pathophysiology

The pathophysiology of AD has been intensely examined; however, the mechanisms of AD remaine unclear. Genetically, AD can be classified into two types first Based on early onset familial AD and other is Late onset sporadic AD. Histopathological study of AD brain suggested that two misfolded proteins of APP are responsible for AD propagation. The first one is β Amyloids (Aβ) are accumulated between the neuronal cells, these accumulated Aβ form plaques and small oligomers. APP was first reported as a genetic cause for early onset familial AD. Many studies targeted this pathway directly or indirectly via small molecules, antibiotics, nanomedicine for reduction of Aβ or clearance of Aβ. The second misfolded protein is TAU which aggregates in neuronal cells (shown in Figure 1) and makes neurofibrillary tangles (Paramanick et al., 2022). However, the majority of the population of AD do not involve mutation of the APP pathway for this population most predictive genetic factor is APO E4. The presence of the APO E4 allele has been observed in about 70% of those diagnosed with AD. Individuals who possess two copies of the E4 allele are at an elevated risk for the development of AD Additionally, it has been observed that there is a heightened susceptibility to cognitive impairment and dementia in elderly adults without AD (Kim et al., 2009). Although the exact method by which it raises the risk for AD is unknown, it is assumed to include changes in the APo E4 protein's synthesis or functionality. More than 50% of patients with frontotemporal dementia have been discovered to have the APO E4 allele. The chance of getting Lewy body dementia is substantially higher in people who carry two E4 alleles (Najm et al., 2019).

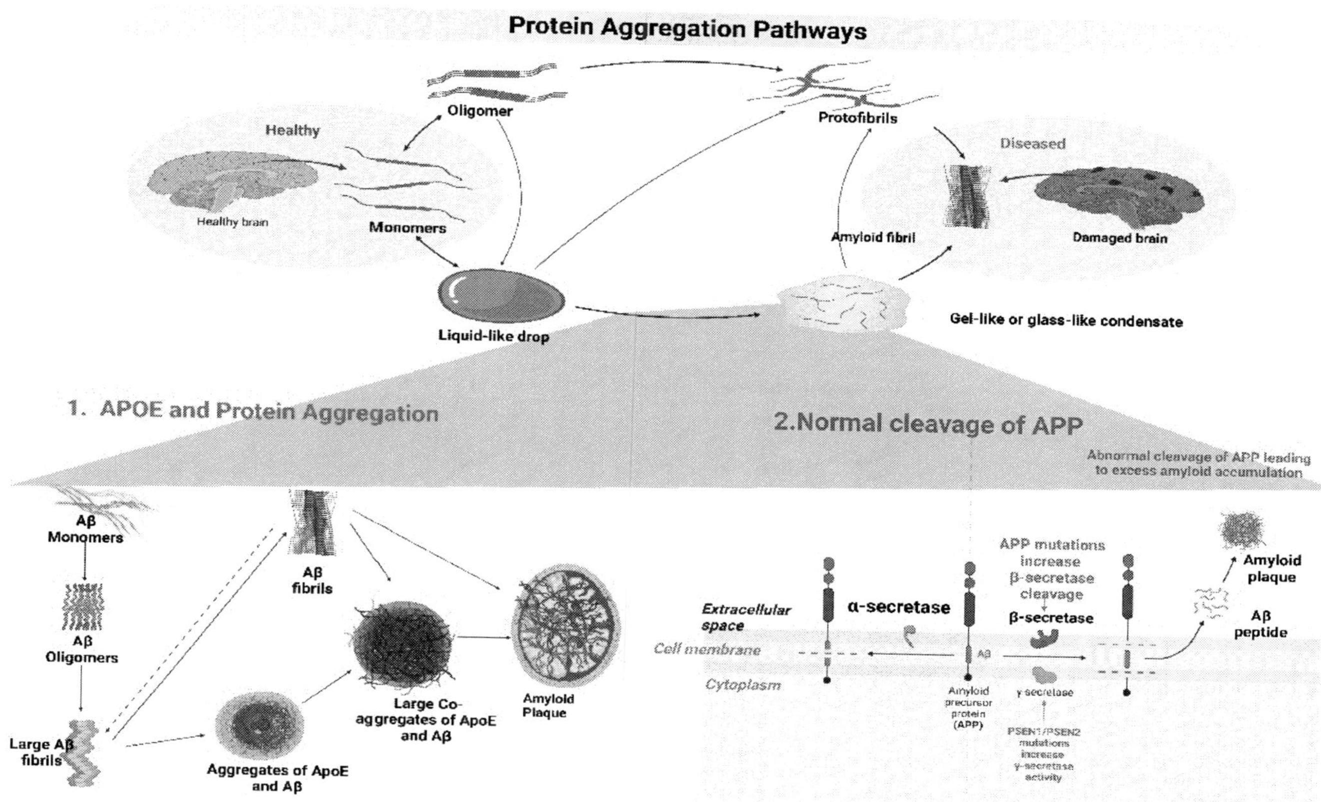

Figure 1. Pathophysiology of Alzheimer disease.

Table 1. Contemporary perspectives on the utilization of nanomedicines as nanocarriers for the targeted delivery of drugs for treatment of AD

S. No.	Type of Nanoparticles	Drug	Method of Preparation	Outcomes	Reference
1.	Polymeric Nanoparticles (PLGA)	Memantine	Ultrasonication	Improved memory impairment	(Kaur et al., 2022)
2.	Liposomes with HCL	Donepezil	Ethanol injection method	Higer drug concentration reached into the brain by intranasal rout	(Rajput & Butani, 2022)
3.	Metal Nanoparticles (Gold)	Curcumin	Solvent casting method	Improved permeability	(Kolathupalayam Shanmugam et al., 2023)
4.	Polymeric Nanoparticles	Curcumin	Single emulsion –solvent evaporation method	Increases its *in vitro* neuronal targeting efficiency	(Mathew et al., 2012)
5.	Solid lipid Nanoparticles	Resveratrol	Sonication	Inhibitory effect	(Loureiro et al., 2017)
6.	Polymeric Nanoparticles	Epigallocatechin-3-gallate	Double emulsion method	Increase drug permeability	(Cano et al., 2019)
7.	Liposome	Rosmaric acid		Effective permeation in BBB	(Kuo et al., 2018)
8.	Micro emulsions	Huperzia	Microemulsion tem plate technique	Efficient promoters for transdermal delivery	(Patel et al., 2013)
9.	Solid Lipid Nanoparticle	Thymoquinone		Efficiently targets the brain and delivers the drug in a controlled manner	(Surekha & Sumathi, 2016)
10.	Solid lipid Nanoparticles	sesamol	Crystallization	Effectively transport in brain	(Sachdeva et al., 2015)
11.	Polymeric nanoparticle	a-mangostin	Emulsion/solvent evaporation	Increased the cellular uptake, improved the biodistribution	(Yao et al., 2016)
12.	nanoemulsion	Naringenin			(Md et al., 2018)
13.	Nano-encapsulation	Quercetin	Controlled De Solvation	Improve its oral bioavailability, prolonged and sustained therapeutic levels	(Moreno et al., 2017)
14.	Polymeric Nanoparticles	Anthocyanins		Enhance the bioavailability and controlled the release	(Ali et al., 2017)

S. No.	Type of Nanoparticles	Drug	Method of Preparation	Outcomes	Reference
15.	Lipid polymer hybrid Nanoparticles	Rutin	Nanoprecipitation	Competency in brain delivery	(Ishak et al., 2017)
16.	Polymeric Nano-carriers	Baicalein	Polymerization	Increase cellular uptake	(Aghajanzadeh et al., 2020)
17.	Solid lipid nanoparticles	Camptothecin	Homogenisation	Penetration through blood brain barrier	(Martins et al., 2012)
18.	Solid lipid Nanoparticles	Bacoside	Homogenization	Prolong the drug release upto 24 hours	(Kumar & Garg, 2020)
19.	High-energy amorphous nano-sized solid dispersion	Nobiletin	Wet-milling	Improve dissolution behavior and pharmacokinetic properties of drug	(Kesharwani et al., 2020)
20.	Chitosen coated Solid-liquid nanoparticles	Ferulic Acid	Homogenization	Superior pharmacodynamic performance	(Saini et al., 2021)
21.	micellar nanocarriers	Morin hydrate	Thin film hydration	Improvement in learning	(Singh et al., 2018)
22.	Carbon nanotubes	Berberine		Effective delivery to brain tissue	(Lohan et al., 2017)
23.	Microemulsions	Alkaloidal extract		Enhancing the ACh levels after transdermal application	(Chaiyana et al., 2013)
24.	Solid lipid nanoparticles	Piperine	Emulsification-Solvent Diffusion	Effective in low dose, effective delivery across blood brain barrier	(Yusuf et al., 2013)
25.	Chitosan nanoparticles	Gallic acid	Ionotropic Gelation	Improve brain targeting	(Nagpal et al., 2013)
26.	Nano-pomegranate seed oil	punicic acid	Sonication		(Mizrahi et al., 2014)
27.	Niosomes	Ginkgo biloba extract	Film dispersion-homogenization	Improved oral bioavailability	(Press, 2013)
28.	Nanocrystal	Hesperetin		Greater permeability	(kheradmand et al., 2018)
29.	Polymeric nano particles	Retinoic acid			(Esteves et al., 2015)
30.	Solid lipid nanoparticles	chrysin	Homogenization	Greater bioavailability	(Vedagiri & Thangarajan, 2016)
31.	Solid lipid nanoparticles	Galantamine	Micro emulsification	Offered approximately twice bioavailability	(Misra et al., 2016) (Raza et al., 2013)
32.	Nanoethosomes	Vinpocetine	Solvent evaporation	Higher drug permeation	(Moghaddam et al., 2015) (Sharma et al., 2016)
33.	Lipid nanoparticulate systems	α-Asarone	Emulsification and ultrasonication	Improve the Uptake of α-Asarone Into the Brain Parenchyma	(Ramalingam et al., 2020) (Zeng et al., 2021)

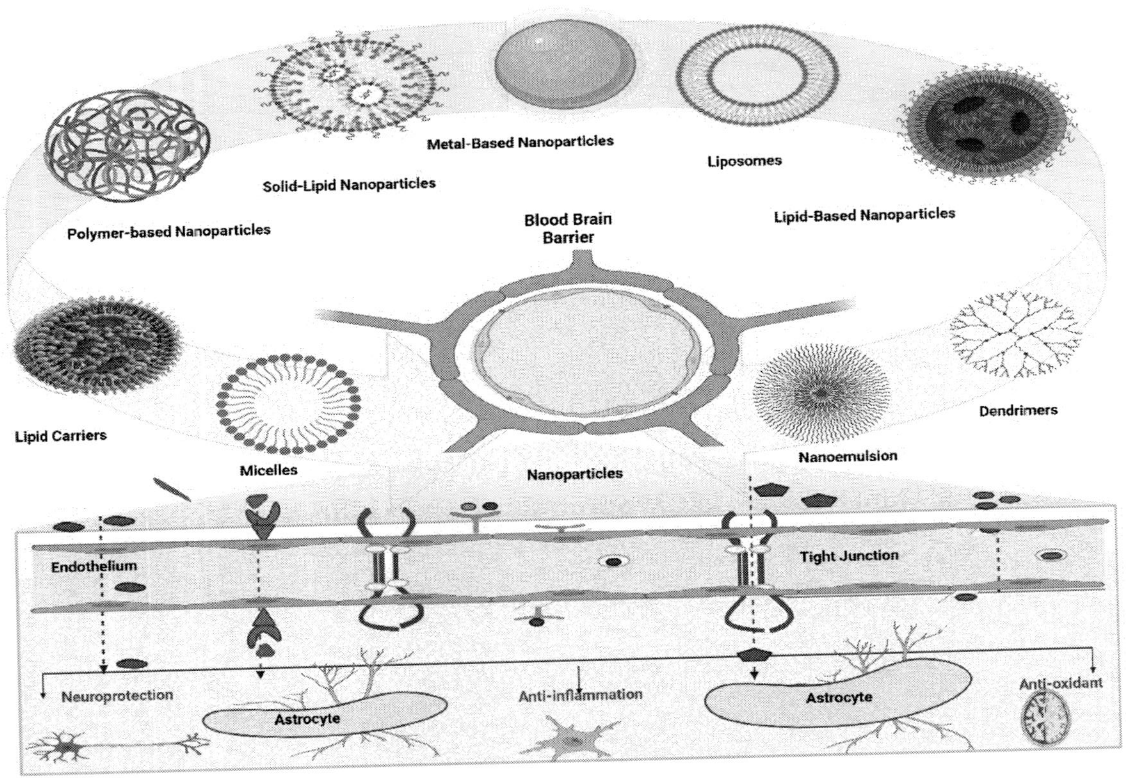

Figure 2. Transport mechanism of Nanoparticles.

The prevalence of the AP3 allele in individuals diagnosed with Alzheimer's disease with Lewy bodies is approximately 25%, while the presence of the APo E2 gene in individuals with Pick's disease is estimated to be around 10%. The prevalence of the APO E4 allele has been observed to exceed 50% in individuals diagnosed with frontotemporal lobar degeneration. Individuals who possess two E4 alleles are at an elevated susceptibility for the development of AD in conjunction with cerebrovascular illness. On the contrary, it is noteworthy that the APo E3 allele is observed in a mere 25% of those diagnosed with dementia with Lewy bodies (Husain et al., 2021). The presence of the APO E4 allele has been observed in over 50% of those diagnosed with frontotemporal lobar degeneration accompanied by AD. Individuals who possess two copies of the E4 allele are at an elevated risk for the development of the disease. In contrast, the prevalence of the AP3 and AP2 alleles is approximately 10% among those diagnosed with Pick's disease and Alzheimer's dementia, respectively.

Transport Pathways Across the Blood-Brain Barrier

The BBB is the barrier by which molecules in the blood can enter and exit the brain through the cerebral parenchyma. Essential substances like nutrients cross the BBB via specialized transcellular pathways (Shown in Figure 2) such as carrier proteins, receptors, and vesiculation transcytosis (Kadry et al., 2020). Drugs are extruded from the brain by special transporters, including ATP-binding cassette, P-glycoprotein and multidrug resistance proteins to deliver them into the brain (Choi & Yu, 2014). Endothelial cells exhibit a variety of receptor types that facilitate the internalization of essential ligands, including growth factors, enzymes, and plasma proteins. The process of ligand-receptor interaction is initiated by the invagination of coated pits, which are specific regions of the endothelial cell membrane housing the receptors. This invagination marks the beginning of vesiculation. Endosomes have the ability to navigate many intracellular destinations through the utilization of microtubule pathways, exhibiting both random and saltatory motion (Mani & Pandey, 2019).

Nano-Formulations for Alzheimer's Disease

Nanotechnology encompasses liposomes, nanoparticles, and dendrimers, which offer significant strategies for drug delivery to the brain. The application has demonstrated reliability due to its extended retention period and lipophilic properties. Nanoparticles have the ability to be administered through several methods, including oral, nasal, and parenteral administration. The size range of nanoparticles is extremely small, often ranging from 1 to 1000 nm, which allows for direct administration to the brain. The medication exhibits target specificity and is formulated with a reduced dosage, hence mitigating the occurrence of systemic adverse effects (Patra et al., 2018). It has been demonstrated by researchers that the utilization of nanoparticles of butyrylcholinesterase, specifically rivastigmine, can effectively target specific areas and mitigate the occurrence of adverse consequences. Curcumin has been demonstrated to boost brain mitochondrial function, hence suggesting its potential utility in the treatment of Alzheimer's disease. Nevertheless, the systemic bioavailability of curcumin is significantly limited. Consequently, research has proposed that the encapsulation of curcumin within nanoparticles can enhance its circulation duration, systemic bioavailability, and target specificity (Abdul Manap et al., 2019). Here in Table 1, we discussed contemporary perspectives on the utilization of nanomedicines as nanocarriers for the targeted delivery of drugs for treatment of AD.

Polymeric Nanoparticles

Polymers present a wide range of possibilities for modifying the characteristics of nanoparticles, hence enabling enhanced regulation of particle interactions in the context of drug administration. Such as Donepezil, Rivastigmine, Galantamine, and memantine are used for the treatment of AD however, it has poor permeability into the brain so to overcome these limitation Cınar E. et al., prepared Donepezil-loaded PLGA-b-PEG Nanoparticles by double emulsion method for improvement of learning and Memory Function. Their results suggested improved permeability of donepezil and improved memory function of AD induced rats (Cinar et al., 2022). In another Study Baysal et al., prepared Donepezil loaded PLGA-PEG nanoparticles dowel emulsion method for reducing effect of β-Amyloid and increased permeability of Donepezil from the BBB. Their finding reported that prepared nanoparticles are smaller in size and easily cross the BBB. It also improved protein expression levels in β-Amyloid (Baysal et al., 2017). Furthermore, Fazil et al., developed rivastigmine loaded chitosan nanoparticles by ionic gelation method for brain drug delivery. Their result reported that Rivastigmine loaded nanoparticles successfully delivered into the brain and reduced effects of AD (Fazil et al., 2012). In another study, Curcumin nanoparticles coated with poly (lactic-co-glycolic acid; PLGA)-poly (ethylene glycol) penetrate and diffuse well into the brain parenchyma, despite the compromised blood-brain barrier. Furthermore, they were found in Alzheimer's disease-affected brain areas and had a protective effect on the damaged newborn brain. Curcumin nanoformulation, which involved modifying the surface of the PLGA polymer and encapsulating selenium nanoparticles, was shown to reduce Aβ burden and inflammation in the brains of AD mice, as well as treating memory loss in the model animals. Furthermore, no misleading anomalies were visible in histological scans of animal tissues (Nance, 2019).

Solid Lipid Nanoparticles

Solid lipid nanoparticles (SLNanoparticles) are widely recognized as highly effective carriers for delivering α-bisabolol to the brain their outcomes suggest that notable inhibitory effects on amyloid aggregation (Sathya et al., 2020). In another study, transferrin nano lipid carriers loaded with P-glycoprotein and breast cancer resistance protein for reducing β-Amyloid in AD. There results find that prepared nano lipid carriers were 120nm in size and its successful delivery into brain along with β-Amyloid clearance (Arduino et al., 2020). Furthermore, Nano lipid carriers with donepezil improved permeability of donepezil into brain via intranasal rout (Yasir et al., 2018). In another study donepezil loaded solid lipid nanoparticles were prepared by using solvent emulsification diffusion method. There result suggested that improved permeability of donepezil as compared to free drug (Yasir et al., 2017). Furthermore, Yavarpour et al., also looked at the neuroprotective effects of curcumin-loaded lipid-core nanocapsules in an AD-induced aged female mouse model. The findings of this study revealed that curcumin-loaded lipid-core nanocapsules provided substantial neuroprotection in a model of Alzheimer's disease against Aβ1-42-induced behavioural and neurochemical alterations (Giacomeli et al., 2019). Recently Sadegh et al., found that nanostructured lipid carriers containing curcumin enhanced memory by targeting oxidative stress markers (ADP/ATP ratio, lipid peroxidation, and ROS production) in the hippocampus tissue. Furthermore, histopathological investigations revealed the ability of nanostructured lipid carriers containing curcumin to inhibit the hallmarks of Alzheimer's disease *in vitro* model (Malvajerd et al., 2019).

Nano-Formulations of Herbal Constituents for Alzheimer's Disease

After 2003 no new drug has approved for the treatment of AD whereas approximately 193 drugs are in pipelines. Herbal drug having potency to treat AD much research proven it however, poor permeability, Slow bioavailability is a major obstacle in herbal drug. Now researchers are focused on nanodrug delivery with herbs which overcome these limitations. Here we discussed some herbal nanocarriers.

Curcumin-Loaded Nanoparticles

Curcumin has neuroprotective properties, however its pharmacokinetics and bioavailability are low due to the blood-brain barrier (interaction with specific efflux transporters) or the presence of hydroxyl groups, β-diketone moiety, and active methylene group in its structure, as well as its lipophilic nature (Farzaei et al., 2018). The presence of hydroxyl groups in curcumin's structure causes it to be quickly metabolized by kidney and liver enzymes, indicating limited absorption (Shabbir et al., 2021). Curcumin is also highly unstable in most bodily fluids, such as water, therefore it's best to combine it with milk or oil before eating it to improve absorption and metabolism (Shabbir et al., 2021, Zhi et al., 2021). As a result of these characteristics, its application is limited, posing a difficulty for disease therapy in *in vivo* investigations as a neuroprotective agent (Naqvi, Panghal and Flora, 2020). Based on the above fact, new curcumin formulations are urgently needed, primarily to enhance curcumin solubility for the treatment of Alzheimer's disease. For improved brain delivery, nano-delivery methods such as polymeric nanoparticles, peptide carriers, micelles, liposomes, cyclodextrins, conjugates, lipidic nanoparticles, emulsions, and solid dispersions have been widely investigated (Gao et al., 2020). Curcumin nanoparticles coated with poly (lactic-co-glycolic acid; PLGA)-poly (ethylene glycol) penetrate and diffuse well into the brain parenchyma, despite the compromised blood-brain barrier. Furthermore, they were found in Alzheimer's disease-affected brain areas and had a protective effect on the damaged newborn brain. Furthermore, no misleading anomalies were visible in histological scans of animal tissues (Nance, 2019). Zhang et al., evaluated the effects of curcumin encapsulated chitosan-coated PLGA nanoparticles and curcumin encapsulated hydroxypropyl-cyclodextrin-encapsulated curcumin complexes through intranasal delivery. Curcumin complexes were shown to be more stable under physiological conditions and to have a greater amount of cellular absorption of curcumin than the chitosan-coated PLGA nanoparticles (Zhang et al., 2020). Another research by Sadegh et al., focused on the neuroprotective effects of nanostructured lipid carriers and solid lipid nanoparticles loaded with curcumin. Both nanoparticle methods had better bioavailability in the brain, according to this study (Sadegh Malvajerd et al., 2019). They discovered that the 2,2-diphenyl-1-picrylhydrazyl free radical scavenging preparation methods had no influence on curcumin's antioxidant efficacy. Furthermore, curcumin nanoparticles containing chitosan and bovine serum albumin substantially increased drug penetration across the blood-brain barrier, expedited Aβ peptide phagocytosis, and promoted microglia activation (Sadegh Malvajerd et al., 2019, Taha et al., 2020).

Withanolides and Withanamides

The valuable medicinal herb Withania somnifera (WS) has been used to treat AD for over 3000 years. Crude extract of this plant produces withanamides and Withanolides which inhibit the production of Amyloid triangle in rat neuronal cells (Narinderpal, Junaid and Raman, 2013). Recently reported that WS have dual inhibitory action against Beta-secretase and Acetylcholinesterase (Huang, Chao and Hu, 2020). The WS ligands (anaferine, anahygrine, cuscohygrine, and isaopelletierine) have been shown to act as agonists at neuronal nicotinic acetylcholine receptors (nAChR) estimated the BBB permeability of withanamides present in W.somnifera fruit extract using an animal model (Remya et al., 2016). They carried out the analysis using high-performance liquid chromatography and a quadrupole period of flight mass spectrometer. The study concluded that four withanamides significantly crossed the BBB and that their major peaks were identical in both brain tissue homogenates and crude plant extracts (Vareed et al., 2014). Singh et al., e investigated the permeability, plasma protein binding of Withanolides. The result indicated that Withanolides have high plasma protein binding and passive permeability. Withaferin-A is a primary constituent which is obtained from traditional medicinal herbs Withania somnifera that has low oral bioavailability (S. K. Singh et al., 2018).

Pipeline-Loaded Nanoparticles

Piperine (1-piperoylpiperidine) is a sour alkaloid found in piper species' fruits. Most data supported Piperine's efficacy on the CNS, which is mostly linked to Piperine's effects on acetylcholine. Piperine has a log P-value of 2.25, indicating that it is a lipophilic molecule with a low water solubility. Furthermore, PIP has low oral bioavailability (Chonpathompikunlert, Wattanathorn and Muchimapura, 2010), (Allameh et al., 1992) so to overcome these limitation Yosra S R Elnaggar et al., developed Intranasal Piperine-Loaded Chitosan Nanoparticles for treatment in Alzheimer's Disease. PIP nasal irritation was greatly reduced by chitosan Nanoparticles, with no evidence of brain damage. Anti-apoptosis and anti-inflammatory properties were also suggested by the findings. Piperine-loaded Nanoparticles are efficacious, safe, non-invasive, and have a higher effectiveness than piperine alone at a lower dose. In Another study Piperine loaded nanoparticles are prepared by emulsification solvent diffusion method with polysorbate 80. There histopathological evulation suggested that reduced plaques and tangles (Elnaggar et al., 2015a). Furthermore, Somasundaram et al., developed piperine nanoparticles by y ionotropic gelation process for improve the bioavailability, minimize the dosing frequency and reduce the toxicity Result Suggested that Piperine as bio enhancer and MAO inhibitors to treat Parkinson's diseases (Kumar and Somasundaram, 2019). In another study Elnaggar et al., developed Tween-integrated monoolein cubosomes loaded with piperine and evaluated their ability to target the Alzheimer brain. In-vivo studies on Wistar rats revealed that therapy improved cognition and slowed the progression of Alzheimer's disease, which was related to its anti-inflammatory and anti-apoptotic properties. Furthermore, no damage was observed in the kidneys or livers of rats when the formulation was used (Elnaggar et al., 2015b). Furthermore, Elnaggar et al., investigated the use of piperine loaded chitosan Nanoparticles for treatment of Alzheimer's disease. Piperine-induced nasal pain in rats was substantially decreased by these chitosan Nanoparticles, with no deleterious effects on the animals' brains.

PIP's anti-apoptotic and anti-inflammatory characteristics were shown to be responsible for the drug's effects in Alzheimer's disease in this study. The authors also succeeded in developing mucoadhesive chitosan Nanoparticles that delivered efficacious, safe, and non-invasive PIP to brains at the same levels as oral treatment but at 5% of the oral dose, thus avoiding PIP's negative effects (Elnaggar et al., 2015a).

Resveratrol-Loaded Nanoparticles

Resveratrol is a polyphenolic phytoalexin from the stilbene family of chemicals. The primary disadvantages of Resveratrol are its rapid metabolism, limited water solubility, and low bioavailability (Salehi et al., 2018). Resveratrol loaded on PS80-coated poly(lactide) Nanoparticles improved the drug's neuroprotective effects against 1-methyl-4-phenyl-1,2,3,6-tetrahydropyridine (MPTP)-induced behavioural and neurochemical changes in a PD mouse model (Lindner et al., 2015). The Aβ-triggered neuroinflammation was regulated *in vitro* by Resveratrol loaded lipid nanoparticles. Resveratrol lipid nanocarriers also reversed Aβ1-42's toxicity in rats (Rahman et al., 2020). A Resveratrol loaded mesoporous nano-selenium delivery device prevented Aβ aggregation, reduced oxidative stress, and corrected memory deficits in another research (Sun et al., 2019). Likewise, *in vitro,* Resveratrol loaded polymeric micelles reduced oxidative stress and apoptosis and thereby decreased Aβ-induced damage (Annaji et al., 2021). In compared to the free medication treated group, the vitamin E loaded RSV nanoemulsion had substantial beneficial benefits in the PD animal model, and a greater concentration of RSV was found in the brain (Sekatskii, Chergui and Dietler, 2003). Resveratrol loaded solid lipid nano system functionalized with apolipoprotein E improved the drug's bioavailability, concentration, and brain penetration in another research (Scioli Montoto, Muraca and Ruiz, 2020). Spinal cord injury in rats, chitosan-coated PLGA nanoparticles of Resveratrol decreased inflammatory cytokines, increased IL-10, improved neuroprotection, and improved functional recovery (Hellenbrand et al., 2019).

Conclusion

The recent advancement of nanotechnology is a promising area in health systems due to its better control over the physical and biological characteristics of the drug compared to conventional therapeutic approaches. Extensive research is being conducted to better understand degenerative disease pathways at molecular and cellular levels. However, preclinical approaches to clinical trials using nanoparticle-based approaches for AD are still limited. The development of biomarkers with nanoparticles may help in the early diagnosis of AD. Nanotechnology applications have the potential to revolutionize drug delivery systems for degenerative diseases. A balance between the development of nanotechnology-based therapeutic approaches and human healthcare safety is a significant concern. The ultimate objectives of nanomedicine are to study the underlying mechanisms of drug-disease interactions and translate findings from bench to bedside with collaboration between scientists and clinicians. Cholinesterase inhibitors have proven their efficacy in the treatment of AD. However, poor permeability, slow bioavailability, and systemic toxicity are major limitations. Currently, researchers are gaining more interest in phytoconstituents and their nano-herbal formulations for the treatment of AD due to their fewer toxic properties. Nowadays, various phytoconstituents have proven their potential to treat AD; however, poor permeability and low bioavailability minimize their potential. The utilization of nanotechnology in neuroscience is a key factor that will be a breakthrough for the effective treatment of AD. Furthermore, nanotechnology can also provide innovative advancements that are related to fundamental and clinical neuroscience. Several studies have reported the beneficial effects of nanoparticles on neurological disorders. Further research is required to make them more essential. Additionally, the clinical efficacy of nanoparticles for AD needs long-term assessments for the design of nano formulations with more specificity for different brain cells.

Disclaimer

None.

References

Abdul Manap, A. S., Wei Tan, A. C., Leong, W. H., Yin Chia, A. Y., Vijayabalan, S., Arya, A., Wong, E. H., Rizwan, F., Bindal, U., Koshy, S., & Madhavan, P. (2019). Synergistic Effects of Curcumin and Piperine as Potent Acetylcholine and Amyloidogenic Inhibitors With Significant Neuroprotective Activity in SH-SY5Y Cells via Computational Molecular Modeling and *in vitro* Assay. In *Frontiers in Aging Neuroscience* (Vol. 11).

Aghajanzadeh, M., Andalib, S., Danafar, H., Rostamizadeh, K., & Shara, A. (2020). *The e ff ect of baicalein-loaded Y-shaped miktoarm copolymer on spatial memory and hippocampal expression of DHCR24 , SELADIN and SIRT6 genes in rat model of Alzheimer. 586*(March). https://doi.org/10.1016/j.ijpharm.2020.119546.

Ali, T., Kim, M. J., Rehman, S. U., Ahmad, A., & Kim, M. O. (2017). Anthocyanin-Loaded PEG-Gold Nanoparticles Enhanced the Neuroprotection of Anthocyanins in an Aβ1–42 Mouse Model of Alzheimer's Disease. *Molecular Neurobiology, 54*(8), 6490–6506. https://doi.org/10.1007/s12035-016-0136-4.

Alzheimer's Association. (2021). 2021 Alzheimer's disease facts and figures special report Race, Ethnicity and Alzheimer's in America. *Alzheimer's & Dementia : The Journal of the Alzheimer's Association, 17*(3), 327–406.

Arduino, I., Iacobazzi, R. M., Riganti, C., Lopedota, A. A., Perrone, M. G., Lopalco, A., Cutrignelli, A., Cantore, M., Laquintana, V., Franco, M., Colabufo, N. A., Luurtsema, G., Contino, M., & Denora, N. (2020). Induced expression of P-gp and BCRP transporters on brain endothelial cells using transferrin functionalized nanostructured lipid carriers: A first step of a potential strategy for the treatment of Alzheimer's disease. *International Journal of Pharmaceutics, 591*, 120011. https://doi.org/10.1016/j.ijpharm.2020.120011.

Baysal, I., Ucar, G., Gultekinoglu, M., Ulubayram, K., & Yabanoglu-Ciftci, S. (2017). Donepezil loaded PLGA-b-PEG nanoparticles: their ability to induce destabilization of amyloid fibrils and to cross blood brain barrier *in vitro. Journal of Neural Transmission, 124*(1), 33–45. https://doi.org/10.1007/s00702-016-1527-4.

Bollen, E., & Prickaerts, J. (2012). Phosphodiesterases in neurodegenerative disorders. *IUBMB Life, 64*(12), 965–970. https://doi.org/10.1002/iub.1104.

Cano, A., Ettcheto, M., Chang, J. H., Barroso, E., Espina, M., Kühne, B. A., Barenys, M., Auladell, C., Folch, J., Souto, E. B., Camins, A., Turowski, P., & García, M. L. (2019). Dual-drug loaded nanoparticles of Epigallocatechin-3-gallate (EGCG)/Ascorbic acid enhance therapeutic efficacy of EGCG in a APPswe/PS1dE9 Alzheimer's disease mice model. *Journal of Controlled Release, 301*, 62–75. https://doi.org/10.1016/j.jconrel.2019.03.010.

Chaiyana, W., Rades, T., & Okonogi, S. (2013). Characterization and *in vitro* permeation study of microemulsions and liquid crystalline systems containing the anticholinesterase alkaloidal extract from Tabernaemontana divaricata. *International Journal of Pharmaceutics, 452*(1–2), 201–210. https://doi.org/10.1016/j.ijpharm.2013.05.005.

Choi, Y., & Yu, A.-M. (2014). ABC Transporters in Multidrug Resistance and Pharmacokinetics, and Strategies for Drug Development. *Current Pharmaceutical Design*, *20*(5), 793–807. https://doi.org/10.2174/138161282005140214165212.

Cinar, E., Mutluay, S. U., Baysal, I., Gultekinoglu, M., Ulubayram, K., Yabanoglu Ciftci, S., Tel, B. C., & Ucar, G. (2022). Donepezil-loaded PLGA-b-PEG Nanoparticles Enhance the Learning and Memory Function of Beta-Amyloid Rat Model of Alzheimer's Disease. *Archives of Neuropsychiatry*. https://doi.org/10.29399/npa.28275.

Colović, M. B., Krstić, D. Z., Lazarević-Pašti, T. D., Bondžić, A. M., & Vasić, V. M. (2013). Acetylcholinesterase inhibitors: pharmacology and toxicology. *Current Neuropharmacology*, *11*(3), 315–335. https://doi.org/10.2174/1570159X11311030006.

Esteves, M., Cristóvão, A. C., Saraiva, T., Rocha, S. M., Baltazar, G., Ferreira, L., & Bernardino, L. (2015). Retinoic acid-loaded polymeric nanoparticles induce neuroprotection in a mouse model for parkinson's disease. *Frontiers in Aging Neuroscience*, *7*(MAR), 1–10. https://doi.org/10.3389/fnagi.2015.00020.

Fazil, M., Md, S., Haque, S., Kumar, M., Baboota, S., Sahni, J. kaur, & Ali, J. (2012). Development and evaluation of rivastigmine loaded chitosan nanoparticles for brain targeting. *European Journal of Pharmaceutical Sciences*, *47*(1), 6–15. https://doi.org/10.1016/j.ejps.2012.04.013.

Giacomeli, R., Izoton, J. C., dos Santos, R. B., Boeira, S. P., Jesse, C. R., & Haas, S. E. (2019). Neuroprotective effects of curcumin lipid-core nanocapsules in a model Alzheimer's disease induced by β-amyloid 1-42 peptide in aged female mice. *Brain Research*, *1721*(June), 146325. https://doi.org/10.1016/j.brainres.2019.146325.

Grossberg, G. T. (2003). Cholinesterase Inhibitors for the Treatment of Alzheimer's Disease: *Current Therapeutic Research*, *64*(4), 216–235. https://doi.org/10.1016/S0011-393X(03)00059-6.

Husain, M. A., Laurent, B., & Plourde, M. (2021). APOE and Alzheimer's Disease: From Lipid Transport to Physiopathology and Therapeutics. *Frontiers in Neuroscience*, *15*. https://doi.org/10.3389/fnins.2021.630502.

Ishak, R. A. H., Mostafa, N. M., & Kamel, A. O. (2017). Stealth lipid polymer hybrid nanoparticles loaded with rutin for effective brain delivery - comparative study with the gold standard (Tween 80): optimization, characterization and biodistribution. *Drug Delivery*, *24*(1), 1874–1890. https://doi.org/10.1080/10717544.2017.1410263.

Ju, I. G., Son, S. Y., Lee, S., Im, H., Huh, E., Eo, H., Choi, J. G., Sohn, M. W., Yim, S.-V., Kim, S. Y., Kim, D.-H., Lee, C. H., & Oh, M. S. (2023). Protective effects of CCL01 against Aβ-induced neurotoxicity in 5xFAD transgenic mouse model of Alzheimer's disease. *Biomedicine & Pharmacotherapy*, *158*, 114105. https://doi.org/10.1016/j.biopha.2022.114105.

Kadry, H., Noorani, B., & Cucullo, L. (2020). A blood–brain barrier overview on structure, function, impairment, and biomarkers of integrity. *Fluids and Barriers of the CNS*, *17*(1), 69. https://doi.org/10.1186/s12987-020-00230-3.

Kaur, A., Nigam, K., Tyagi, A., & Dang, S. (2022). A Preliminary Pharmacodynamic Study for the Management of Alzheimer's Disease Using Memantine-Loaded PLGA

Nanoparticles. *AAPS PharmSciTech, 23*(8), 298. https://doi.org/10.1208/s12249-022-02449-9.

Kesharwani, S. S., Mallya, P., Kumar, V. A., Jain, V., Sharma, S., & Dey, S. (2020). Nobiletin as a Molecule for Formulation Development: An Overview of Advanced Formulation and Nanotechnology-Based Strategies of Nobiletin. *AAPS PharmSciTech, 21*(6). https://doi.org/10.1208/s12249-020-01767-0.

kheradmand, E., Hajizadeh Moghaddam, A., & Zare, M. (2018). Neuroprotective effect of hesperetin and nano-hesperetin on recognition memory impairment and the elevated oxygen stress in rat model of Alzheimer's disease. *Biomedicine & Pharmacotherapy, 97*, 1096–1101. https://doi.org/https://doi.org/10.1016/j.biopha.2017.11.047.

Kim, J., Basak, J. M., & Holtzman, D. M. (2009). The Role of Apolipoprotein E in Alzheimer's Disease. *Neuron, 63*(3), 287–303. https://doi.org/10.1016/j.neuron.2009.06.026.

Kolathupalayam Shanmugam, B., Rajendran, N., Arumugam, K., Rangaraj, S., Subramani, K., Srinivasan, S., Nayagam, L., Aicher, W. K., & Venkatachalam, R. (2023). Curcumin loaded gold nanoparticles–chitosan/sodium alginate nanocomposite for nanotheranostic applications. *Journal of Biomaterials Science, Polymer Edition, 34*(7), 875–892. https://doi.org/10.1080/09205063.2022.2151819.

Kumar, R., & Garg, R. (2020). Bacoside rich extract loaded solid lipid nanoparticles for Alzheimer's disease. *Plant Archives, 20*, 247–252.

Kuo, Y. C., Chen, I. Y., & Rajesh, R. (2018). Use of functionalized liposomes loaded with antioxidants to permeate the blood–brain barrier and inhibit β-amyloid-induced neurodegeneration in the brain. *Journal of the Taiwan Institute of Chemical Engineers, 87*, 1–14. https://doi.org/10.1016/j.jtice.2018.03.001.

Lohan, S., Raza, K., Mehta, S. K., Bhatti, G. K., Saini, S., & Singh, B. (2017). Anti-Alzheimer's potential of berberine using surface decorated multi-walled carbon nanotubes: A preclinical evidence. *International Journal of Pharmaceutics, 530*(1), 263–278. https://doi.org/10.1016/j.ijpharm.2017.07.080.

Loureiro, J. A., Andrade, S., Duarte, A., Neves, A. R., Queiroz, J. F., Nunes, C., Sevin, E., Fenart, L., Gosselet, F., Coelho, M. A. N., Pereira, M. C., & Latruffe, N. (2017). Resveratrol and grape extract-loaded solid lipid nanoparticles for the treatment of Alzheimer's disease. *Molecules, 22*(2), 1–16. https://doi.org/10.3390/molecules22020277.

Malvajerd, S. S., Izadi, Z., Azadi, A., Kurd, M., Derakhshankhah, H., Zadeh, M. S., Javar, H. A., & Hamidi, M. (2019). Neuroprotective Potential of Curcumin-Loaded Nanostructured Lipid Carrier in an Animal Model of Alzheimer's Disease: Behavioral and Biochemical Evidence. *Journal of Alzheimer's Disease, 69*(3), 671–686. https://doi.org/10.3233/JAD-190083.

Mani, I., & Pandey, K. N. (2019). Emerging concepts of receptor endocytosis and concurrent intracellular signaling: Mechanisms of guanylyl cyclase/natriuretic peptide receptor-A activation and trafficking. *Cellular Signalling, 60*, 17–30. https://doi.org/10.1016/j.cellsig.2019.03.022.

Martins, S., Tho, I., Reimold, I., Fricker, G., Souto, E., Ferreira, D., & Brandl, M. (2012). Brain delivery of camptothecin by means of solid lipid nanoparticles: Formulation design, *in vitro* and *in vivo* studies. *International Journal of Pharmaceutics, 439*(1–2), 49–62. https://doi.org/10.1016/j.ijpharm.2012.09.054.

Mathew, A., Fukuda, T., Nagaoka, Y., Hasumura, T., Morimoto, H., Yoshida, Y., Maekawa, T., Venugopal, K., & Kumar, D. S. (2012). Curcumin loaded-PLGA nanoparticles conjugated with Tet-1 peptide for potential use in Alzheimer's disease. *PLoS ONE, 7*(3). https://doi.org/10.1371/journal.pone.0032616.

Md, S., Gan, S. Y., Haw, Y. H., Ho, C. L., Wong, S., & Choudhury, H. (2018). *In vitro* neuroprotective effects of naringenin nanoemulsion against β-amyloid toxicity through the regulation of amyloidogenesis and tau phosphorylation. *International Journal of Biological Macromolecules, 118*, 1211–1219. https://doi.org/10.1016/j.ijbiomac.2018.06.190.

Misra, S., Chopra, K., Sinha, V. R., & Medhi, B. (2016). Galantamine-loaded solid–lipid nanoparticles for enhanced brain delivery: preparation, characterization, *in vitro* and *in vivo* evaluations. *Drug Delivery, 23*(4), 1434–1443. https://doi.org/10.3109/10717544.2015.1089956.

Mizrahi, M., Friedman-Levi, Y., Larush, L., Frid, K., Binyamin, O., Dori, D., Fainstein, N., Ovadia, H., Ben-Hur, T., Magdassi, S., & Gabizon, R. (2014). Pomegranate seed oil nanoemulsions for the prevention and treatment of neurodegenerative diseases: The case of genetic CJD. *Nanomedicine: Nanotechnology, Biology, and Medicine, 10*(6), 1353–1363. https://doi.org/10.1016/j.nano.2014.03.015.

Moghaddam, A. A., Aqil, M., Ahmad, F. J., Ali, M. M., Sultana, Y., & Ali, A. (2015). Nanoethosomes mediated transdermal delivery of vinpocetine for management of Alzheimers disease. *Drug Delivery, 22*(8), 1018–1026. https://doi.org/10.3109/10717544.2013.846433.

Moreno, L. C. G. e. I., Puerta, E., Suárez-Santiago, J. E., Santos-Magalhães, N. S., Ramirez, M. J., & Irache, J. M. (2017). Effect of the oral administration of nanoencapsulated quercetin on a mouse model of Alzheimer's disease. *International Journal of Pharmaceutics, 517*(1–2), 50–57. https://doi.org/10.1016/j.ijpharm.2016.11.061.

Nagpal, K., Singh, S. K., & Mishra, D. N. (2013). Nanoparticle mediated brain targeted delivery of gallic acid: *in vivo* behavioral and biochemical studies for protection against scopolamine-induced amnesia. *Drug Delivery, 20*(3–4), 112–119. https://doi.org/10.3109/10717544.2013.779330.

Najm, R., Jones, E. A., & Huang, Y. (2019). Apolipoprotein E4, inhibitory network dysfunction, and Alzheimer's disease. *Molecular Neurodegeneration, 14*(1), 24. https://doi.org/10.1186/s13024-019-0324-6.

Nance, E. (2019). The Role of Nanoparticles in Neuroscience. *Scientia*. https://doi.org/10.33548/scientia383.

Paramanick, D., Singh, V. D., & Singh, V. K. (2022). Neuroprotective effect of phytoconstituents via nanotechnology for treatment of Alzheimer diseases. *Journal of Controlled Release, 351*, 638–655. https://doi.org/10.1016/j.jconrel.2022.09.058.

Patel, P. A., Patil, S. C., Kalaria, D. R., Kalia, Y. N., & Patravale, V. B. (2013). Comparative *in vitro* and *in vivo* evaluation of lipid based nanocarriers of Huperzine A. *International Journal of Pharmaceutics, 446*(1–2), 16–23. https://doi.org/10.1016/j.ijpharm.2013.02.014.

Patra, J. K., Das, G., Fraceto, L. F., Campos, E. V. R., Rodriguez-Torres, M. del P., Acosta-Torres, L. S., Diaz-Torres, L. A., Grillo, R., Swamy, M. K., Sharma, S., Habtemariam, S., & Shin, H.-S. (2018). Nano based drug delivery systems: recent developments and future prospects. *Journal of Nanobiotechnology, 16*(1), 1–33. https://doi.org/10.1186/s12951-018-0392-8.

Press, D. (2013). *Development of a novel niosomal system for oral delivery of Ginkgo biloba extract*. 421–430.

Rajput, A., & Butani, S. (2022). Donepezil HCl Liposomes: Development, Characterization, Cytotoxicity, and Pharmacokinetic Study. *AAPS PharmSciTech, 23*(2), 74. https://doi.org/10.1208/s12249-022-02209-9.

Ramalingam, P., Ganesan, P., Prabakaran, D. S., Gupta, P. K., Jonnalagadda, S., Govindarajan, K., Vishnu, R., Sivalingam, K., Sodha, S., Choi, D. K., & Ko, Y. T. (2020). Lipid Nanoparticles Improve the Uptake of α-Asarone Into the Brain Parenchyma: Formulation, Characterization, *In Vivo* Pharmacokinetics, and Brain Delivery. *AAPS PharmSciTech, 21*(8). https://doi.org/10.1208/s12249-020-01832-8.

Raza, K., Katare, O. P., Setia, A., Bhatia, A., & Singh, B. (2013). Improved therapeutic performance of dithranol against psoriasis employing systematically optimized nanoemulsomes. *Journal of Microencapsulation, 30*(3), 225–236. https://doi.org/10.3109/02652048.2012.717115.

Sachdeva, A. K., Misra, S., Pal Kaur, I., & Chopra, K. (2015). Neuroprotective potential of sesamol and its loaded solid lipid nanoparticles in ICV-STZ-induced cognitive deficits: Behavioral and biochemical evidence. *European Journal of Pharmacology, 747*, 132–140. https://doi.org/10.1016/j.ejphar.2014.11.014.

Saini, S., Sharma, T., Jain, A., Kaur, H., Katare, O. P., & Singh, B. (2021). Systematically designed chitosan-coated solid lipid nanoparticles of ferulic acid for effective management of Alzheimer's disease: A preclinical evidence. *Colloids and Surfaces B: Biointerfaces, 205*(May), 111838. https://doi.org/10.1016/j.colsurfb.2021.111838.

Sathya, S., Shanmuganathan, B., & Devi, K. P. (2020). Deciphering the anti-apoptotic potential of α-bisabolol loaded solid lipid nanoparticles against Aβ induced neurotoxicity in Neuro-2a cells. *Colloids and Surfaces B: Biointerfaces, 190*, 110948. https://doi.org/10.1016/j.colsurfb.2020.110948.

Schönecker, S., Neuhofer, C., Otto, M., Ludolph, A., Kassubek, J., Landwehrmeyer, B., Anderl-Straub, S., Semler, E., Diehl-Schmid, J., Prix, C., Vollmar, C., Fortea, J., Huppertz, H.-J., Arzberger, T., Edbauer, D., Feddersen, B., Dieterich, M., Schroeter, M. L., Volk, A. E., … Levin, J. (2018). Atrophy in the Thalamus But Not Cerebellum Is Specific for C9orf72 FTD and ALS Patients – An Atlas-Based Volumetric MRI Study. *Frontiers in Aging Neuroscience, 10*. https://doi.org/10.3389/fnagi.2018.00045.

Sehar, U., Rawat, P., Reddy, A. P., Kopel, J., & Reddy, P. H. (2022). Amyloid Beta in Aging and Alzheimer's Disease. *International Journal of Molecular Sciences, 23*(21), 12924. https://doi.org/10.3390/ijms232112924.

Sharma, D., Bansal, P. K., & Mishra, N. (2016). Role of lipidic nanoparticles for management of Alzheimer's disease. *Asian Journal of Biomaterial Research*, *2*(1), 1–8.

Singh, M., Thakur, V., Deshmukh, R., Sharma, A., Rathore, M. S., Kumar, A., & Mishra, N. (2018). Development and characterization of morin hydrate-loaded micellar nanocarriers for the effective management of Alzheimer's disease. *Journal of Microencapsulation*, *35*(2), 137–148. https://doi.org/10.1080/02652048.2018.1441916.

Surekha, R., & Sumathi, T. (2016). An efficient encapsulation of thymoquinone using solid lipid nanoparticle for brain targeted drug delivery: Physicochemical characterization, pharmacokinetics and bio-distribution studies. *International Journal of Pharmaceutical and Clinical Research*, *8*(12), 1616–1624.

Tahami Monfared, A. A., Byrnes, M. J., White, L. A., & Zhang, Q. (2022). Alzheimer's Disease: Epidemiology and Clinical Progression. *Neurology and Therapy*, *11*(2), 553–569. https://doi.org/10.1007/s40120-022-00338-8.

Theerasri, A., Janpaijit, S., Tencomnao, T., & Prasansuklab, A. (n.d.). Beyond the classical amyloid hypothesis in Alzheimer's disease: Molecular insights into current concepts of pathogenesis, therapeutic targets, and study models. *WIREs Mechanisms of Disease*, *n/a*(n/a), e1591. https://doi.org/https://doi.org/10.1002/wsbm.1591.

Vedagiri, A., & Thangarajan, S. (2016). Mitigating effect of chrysin loaded solid lipid nanoparticles against Amyloid β25–35 induced oxidative stress in rat hippocampal region: An efficient formulation approach for Alzheimer's disease. *Neuropeptides*, *58*, 111–125. https://doi.org/10.1016/j.npep.2016.03.002.

Yao, L., Gu, X., Song, Q., Wang, X., Huang, M., Hu, M., Hou, L., Kang, T., Chen, J., Chen, H., & Gao, X. (2016). Nanoformulated alpha-mangostin ameliorates Alzheimer's disease neuropathology by elevating LDLR expression and accelerating amyloid-beta clearance. *Journal of Controlled Release*, *226*, 1–14. https://doi.org/10.1016/j.jconrel.2016.01.055.

Yasir, M., Chauhan, I., Haji, M. J., Tura, A. J., & Saxena, P. K. (2018). Formulation and Evaluation of Glyceryl Behenate based Solid Lipid Nanoparticles for the Delivery of Donepezil to Brain through Nasal Route. *Research Journal of Pharmacy and Technology*, *11*(7), 2836. https://doi.org/10.5958/0974-360X.2018.00523.1.

Yasir, M., Sara, U. V. S., Chauhan, I., Gaur, P. K., Singh, A. P., Puri, D., & Ameeduzzafar. (2017). Solid lipid nanoparticles for nose to brain delivery of donepezil: formulation, optimization by Box–Behnken design, *in vitro* and *in vivo* evaluation. *Artificial Cells, Nanomedicine, and Biotechnology*, 1–14. https://doi.org/10.1080/21691401.2017.1394872.

Yusuf, M., Khan, M., Khan, R. A., & Ahmed, B. (2013). Preparation, characterization, *in vivo* and biochemical evaluation of brain targeted Piperine solid lipid nanoparticles in an experimentally induced Alzheimer's disease model. *Journal of Drug Targeting*, *21*(3), 300–311. https://doi.org/10.3109/1061186X.2012.747529.

Zeng, L., Zhang, D., Liu, Q., Zhang, J., Mu, K., Gao, X., Zhang, K., Li, H., Wang, Q., Zheng, Y., & Mao, S. (2021). Alpha-asarone Improves Cognitive Function of APP/PS1 Mice and Reducing Aβ42, P-tau and Neuroinflammation, and Promoting Neuron Survival in the Hippocampus. *Neuroscience*, *458*, 141–152. https://doi.org/10.1016/j.neuroscience.2020.12.026.

Index

B

D

E

M

N

O

P

Q

R

S

T